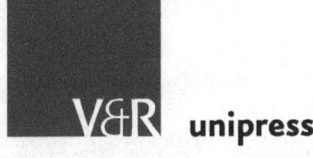

Pflegewissenschaft und Pflegebildung

Band 23

Herausgegeben von
Prof. Dr. Manfred Hülsken-Giesler

Jette Lange

The Nursing Process as a Strategy for a (De-)Professionalization in Nursing

A Critical Analysis of the Transformation of Nursing in Germany in the 1970s and 1980s

With a foreword by Thomas Foth, PhD

V&R unipress

Universitätsverlag Osnabrück

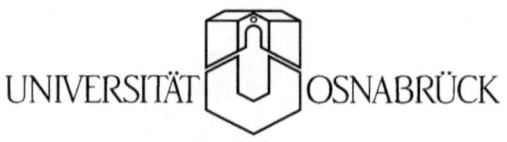

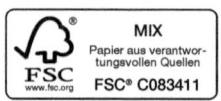

Bibliografische Information der Deutschen Nationalbibliothek
Die Deutsche Nationalbibliothek verzeichnet diese Publikation in der Deutschen
Nationalbibliografie; detaillierte bibliografische Daten sind im Internet über
https://dnb.de abrufbar.

**Veröffentlichungen des Universitätsverlags Osnabrück
erscheinen bei V&R unipress.**

© 2024 Brill | V&R unipress, Robert-Bosch-Breite 10, D-37079 Göttingen, ein Imprint der Brill-Gruppe
(Koninklijke Brill NV, Leiden, Niederlande; Brill USA Inc., Boston MA, USA; Brill Asia Pte Ltd,
Singapore; Brill Deutschland GmbH, Paderborn, Deutschland; Brill Österreich GmbH, Wien,
Österreich)
Koninklijke Brill NV umfasst die Imprints Brill, Brill Nijhoff, Brill Schöningh, Brill Fink, Brill mentis,
Brill Wageningen Academic, Vandenhoeck & Ruprecht, Böhlau und V&R unipress.
Wo nicht anders angegeben, ist diese Publikation unter der Creative-Commons-Lizenz
Namensnennung-Nicht kommerziell-Keine Bearbeitungen 4.0 lizenziert (siehe https://creative
commons.org/licenses/by-nc-nd/4.0/) und unter dem DOI 10.14220/9783737015868 abzurufen.
Jede Verwertung in anderen als den durch diese Lizenz zugelassenen Fällen bedarf der vorherigen
schriftlichen Einwilligung des Verlages.

Druck und Bindung: CPI books GmbH, Birkstraße 10, D-25917 Leck
Printed in the EU.

Vandenhoeck & Ruprecht Verlage | www.vandenhoeck-ruprecht-verlage.com

ISSN 2198-6193
ISBN 978-3-8471-1586-1

Contents

Foreword 9

Abstract 13

Abbreviations 15

Acknowledgements 17

Chapter 1: Introduction 19
   1.1 Research Objectives 26
   1.2 Research Questions 26
   1.3 Organization and Structure 27

Chapter 2: Background 29
   2.1 Societal Transformations in Germany "After the Boom" 30
   2.2 The Transformation of the Healthcare System 33

Chapter 3: Studies on Developments in German Nursing and on the
Nursing Process 37
   3.1 Historiography 38
   3.2 Critiques on the Nursing Process 46

Chapter 4: Methodological Considerations 53
   4.1 The History of the Present 53
   4.2 Historical Discourse Analysis 60
   4.3 Data Collection and Data Analysis 61

Chapter 5: Theoretical Framework 71
   5.1 Biopower and the Development of Expertise in Healthcare 72

5.2 Governmentality and the Issue of Professionalism 77
    5.2.1 The Neoliberal Rationale and Professions 79
    5.2.2 De-professionalization or the Concept of New Professionalism   88
5.3 Critical Accounting and its Application in Healthcare 93
5.4 Summary 97

Chapter 6: The Nursing Process and Its Way into German Nursing . . . 99
6.1 Introductory Explanation 99
6.2 The Nursing Process 101
6.3 The WHO's Role in the Implementation of the Nursing Process . . 107
    6.3.1 The WHO's Construction of Health as an Economic Product . 109
    6.3.2 The Nursing Process as an Instrument to Transform
        Healthcare Services 112
6.4 The German Debate over the Medium-Term Program of the WHO . 120

Chapter 7: The Benefit of the Nursing Process to the Economization
of Healthcare 129
7.1 Reorganization of Nursing Care in the Hospital 133
    7.1.1 Patients' Needs as Foundation for the Reorganization of
        Healthcare Services 134
    7.1.2 Focusing on Health 140
    7.1.3 Economizing Subjects in Hospital Care 143
7.2 Making Nursing Service Traceable 147
    7.2.1 Transparency 148
    7.2.2 Control 156
    7.2.3 Quality 159
7.3 Digitalization 161
7.4 Accountable Nursing – A Summary 165

Chapter 8: The Impact of the Nursing Process on the Concept of
Professionalism in Nursing 167
8.1 Autonomy Via a Distinct Scope of Practice 170
    8.1.1 Stepping Away from the Medical Profession: The Focus on
        Health and Basic Nursing Care 171
    8.1.2 Influencing the Patient: The Focus on Cybernetic Holism . . . 177
    8.1.3 Becoming Autonomous: The Focus on Rationality and
        Accountability 181
    8.1.4 Establishing Nursing Research: The Focus on
        Cost-Containment 187

 8.2 Professionalization or De-professionalization – A Summary 192
  8.2.1 Implementation of Mechanisms of Mistrust 193
  8.2.2 The Decline of Monopolized Knowledge 194
  8.2.3 Subordination Under Economic Premises 196

Chapter 9: Conclusion 199
 9.1 Summary 200
 9.2 Limitations 205
 9.3 Relevance and Implication 206

Bibliography 207

Foreword

Since the second half of the twentieth century, healthcare systems globally have been undergoing continuous and dramatic transformations. These transformations have always been justified by invoking a menacing crisis. Since the 1960s and 70s politicians and economist have warned about the increasing costs of healthcare systems and the need to make them more efficient and effective. Healthcare, we have been told again and again, is not sustainable if it isn't subjected to strict austerity measures. Decreasing the costs of healthcare delivery has led to an increasing precarity in large parts of populations. To break what the proponents of these transformations have called "welfare dependency," governments have systematically rolled back support for the vulnerable, and healthcare services have increasingly been privatized.

This change has had consequences for the nursing profession as a whole. Registered nurses have often been laid off or replaced by lower-trained assistant nurses or support workers and many hospitals have closed. The work environment for nurses has also changed dramatically with the implementation of different managerial technologies embodied in neoliberalism. We are witnessing endless reform cycles and practices that are often transferred from industrial organizations.. Examples are Best Practices, Evidence Based Medicine and Nursing, Quality Management, Diagnosis Related Groups, etc. The latest example is the implementation of the LEAN management concept in hospitals, originally developed by Toyota in the 1960s for more efficient car production. The delivery of healthcare is construed as no different from the production of a car, assuming that there is an unquestionable claim for efficiency on which all these technologies are based. Patients are treated according to standardized pathways that predetermine their hospital stay and the steps they will traverse from admission to discharge. The hospital resembles more and more a logistical operation in which every action and intervention is calculated in monetary terms. Furthermore, healthcare has become a data-driven business.

Entering a hospital today, one is confronted with Electronic Patient Records, digitalized management technologies, like EPIC, and endless algorithms in the organization of the neoliberal hospital. The US National Academies of Science, Engineering and Medicine report that the digitalization of hospitals is a major contributor to clinician burnout. Nurses and physicians spend more time on electronic charting than with patients. The average hospital in the US produces roughly 50 petabytes of data every year, more than twice the amount of data stored in the Library of Congress. Healthcare is not structured around patient needs but rather has become a lucrative business prioritizing profits, whether in privatized healthcare system such as in the US, universal healthcare system as in Germany, or publicly funded healthcare systems as in Canada. Healthcare and nursing care have developed into global commodities promising large profit margins. However, despite all these "innovations" that promised the amelioration of healthcare services for all, we are confronted with a deepening of the "crisis." This became particularly clear during the Covid pandemic and the subsequent collapse of entire health care systems, demonstrating the unpreparedness and vulnerability of LEAN healthcare systems. Many nurses either decide to leave the profession or they suffer from burnout due to unbearable working conditions. How did we get here? And is there any alternative?

Lange's ground-breaking genealogical study provides some answers to these questions. Her history of the present asks how power emerges in relations and how power relations change according to different constellations. It is a history that rests on the analysis of historical documents to understand how they contributed to the constitution of past and present realities – how truth and particular forms of knowledge were solidified in the past, and how realities in the present are formed. Lange's historical inquiry disturbs our taken-for-granted conceptualizations and opens a critical perspective on our present. This is a rather unusual perspective in nursing science because nursing practice is often considered ahistorical, and there is little questioning about the assumptions that underpin contemporary practices. This is particularly the case for the Nursing Process, the subject of Lange's study. Her understanding of critique is close to that of Theodor W. Adorno (1967), "[f]or critique to operate as part of a praxis is for it to apprehend the ways in which categories are themselves instituted, how the field of knowledge is ordered, and how what it suppresses returns, as it were, as its own constitutive occlusion."

Lange has chosen the implementation of the Nursing Process in the German healthcare system as the starting point of her analysis. This choice is interesting in several respects. First, the Nursing Process is considered a rather mundane instrument compared to management strategies like the aforementioned LEAN management or Quality Management, etc. However, Lange demonstrates that all these management strategies could not have been implemented without the Nursing Process in place. The Nursing Process is today considered the decisive quality characteristic of nursing care and the foundation of planned care. It has become a global concept and a taken-for-granted instrument as the Standard of Practice for nurses worldwide that has been disseminated by the WHO and the ICN and other global organizations. Even though the Nursing Process collided with "traditional" core values of nursing (like compassion, care, or emotional dimensions of nursing actions, etc.), the majority of nurses welcomed it enthusiastically as a chance to make their work visible and valuable, and to demonstrate their professionalism. However, Lange demonstrates that underlying the Nursing Process is a rationality to organizing nursing knowledge that is deeply antithetical to how nurses saw themselves and how nursing was conceptualized before.

Second, Lange chose the German context for her genealogy, which is in itself an interesting choice. Even though the Nursing Process originated in the US, Germany had a significant role in the development of what she calls a neoliberal rationale, because it was here that Ordoliberalism, a particular variety of neoliberalism, emerged that became the leading paradigm for the construction of the European Union. Lange's analysis enables us to understand how the neoliberal rationale has been adopted and incorporated by the nursing profession.

Whereas the Nursing Process promised better accuracy, streamlined patient-centred care, and the empowerment of patients, it became a decisive technology in changing the way nursing care was imagined and provided.

Significantly, the neoliberal conceptualization of humans as rational decision makers – or *homo oeconomicus* – also changed the way the patient was construed. That is, by emphasizing patients' active participation in the planning of their care, the nursing process became a means to realize the neoliberal idea of self-responsibility and the entrepreneurial decision-making of both nurses and patients. It was the foundation that enabled the implementation of Evidence Based Nursing (EBN), Best Practices (BP), quality management (QM), and other technologies – the building blocks of the neoliberal transformation of nursing and healthcare. This aspect of Lange's analysis is another reason why her study is so unique. Her critical historical analysis seriously engages with Foucault's concept of governmentally, neoliberalism, critical accounting, and nursing theory.

Finally, Lange uses accounting history in a very innovative way. Inspired by Foucault and accounting scholars like Peter Miller, she deconstructs the general perception of accounting as a neutral, non-intervening activity. In general, accounting is construed as concerned simply with the calculation of budgets and the representation of the economic situation of an enterprise or organization. Lange understands accounting as a mechanism by which organizations implement rational ways of organizing, providing techniques to monitor activities and a language with which to define and delineate organizational goals, procedures, and policies. From this perspective, the term "economization" is thus not so much about costs and ways of increasing profits as it is about processes and practices that mold individuals, organize activities, and constitute organizations, transforming them as economic entities or activities. Accordingly, Lange defines the Nursing Process as a calculative device that incorporates or materializes neoliberal programs of governing. The Nursing Process helped to develop a standardized vocabulary that allows thinking about hospital and nursing care as economic or financial entities. Accounting in (nursing) management provided important preconditions to transforming nursing and hospitals into calculative spaces. This book is a must-read for every nurse, nursing student, and anyone interested in understanding how a neoliberal rationale materializes in concrete technologies and practices.

Ottawa March 22, 2024   Thomas Foth

Abstract

In this study, I analyze a discourse that emerged during the 1970s and 1980s in German nursing. At that time, the German healthcare system underwent dramatic changes and economic reorganization, which can be understood as the emergence of the neoliberal rationale in Germany. The argument of cost explosion was used to restructure hospitals into enterprises that were to operate based on the logic of the market. At the same time, the nursing process was introduced into German nursing. The nursing process is a cybernetic, problem-solving cycle containing distinct steps of assessing the patient, planning nursing goals, executing and documenting nursing interventions, and evaluating performance. German nurses valued the nursing process as a central component of the professionalization of the nursing vocation. However, in neoliberalism, professions are seen as obstacles to free competition in marketized areas, and thus strategies such as accounting mechanisms were implemented to decrease their power.

Using the historical approach of the history of the present, the perspective of governmentality and insights from critical accounting, this study analyzes the impact of the nursing process on the German nursing vocation. The nursing process needs to be understood as an accounting tool and hence, as a component of neoliberal strategies to make formerly intangible fields of work like nursing service calculable. As an accounting tool, the nursing process does not represent reality in a neutral manner but affects the areas to which it is applied in a constitutive way. As this study shows, the implementation of the nursing process led to reconstituting the nursing vocation into a calculable entity. And while German nurses valued the potential that the call for increased accountability and transparency in nursing care held for their professionalization, the findings suggest that a newly constituted accountable nursing vocation can instead be considered as de-professionalizing.

Abbreviations

AEDL	Aktivitäten und existentielle Erfahrungen des Lebens [Activities and Existential Experiences of Life]
AKV	Agnes-Karll-Verband [Agnes-Karll-Association]
BMG	Bundesministerium für Gesundheit [Federal Ministry of Health]
B.O.K.D.	Berufsorganisation der Krankenpflegerinnen Deutschlands [Vocational Organization of the Female Nurses of Germany]
CICIAMS	Comité International Catholique des Infirmières et Assistantes Médico-Sociales [The International Catholic Committee of Nurses and Medico-Social Assistants]
DBfK	Deutscher Berufsverband für Krankenpflege [German Nursing Association]
DKG	Deutsche Krankenhausgesellschaft [German Hospital Society]
DKI	Deutsches Krankenhausinstitut [German Hospital Institute]
DM	Deutsche Mark [German Mark]
DRGs	Diagnostic Related Groups
EBM	Evidence-based medicine
EBN	Evidence-based nursing
EFN	European Federation of Nurses Associations
ENG	European Nursing Group
ICN	International Council of Nurses
IDM	International Confederation of Midwives
IHD	International Health Division
LNHO	League of Nations Health Organization
NIC	Nursing Interventions Classification
NOC	Nursing Outcomes Classification
OIHP	Office International d'Hygiene Publique
ÖTV	Gewerkschaft Öffentliche Dienste, Transport und Verkehr [Public Services, Transport and Traffic Union]
PSI	Public Service International
RCT	Randomized controlled trial
UK	United Kingdom
USA	United States of America
Ver.di	Vereinigte Dienstleistungsgewerkschaft [United Services Trade Union]

WCPT   World Confederation for Physical Therapy
WHO   World Health Organization
WWII   World War Two

Acknowledgements

The book in your hands is the outcome of my PhD project that took place from 2015 to 2020 at the University of Ottawa and the FH Münster University of Applied Science. Before, during, and after that time, I was supported by several friends, colleagues, and academics.

The greatest thank-yous go to my supervisors Dr Thomas Foth and Dr Susanne Kreutzer. Without them, this PhD project would not have been possible. Not only have they been on my side for many years, working hard to organize and financially enable this international PhD project, they were also an immense support during the research and writing process: they challenged me and stretched my horizons to gain understandings I never could imagine, they helped me to navigate complex approaches, problems, and perspectives, and encouraged me over and over again to keep on working. I am grateful for our countless discussions, for them sharing their knowledge, and for their patience with me.

I am thankful also to the members of my committee who accompanied my research journey over the years and encouraged me in my undertaking. I thank Dr Cheryl McWatters, Dr Amélie Perron, Dr Jayne Elliott, and Dr Dave Holmes, as well as Dr Laurence Bernard, for giving me inspiring information and helpful recommendations.

Writing in a second language poses problems on how to express thoughts and make them understandable. Right from the beginning and throughout the PhD process, Dr Jayne Elliott was an invaluable help. She fought with me in my struggles through the English language and helped me to get my arguments through. I thank her for her amazing editing work and for being approachable at all times even when the time was short (which happened quite often), and for her criticism.

I want to thank the University of Ottawa School of Nursing and especially the members of the Nursing History Research Unit who not only gave me professional support but also financial aid throughout my PhD project. At the FH Münster University of Applied Science, I found my "professional home," space, atmosphere, and resources to gain academic competence.

Several friends accompanied me during my research and my writing. I am grateful that I could always count on them. Many thanks go to Bärbel Wegner, Dorothe Wiening, Dr Anja Fiori, Dr Shokoufeh Modanloo, Dr Michelle Crick, and Dr Jiale Hu for many talks and intellectual discussions, for encouraging me and supporting me emotionally, for spending time together to relax and have fun. I also want to thank Renée Blouin. She welcomed me in Ottawa, provided me with my Canadian home, and adopted me into her family. I am grateful to Dr Nadin Dütthorn for her constant support and for giving me probably the most important advice for my PhD time: "Doing a PhD is all about not giving up."

Many thanks go to my family who made sure that I did not forget where I come from. I thank my sister Kelly for her ongoing and unconditional support. My mom was always by my side and constantly reminded me to think about my happiness when making decisions. I thank her for giving me wings and for educating me on how to manoeuvre through difficult times.

Chapter 1:
Introduction

Today, professional nursing in the Western world in general, and Germany in particular, is thought of as a practice based on a net of nursing standards, guidelines, and evidence-based nursing (EBN), etc. These tools should guarantee quality in nursing care and should make professional care transparent. At the same time, German nurses experience financial constraints, shortages in nursing personnel, a decreasing quality in nursing care, an increasing level of emotional stress leading to diseases such as burnout, and lack of time in daily nursing care.[1] While German nursing scholars ascribe a steadily increasing professional level to the German nursing vocation,[2] the situation in German nursing care became so serious that political leaders started a concerted action [*konzertierte Aktion*] in support of nursing care. This political campaign is administered by the Federal

---

1 E.g. Michael Isfort et al., "Pflege-Thermometer 2009. Eine bundesweite Befragung von Pflegekräften zur Situation der Pflege und Patientenversorgung im Krankenhaus [The NursingThermometer: A Federal Survey of Nurses on the Situation of Nursing and Patient Care in the Hospital]," (Deutsches Institut für angewandte Pflegeforschung e.V. (dip), 2010), https://www.researchgate.net/profile/Michael_Isfort/publication/288897767_Zur_Situation_des_Pflegepersonals_in_deutschen_Krankenhausern_-_Ergebnisse_des_Pflege-Thermometers_2009/links/56b47c6608aecddf26b573a9.pdf; Kerstin Hämel and Doris Schaeffer, "Who Cares? Fachkräftemangel in der Pflege [Who Cares? Shortage of Professional Nurses]," *Zeitschrift für Sozialreform* 59, no. 4 (2013), 413–31; Stephanie Kraft and Matthias Drossel, "Untersuchung des sozialen, beruflichen und gesundheitlichen Erlebens von Pflegekräften in stationären Krankenpflegeeinrichtungen – Eine qualitative Analyse [A Study on the Social, Vocational, and Health-Related Experiences of Nurses in Stationary Nursing Care Organizations]," *HeilberufeScience* 10, no. 3 (2019), 39–45.
2 E.g. Marita Neumann, "Berufsspezifische Entwicklung der Pflege – Vom Helfer zur Profession [Vocational Development of Nursing: From Assistant to Profession]," in *Case Management: Praktisch und Effizient*, ed. Christine von Reibnitz (Berlin, Heidelberg: Springer Berlin Heidelberg, 2009), 3–18; Irmgard Hofmann, "Die Rolle der Pflege im Gesundheitswesen. Historische Hintergründe und heutige Konfliktkonstellationen [The Role of the Nursing Vocation in the Healthcare System: Historical Background and Recent Conflicts]," *Bundesgesundheitsblatt - Gesundheitsforschung - Gesundheitsschutz* 55, no. 9 (2012), 1161–67; Martin Moers and Doris Schaeffer, "Pflegetheorien [Nursing Theories]," in *Handbuch Pflegewissenschaft*, ed. Doris Schaeffer and Klaus Wingenfeld (Weinheim und Basel: Beltz Juventa, 2014), 37–66.

Ministry of Health [*Bundesministerium für Gesundheit (BMG)*] and aims to improve the recognition of nursing as an occupation, the working conditions in healthcare organizations, and the autonomy of nurses.[3] During the COVID-19 pandemic, the situation worsened resulting in a severe nursing shortage in Germany.[4]

In this study, I will analyze how the existence of these contradictory phenomena of professionalization and inadequate working conditions became possible and how they are even interconnected. In order to undertake such a complex analysis, I will use the example of the nursing process, which was introduced in the 1970s, arguing that the above-described developments were only possible because the nursing process enabled the ability to think about nursing differently and consequently restructure nursing service.

The focus of my thesis, therefore, is on the developments in German nursing in the second half of the 20th century. The 1960s and 1970s are considered the beginning decades of the professionalization of German nursing.[5] However, contrary to many other countries like the United States of America (US), Canada, and the United Kingdom (UK), German nursing still struggles with being fully acknowledged as a profession.[6] This might be due to the lack of a general aca-

---

3 BMG, "Konzertierte Aktion Pflege [Concerted Action Nursing]," (Bundesministerium für Gesundheit, 2019), https://www.bundesgesundheitsministerium.de/en/service/begriffe-von-a-z/k/konzertierte-aktion-pflege.html.
4 Anke Begerow and Uta Gaidys, "COVID-19 Pflege Studie. Erfahrung von Pflegenden während der Pamdemie – erste Teilergebnisse [COVID-19 Nursing Study. Experiences of Nurses during the Pandemic – First Results]," *Pflegewissenschaft Sonderausgabe*, April (2020), 33–36; Norbert Grote and Bernd Tews, "Der Pflegenotstand ist längst da. Die Sicherstellung der pflegerischen Versorgung muss wieder gewährleistet werden [The Nursing Shortage already exists. Ensuring Nursing Care Needs to be Guaranteed]," *bpa Magazin* 12 (2022), no. 4, 12–14.
5 E. g. Martin Albert, "Krankenpflege auf dem Weg zur Professionalisierung [Nursing on Its Way to Professionalization]," 1998), http://phfr.bsz-bw.de/files/12/93_1.pdf; Renate Fischer, *Berufliche Identität als Dimension beruflicher Kompetenz: Entwicklungsverlauf und Einflussfaktoren in der Gesundheits- und Krankenpflege [Vocational Identity as Dimension of Vocational Competence: Development and Influencing Factors in Nursing]* (Bielefeld: Bertelsmann, 2013); Hilde Steppe, "Das Selbstverständnis der Krankenpflege in ihrer historischen Entwicklung [Self-Conception of Nursing in Its Historical Development]," *Pflege – Die wissenschaftliche Zeitschrift für Pflegeberufe* 13 (2000), 77–83; Johanna Taubert, *Pflege auf dem Weg zu einem neuen Selbstverständnis: Berufliche Entwicklung zwischen Diakonie und Patientenorientierung [Nursing on Its Way to a New Self-Concept: Occupational Development between Diaconry and Patient Orientation]*, 2nd ed. (Frankfurt am Main: Mabuse-Verlag, 1994); Horst-Peter Wolff and Jutta Wolff, *Geschichte der Krankenpflege: Mit 5 Tabellen [History of Nursing: With 5 Charts]* (Basel [u. a.]: RECOM-Verlag, 1994); Marianne Schmidbaur, *Vom "Lazaruskreuz" zu "Pflege Aktuell": Professionalisierungsdiskurse in der deutschen Krankenpflege 1903–2000 [From "Lazaruskreuz" to "Pflege Aktuell": Discourses on Professionalization in German Nursing Care 1903–2000]* (Königstein: Helmer, 2002).
6 Ingrid Darmann-Finck and Heiner Friesacher, "Editorial zu Professionalisierung in der Pflege [Editorial on the Professionalization in Nursing]," *ipp info* 5, no. 07 (2009), 1–2.

demic education for nurses, to the inability of German nurses to unionize, or maybe even to a different understanding of the term "profession."[7] Even today general education for nurses in Germany still takes place mainly outside academia. Nursing research in Germany is a relatively young science; the first nursing professor was appointed only in 1987. In was not until 2003 that an academic level as entry to the vocation became possible, although it remains as a parallel educational program to those already established outside academia. Although the main German nursing association was established in 1903, there is still no self-regulation of the profession. Colleges of nursing have emerged just recently.[8]

---

7 In Germany the term "profession" was and still is clearly linked to an academic education. This is somewhat different from Canada, for example, where nursing was called a "profession" before an academic education became legally necessary (see for example George Moir Weir, *Survey of Nursing Education in Canada* (Toronto: University of Toronto Press, 1932); Isabel Hampton-Robb, "The Nurse and the Public," *The Canadian Nurse* 1, no. 1 (1905), 9–11.). In order to prepare for the workforce two main strands of education are institutionalized in Germany: academic study programs, which traditionally prepare students for a profession, and vocational education and training which prepare them for vocations. 'Vocation' in this thesis is not referring to a calling, as it is understood traditionally, but rather is used for occupations that require a standardized vocational education and training. Vocational education and training is highly regulated through a combination of federal and provincial laws and many vocations have institutions for self-regulation such as the *Handwerkskammer* [*Chamber of Handicraft*]. The term "vocation" [*Beruf*] is highly significant in the German workforce and comes not only with a specific perception but also with a standardized education and a certain level of autonomy, identity, and status. However, the German understanding of profession is connected to a university education and enjoys a much higher status in society (Geoffrey Cocks and Konrad Hugo Jarausch, *German Professions, 1800–1950* (New York: Oxford University Press, 1990); Helga Krüger, "Professionalisierung von Frauenberufen – Oder Männer für Frauenberufe interessieren? Das Doppelgesicht des arbeitsmarktlichen Geschlechtersystems [Professionalization of Female Vocations, or Making Men Interested in Female Vocations?]," in *Feministische Forschung — Nachhaltige Einsprüche*, ed. Kathrin Heinz and Barbara Thiessen, Studien Interdisziplinäre Geschlechterforschung (Wiesbaden: VS Verlag für Sozialwissenschaften, 2003), 123–43). Although nursing emerged as a female occupation in Germany, despite differences in how nursing education has been regulated, it has been since the 1960s considered a vocation in the German sense, with a specific perception and a standardized education (Susanne Kreutzer, *Vom "Liebesdienst" zum modernen Frauenberuf: Die Reform der Krankenpflege nach 1945 [From "Labor of Love" to a Modern Female Profession: Nursing Reform after 1945]*, vol. 45, Reihe Geschichte und Geschlechter (Frankfurt am Main u. a.: Campus-Verlag, 2005).
8 Claudia Bischoff-Wanner, "Pflege im historischen Vergleich [Nursing in Historical Comparison]," in *Handbuch Pflegewissenschaft*, ed. Doris Schaeffer and Klaus Wingenfeld (Weinheim und Basel: Beltz Juventa, 2014), 19–36; Uta Oelke, *Projektbericht – Akademisierung von Pflege [Project Report – Academization of Nursing]*, vol. 2015 (1994); Horst-Peter Wolff and Jutta Wolff, *Krankenpflege: Einführung in das Studium ihrer Geschichte [Nursing Care: Introduction to the Study of Its History]*, vol. 2nd (Frankfurt am Main: Mabuse-Verlag, 2011); KrPflG, "Krankenpflegegesetz vom 16. Juli 2003 (Bgbl. I S. 1442), das zuletzt durch Artikel 1a des Gesetzes vom 17. Juli 2017 (Bgbl. I S. 2581) geändert worden ist [Nursing Act 2003]," (2003).

The start of this so-called professionalization[9] coincided with the transformation of social services in general, including the healthcare system, in the second half of the 20th century, particularly in the 1970s and 1980s. Characteristically for this transformation process was the introduction of an economic logic based on a neoliberal political rationale, a process that can be found all over the (Western) world.[10] As I will discuss in more detail later, this rationale construes individuals and organizations as economic actors or enterprises who follow their self-interest and are in competition with each other. Society as a whole is perceived as driven by economic interests and successful governments are those which are able to increase "efficiency" and make maximal use of "resources." In these transformations, management and accounting techniques played a decisive role because they were and still are considered objective and politically neutral ways of knowing and intervening in society.[11]

Transformation of Healthcare Services

Beginning in the 1970s, the German "universal" healthcare system underwent dramatic changes, providing all citizens free medical care based upon mandatory health insurance (and, since 1995, upon a mandatory nursing care insurance [*Pflegeversicherung*]). Most German citizens have statutory health insurance which pays healthcare costs directly to the provider; only a few, such as self-employed workers or public servants, possess private health insurance.[12] The German government was and still is responsible for the regulation of the healthcare system though regulation is mostly negotiated and executed by the payers (e.g. statutory and private health insurance companies) and the service providers (e.g. hospital managers or professional healthcare associations).

---

9 Professionalization in this study is understood as a process of development of a vocation towards a profession (Harald A. Mieg, "Professionalisierung [Professionalization]," in *Handbuch Berufsbildungsforschung*, ed. Felix Rauner (Bielefeld: Bertelsmann, 2005), 342–49). What a profession is seems to be seen differently in different contexts and countries. The chosen strategies to push a vocation towards professional status depend on a certain understanding of what 'profession' means and how professionalization processes are characterized.
10 Wendy Brown, *Undoing the Demos: Neoliberalism's Stealth Revolution* (New York: Zone Books, 2015).
11 Michel Foucault, *The Birth of Biopolitics: Lectures at the Collège De France, 1978–79* (Basingstoke, New York: Palgrave Macmillan, 2008); Peter Miller and Michael Power, "Accounting, Organizing, and Economizing: Connecting Accounting Research and Organization Theory," *Academy of Management Annals* 7, no. 1 (2013), 557–605.
12 Goran Ridic, Suzanne Gleason, and Ognjen Ridic, "Comparisons of Health Care Systems in the United States, Germany and Canada," *Materia socio-medica* 24, no. 2 (2012), 112–20.

Health insurance is financed by contributions from employers and employees equally.[13]

The German social insurance system has its origins in the 19th century. As the first plank of statesman Otto von Bismarck's social policy agenda, health insurance was founded in 1883. At first it covered only employed workers but it steadily broadened to include most German citizens. According to the recent regulations of health insurance, which took effect in 1989, the German healthcare system has to function according to three profound principles: the principle of need [*Bedarfsprinzip*], the principle of solidarity [*Solidaritätsprinzip*], and the principle or dictate of efficiency [*Wirtschaftlichkeitsgebot*]. The first principle means that the insured, when in need, are entitled to receive appropriate care for their specific healthcare need or problem regardless of what they have paid. The principle of solidarity acknowledges a community of solidarity in which all insured help each other indirectly through their financial contribution to health insurance. The dictate of efficiency means that healthcare services have to be sufficient and expedient, have to be provided in an efficient manner, and must not exceed the necessary.[14]

The emergence of this kind of economic thinking in healthcare can be dated to a time when many in Western societies began to criticize "big government" and neoliberals started their attacks on the welfare state. In Germany, the perceived increasing costs of healthcare were characterized as an important economic liability and a societal burden that needed to be addressed. Healthcare was no longer automatically understood as a right but was rather dependent on cost calculations and available resources.[15]

Health came to be understood as an economic product produced by different healthcare services and providers, thus turning healthcare professionals such as nurses into (service) producers. With these transformations came the implementation of accounting technologies in institutions, such as hospitals, that were previously understood as non-profit organizations aimed solely at protecting or improving the health of the population. As my research will demon-

---

13 Michael Simon, *Das Gesundheitssystem in Deutschland. Eine Einführung in Struktur und Funktionsweise [The Healthcare System in Germany. An Introduction in Structure and Functionality]*, 4th ed. (Bern: Verlag Hans Huber, 2013).
14 Rolf Rosenbrock and Thomas Gerlinger, *Gesundheitspolitik. Eine systematische Einführung [Health Policy: A Systematic Introduction]*, 3rd. ed. (Bern: Verlag Hans Huber, 2014); SGB V, "Sozialgesetzbuch. Fünftes Buch. Gesetzliche Krankenversicherung [Social Legislation Book. Book Five. Statutory Health Insurance]," (2019); Simon, *Das Gesundheitssystem in Deutschland*.
15 Monika Elisabeth Radek, *Weltkultur am Werk? Das globale Modell der Gesundheitspolitik und seine Rezeption im nationalen Reformdiskurs am Beispiel Polens [World Culture at Work? The Global Model of Health Policy and Its Reception in the National Reform Discourse – the Example of Poland]* (Bamberg: University of Bamberg Press, 2011).

strate, these accounting technologies, like the nursing process, which is the focus of this research project, had and still have a huge impact on those working in these institutions, because they have led to increased visibility and controllability of the nursing workforce. By making nursing actions visible and calculable in economic terms, nurses had from then on to justify their actions in economic terms and to constantly demonstrate the efficiency and effectiveness of their interventions. The introduction of accounting techniques into an institution, such as a hospital, makes its members, such as nurses, accountable for their work, meaning that nursing activities need to be justified by the rationale of economy. In order to be able to show the efficiency and effectiveness of nursing interventions and to make them calculable, nursing actions had to be understood as following a logic of means-end analysis, in which a defined target state would determine the means needed to achieve this target. The result of the nursing intervention could then be compared to the target set in advance in order to evaluate the effectiveness/efficiency of the nursing intervention. The nursing process as an input-output-process with a cybernetic logic is a paradigmatic example of how this logic has been implemented in healthcare and how an accounting tool such as the nursing process successfully transformed the way we understand nursing.

The Nursing Process

In most Western countries today the nursing process is an important component of what is considered professional nursing care. It was defined as "The Standard of Practice" by the American Nurses Association[16] and in Germany, the nursing process is the central characteristic of professional nursing as defined in the new German law, the nursing act [*Pflegeberufegesetz*] and – besides the steps of nursing performance and reporting – is reserved for fully educated nurses.[17] Thus, the nursing process is considered *the* quality indicator of nursing care and the basis of planned care.[18] This is why nursing scholars Monika Habermann and

---

16 American Nurses Association, *Nursing: Scope and Standards of Practice*, ed. Inc Ovid Technologies, 2 ed. (Silver Spring, Md.: American Nurses Association, 2010), 3.
17 PflBRefG, "Gesetz zur Reform der Pflegeberufe (Pflegeberufereformgesetz) vom 17. Juli 2017 [Law for the Reformation of the Occupations in Nursing from July 17th, 2017]," in *Teil I Nr. 49,*, ed. Bundesgesetzblatt (ausgegeben zu Bonn am 24. Juli 20172017); Rainer Ammende et al., "Rahmenpläne der Fachkommission nach § 53 PflBG [Frameworks for Nursing Education]," 2019), https://www.bibb.de/dokumente/pdf/geschst_pflgb_rahmenplaene-der-fachkommission.pdf.
18 Dorothy C. Hall, "Probleme der Krankenpflegeausbildung in Europa [Problems of the Nursing Education in Europe]," *Krankenpflege* 29, no. 10 (1976), 292, 301–03; Dorothy C. Hall, "Überlegungen zum Krankenpflegeberuf [Considerations About the Nursing Vocation]," *Krankenpflege* 31, no. 2 (1977), 40–42.

Leana R. Uys called the nursing process a "global concept;"[19] it has become a taken-for-granted instrument.

Most critical analyses of the nursing process are related to the situation in the USA and the UK. Germany, however, is particularly interesting, because the introduction of the nursing process happened at a time when nursing in Germany had been affected by a steadily decreasing Christian influence that had formerly been its foundation. Hence, from the 1960s on, German nursing began to transform its very substance. The introduction of the nursing process further limited the influence of the Christian sisterhoods in German nursing and transformed nursing into a secularized and rational activity.[20] An analysis of the development of the German nursing process helps to understand how the neoliberal rationale has been adopted by the nursing profession more broadly. The nursing process is understood as a decisive technology for changing the way nursing care is imagined and provided, and consequently, how the patient is perceived.

The nursing process is a four- to six-step problem-solving process that contains the assessment of the patient, the planning of nursing goals and interventions in order to meet the patient's needs, the performance of the planned nursing care and its documentation, as well as the evaluation of the output of the nursing interventions. With this rationality and the cybernetic structure of the nursing process, as I will show in this study, it is a powerful technology which enabled significant changes in German nursing. The structure allows linking certain single nursing tasks to specific nursing problems, and planned nursing goals to the actual outcome of patient care. This visualization of nursing care and the use of standardized language that is based on input, process, and output enables the manipulation of nursing actions by nursing colleagues but also by others who do not belong to the nursing vocation.

The majority of nursing scholars in Germany and abroad saw the implementation of the nursing process as a historic chance to strengthen processes of professionalization. This was particularly the case for the German context with nursing professionalization lagging far behind Anglo-American and other European countries. Nursing scholars welcomed the nursing process as an oppor-

---

19 Monika Habermann and Leana R. Uys, *The Nursing Process: A Global Concept* (Edinburgh; New York: Elsevier/Churchill Livingstone, 2006).
20 Susanne Kreutzer, "Conflicting Christian and Scientific Nursing Concepts in West Germany, 1945–1970," in *Routledge Handbook on the Global History of Nursing*, ed. Patricia D'Antonio, Julie A. Fairman, and Jean C. Whelan (London, New York: Routledge, 2016), 151–64; Susanne Kreutzer, "Rationalization of Nursing in West Germany and the United States, 1945–1970," in *Critical Approaches in Nursing Theory and Nursing Research*, ed. Thomas Foth, et al. (Göttingen: Universitätsverlag Osnabrück im V&R unipress GmbH, 2017), 209–27.

tunity to demonstrate the importance of nursing and to eventually professionalize it.[21]

However, it is noteworthy that discussions on the professionalization of the nursing vocation in Germany started at the same time as the neoliberal rationale and an economic logic became dominant. Using the nursing process and its impact on German nursing as my empirical focus, I will critically question the assumption that the nursing process was a successful tool in the professionalization of German nursing. This is the reason why the thesis title plays with the terms "professionalization" versus "de-professionalization." Whereas most nurses perceived the nursing process as a means to advance the professionalization process in Germany, it effectively contributed to the transformation of nursing actions into calculable, controllable, and technical actions that could rather be understood as a form of de-professionalization. This project follows the tensions around the implementation of the nursing process and I want to emphasize or "visualize" the contradictory consequences of the nursing process in the professionalization of nursing in the German context.

1.1 Research Objectives

To analyze the tension between the arguments praising the nursing process as an instrument of professionalization and the potential of the nursing process to consequently transform nursing into a calculable activity, leading instead to a form of de-professionalization.

1.2 Research Questions

1) What was the rationale that led to the perception that professional nursing must be based on economic thinking?
2) How did the introduction of the nursing process reconstitute the nursing vocation?
3) How can the paradox be described in which German nurses believed in the professionalization of nursing while at the same time the nursing vocation showed characteristics of a de-professionalization?

---

21 Hall, "Probleme der Krankenpflegeausbildung," 292, 301–03; Renate Reimann, "Pflegeplanung – Was bedeutet geplante Pflege in der Berufspraxis [The Nursing Care Plan: the Meaning of Planned Nursing Care in Daily Professional Practice]," *Krankenpflege* 33, no. 5 (1979), 154–57.

1.3 Organization and Structure

With the focus on German nursing I need to specify the following: (1) The transformations I analyze happen at a time when Germany was still divided into the Federal Republic of Germany (West Germany) and the German Democratic Republic (East Germany). With the unification of Germany in 1990, the system and regulations of East German nursing were dissolved and West German nursing became the model of nursing for a united Germany. Therefore, I will analyze the transformation of the West German model of nursing and I am referring to this model when I use the phrases "German nursing" or "nursing in Germany." (2) The German nursing vocation is split into three different types: pediatric nursing, nursing for ill adults (general nursing), and geriatric nursing. In my study, I will focus only on general nursing because it contains the largest group of nurses in Germany, especially in my time frame, and developments in general nursing have had a huge impact on developments in the other types of nursing.

In chapter 2, the "Background" section, I introduce developments in Germany in the second half of the 20th century with a special focus on the 1970s and 1980s. These decades witnessed many changes in the economic and societal spheres. Of special interest are those developments that occurred in the healthcare sector. I will present the arguments which led to strategies of cost control and cost consciousness.

Chapter 3 contains the historiography and a literature review. First, I present historical studies of the developments in German nursing in the 20th century, with a particular focus on the second half of the century. Although several nursing scholars have emphasized the narrative of the professionalization of nursing, critical perspectives, questioning this image of progress in German nursing, can be found. My study is built on those critical approaches. Second, I also review the few critical studies concerning the nursing process. While most critics of the nursing process focus on its weak implementation and poor reception in practical nursing, the critical analyses I present discuss the nature of the nursing process, the arguments surrounding the process, and its impact on practical nursing. These studies are related not only to the German context but analyze the implementation of the nursing process in other countries, although I have only considered those written in English and German.

In chapter 4, I present my methodological framework, where I first introduce my epistemic stance as the history of the present. This historical approach will help me to question the established narrative of professionalization in nursing and view it from another perspective. I follow with an overview of my empirical material and the way I analyzed it discursively.

Chapter 5 contains my theoretical framework. In order to acknowledge the neoliberal rationale and its impact on healthcare, and particularly in nursing, I will use the perspective of governmentality. Understanding neoliberalism with the concept of governmentality reveals a contradiction: In the neoliberal rationale, professions are seen as unnecessary and even obstacles for the government of people. I will analyze this contradiction by using concepts from critical accounting, which will help me to understand the impact of the nursing process as an accounting tool.

The empirical section begins in chapter 6 and introduces the broader setting in which the implementation of the nursing process took place. I will present the role of the World Health Organization (WHO) in the transformation of healthcare settings, particularly in Germany. From the empirical data, I outline the overall discussions around the implementation of the nursing process in Germany. It is interesting to note that resistance to the introduction of the nursing process can barely be found.

Chapter 7 focuses on the reconstruction of nursing care within the hospital sector on the basis of the nursing process. In published articles, nurses showed their enthusiasm in applying the nursing process and in developing a new hospital organization. Chapter 8 contains the analysis and discussion around the issue of professionalization in nursing. The logic of the accounting tool "nursing process" seems to have framed the understanding of nursing as a profession. The summary and the answers to my research questions can be found in chapter 9 together with the limitations and implications of my study.

Chapter 2:
Background

The 1970s have been and still are analyzed from different perspectives in regard to their importance for societal, political, and economic developments in Germany. This decade is now mostly constructed as a time of societal and economic disturbances, often summarized in notions like "change in values," "structural change," or even "structural upheaval."[22] German historians Anselm Doering-Manteuffel and Lutz Raphael were primarily responsible for the slogan "after the boom," [*nach dem Boom*][23] which has since been used in historical analyses concerning the decades after the 1960s. However, an economic boom could only be constituted when compared with the time of World War Two (WWII) and the economic breakdown thereafter. The reestablishment of the industrial economy and the financial help of the USA with the Marshal Plan were dominant factors for the perception of economic prosperity.[24] It seems that several developments and shifts – and their consequences – came together in the decade of the 1970s.

Historians Anselm Doering-Manteuffel and Lutz Raphael discuss the importance of the years 1968 and 1973 in determining a chronological period in which shifts in the economic rationale and societal discourses can be recognized.[25] In these years, changes in the narrative regarding the economy become

---

22 Knut Andresen, Ursula Bitzegeio, and Jürgen Mittag, "Arbeitsbeziehungen und Arbeitswelt(en) im Wandel: Problemfelder und Fragestellungen [Work Relations and Working Environment(s) in Transition: Problems and Questions]," in *"Nach dem Strukturbruch"? Kontinuität und Wandel von Arbeitsbeziehungen und Arbeitswelt(en) seit den 1970er Jahren*, ed. Knut Andresen, Ursula Bitzegeio, and Jürgen Mittag (Bonn: Verlag J. H. W. Dietz Nachf. GmbH, 2011), 7–23; Konrad H. Jarausch, "Verkannter Strukturwandel [Misunderstood Structural Change]," in *Das Ende der Zuversicht? Die siebziger Jahre als Geschichte*, ed. Konrad H. Jarausch (Göttingen: Vandenhoeck & Ruprecht, 2008), 9–26.
23 Anselm Doering-Manteuffel and Lutz Raphael, *Nach dem Boom. Perspektiven auf die Zeitgeschichte seit 1970 [After the Boom: Perspectives on Contemporary History since 1970]*, 3rd ed. (Göttingen: Vandenhoeck & Ruprecht, 2012).
24 Ralph Jessen, "Bewältigte Vergangenheit – Blockierte Zukunft? [Mastered Past – Blocked Future?]," in *Das Ende der Zuversicht? Die siebziger Jahre als Geschichte*, ed. Konrad H. Jarausch (Göttingen: Vandenhoeck & Ruprecht, 2008), 177–95.
25 Doering-Manteuffel and Raphael, *Perspektiven auf die Zeitgeschichte seit 1970*.

obvious as well as other societal changes such as the growing trends of female emancipation and individualization. Demands for competitive markets and for the flexibility of employees increased in order to assure competition. This was connected with an ever-strengthening shift of focus from industrial work to the service industry.[26] In this chapter, I describe the changes that occurred from the 1960s on in Germany, with a special focus on changes in the German healthcare system, since they provide the background in which nursing became restructured and rethought.

2.1 Societal Transformations in Germany "After the Boom"

By the end of the 1960s, the consequences of the welfare system – rising social costs, bureaucracy, enclosures of professions and their paternalism – were increasingly problematized by economists.[27] Furthermore, discussions were raised about the potential inability of the government to govern society.[28] Named a "cultural revolution" [*Kulturrevolution*][29] the changes following the year 1968 affected the economic sphere as well as the societal and individual spheres. German historians often use the notions of Fordism and Post-Fordism to describe the shift in the mode of production.[30] However, as philosopher Nancy Fraser argues, Fordism is "a multifaceted social formation. A historically specific

---

26 Anselm Doering-Manteuffel, "Langfristige Ursprünge und dauerhafte Auswirkungen [Long-Term Origins and Lasting Effects]," in *Das Ende der Zuversicht? Die siebziger Jahre als Geschichte*, ed. Konrad H. Jarausch (Göttingen: Vandenhoeck & Ruprecht, 2008), 313–29; Gabriele Metzler, "Staatsversagen und Unregierbarkeit in den Siebziger Jahren? [Government Failure and Ungovernability in the 1970s?]," in *Das Ende der Zuversicht? Die siebziger Jahre als Geschichte*, ed. Konrad H. Jarausch (Göttingen: Vandenhoeck & Ruprecht, 2008), 243–60; Dietmar Süß, "Der Sieg der Grauen Herren? [The Victory of the Men in Grey]," in *Vorgeschichte der Gegenwart*, (Vandenhoeck & Ruprecht, 2016), 109–28.
27 Matthias Wismar, *Gesundheitswesen im Übergang zum Postfordismus [The Healthcare System in Transition to Post-Fordism]* (Frankfurt am Main: VAS – Verlag für akademische Schriften, 1996); Winfried Süß, "Der bedrängte Wohlfahrtsstaat. Deutsche und Europäische Perspektiven auf die Sozialpolitik der 1970er-Jahre," *Archiv für Sozialgeschichte* 47 (2007), 95–126; Winfried Süß, "Umbau am "Modell Deutschland". Sozialer Wandel, ökonomische Krise und wohlfahrtsstaatliche Reformpolitik in der Bundesrepublik "nach dem Boom" [Rebuilding a "Model Germany": Social Change, Economic Crisis and Reform Policy of the Welfare State of the Federal Republic "after the Boom"]," *Journal of Modern European History* 9, no. 9 (2011), 215–40.
28 Metzler, "Staatsversagen und Unregierbarkeit," 243–60.
29 Doering-Manteuffel and Raphael, *Perspektiven auf die Zeitgeschichte seit 1970*, 51.
30 E.g. Dieter Sauer, "Permanente Reorganisation [Permanent Re-Organization]," in *Vorgeschichte der Gegenwart. Dimensionen des Strukturbruchs nach dem Boom*, ed. Anselm Doering-Manteuffel, Lutz Raphael, and Thomas Schlemmer (Göttingen: Vandenhoeck & Ruprecht, 2016), 37–56; Jarausch, "Verkannter Strukturwandel," 9–26; Doering-Manteuffel and Raphael, *Perspektiven auf die Zeitgeschichte seit 1970*.

phase of capitalism, yet not simply an economic category, Fordism was an international configuration that embedded mass production and mass consumption in national frames."[31] Fordism was based on a certain political, cultural, societal, and social constitution of nation-states in Western society as well as on colonial exploitation of the Third World. And it also reached far into the area of the individual. Fraser describes it as a disciplinary power (see chapter 4.1), as "fordist discipline [it] was totalizing,"[32] directing the behaviour and private lives of workers as well as society in general. Hence, instead of a mode of production, Fordism, from a Foucauldian perspective, needs rather to be understood as a mode of social regulation.[33] This disciplinary power structured and regulated the working environment, with assembly-line work as one of its prominent manifestations. The standard of employment in Fordism was characterized by predominantly male employees working full-time in an open-ended working relationship with their employer from the time of their vocational education on (or shortly after their training) until their retirement.[34]

The Fordist disciplinary society demanded that citizens had to follow strict rules and regulations. In the productive field, this mode of regulation became increasingly criticized as repressive, inflexible, and authoritarian, in which the worker was only a receiver of orders without any focus on individuality.[35] With the notion of post-Fordism, market mechanisms become the foundation of regulation. The individual became "[a] subject of (market) choice and a consumer of services ... obligated to enhance her quality of life through her own decisions" and "responsible for managing her own human capital to maximal effect."[36] The field of work demanded active employees who could make their own decisions based on means-ends analyses. Workers had more autonomy in and responsibility for the production process. Shifting the administration and organization of performances from the level of the enterprise to the level of the individual worker caused additional but mostly invisible work.[37] Accompanying

---

31 Nancy Fraser, "From Discipline to Flexibilization? Rereading Foucault in the Shadow of Globalization," *Constellations* 10, no. 2 (2003), 160–71: 162.
32 Fraser, "From Discipline to Flexibilization?," 163.
33 Fraser, "From Discipline to Flexibilization?," 160–71.
34 Andresen, Bitzegeio, and Mittag, "Arbeitsbeziehungen und Arbeitswelt(en) im Wandel," 7–23; Doering-Manteuffel and Raphael, *Perspektiven auf die Zeitgeschichte seit 1970*.
35 Doering-Manteuffel and Raphael, *Perspektiven auf die Zeitgeschichte seit 1970*; Dennis Eversberg, "Destabilisierte Zukunft [The De-Stabilized Future]," in *Vorgeschichte der Gegenwart*, ed. Anselm Doering-Manteuffel and Lutz Raphael, (Göttingen: Vandenhoeck & Ruprecht, 2016), 451–74; Andresen, Bitzegeio, and Mittag, "Arbeitsbeziehungen und Arbeitswelt(en) im Wandel," 7–23.
36 Fraser, "From Discipline to Flexibilization?" 168.
37 Sauer, "Permanente Reorganisation," 37–56.

this trend was automatization as well as a slowly growing computerization, especially in the administrative and bureaucratic areas.[38]

The working subject was framed within the economic demands of the enterprise: only by following the logic and objectives of the enterprise was the individual able to gain autonomy and responsibility. The organization of work was restructured as mechanisms of control that included such things as benchmarks and the documentation of time were increasingly introduced in order to measure the outcome of work processes and hence, the performance of the worker.[39] The idea of performance itself was redefined throughout the 1970s and 1980s from the notion of what could be achieved to that which needs to be achieved. Hence, the evaluation of worker performance shifted. It was not compared anymore to a feasible aim but to an aim that was constituted as necessary. It thus became more likely that aims could not be achieved.[40]

Also, workspaces themselves changed: "Timely measured work with lower physical but often higher mental burdens led to completely new forms of work – whether in public or in private circumstances."[41] This problem of time, as in judging the quality of nursing work (at least partly) based on time, and the increase of time control, could also be found in the healthcare sector and especially in the nursing field, as I will show in my study.[42]

Over the course of the 1970s, the shape of employment changed. While an increasing unemployment rate was declared a serious problem,[43] the employment rate of women increased dramatically from the 1960s on, especially with the growing field of service vocations. Historian Axel Schildt calls this the "'feminization' of the tertiary sector."[44] However, this should not be understood as a trouble-free process. Employed women, especially those who were mothers, primarily worked in part-time, low-paid jobs. Moreover, the difference in wages

---

38 Andreas Rödder, *Die Bundesrepublik Deutschland 1969–1990 [The Federal Republic of Germany 1969–1990]*, ed. Lothar Gall, Karl-Joachim Hölkeskamp, and Hermann Jakobs, vol. 19 A, Oldenbourg Grundriss der Geschichte (München: R. Oldenbourg Verlag, 2004).
39 Sauer, "Permanente Reorganisation," 37–56.
40 Sauer, "Permanente Reorganisation," 37–56.
41 Andresen, Bitzegeio, and Mittag, "Als zeitlich gemessene Arbeit mit geringer physischer, aber oft erheblicher psychischer Belastung hat sie zu völlig neuen Arbeitsformen geführt – ob öffentlichen oder privaten Charakters," "Arbeitsbeziehungen und Arbeitswelt(en) im Wandel," 15; my translation.
42 See also Thomas Foth, Jette Lange, and Kylie Smith, "Nursing History as Philosophy: Towards a Critical History of Nursing," *Nursing Philosophy* 19, no. 3 (2018), e12210.
43 Andresen, Bitzegeio, and Mittag, "Arbeitsbeziehungen und Arbeitswelt(en) im Wandel," 7–23.
44 Axel Schildt, 'Feminisierung' des tertiären Sektors, *Die Sozialgeschichte der Bundesrepublik Deutschland bis 1989/90 [The Social History of the Federal Republic of Germany until 1989/90]*, ed. Lothar Gall, vol. 80, Enzyklopädie Deutscher Geschichte (München: R. Oldenbourg Verlag, 2007), 36; my translation.

of female employees compared with their male colleagues decreased only slightly. In the 1980s, women continued to earn two-thirds of what men earned, thus not disturbing the traditional economic relationship between men and women, which ascribed men to the economic sphere with paid jobs and professional careers and women to the familial sphere.[45]

For German historians, the 1980s are the decade in which "Post-Fordism" and the neoliberal change became more visible.[46] The women's movement grew stronger and put a strong focus on the assumed naturalism of gratuitous household-work. The call for paid household work was connected to the hope of equality with men.[47] Also in the 1980s, the trend towards digitalization, individualization, and the establishment of the individual as entrepreneur strengthened and became more pertinent, raising discussions about privatization.[48]

2.2 The Transformation of the Healthcare System

Criticism of the German Social Security System

The German social security system, particularly healthcare, was and still is financed by contributions from employers and employees, with the prices of pharmaceuticals regulated, etc. However, by the 1960s, Ordoliberals were criticizing the social security and healthcare system for its cost intensity and authoritarian style in governing the population, meaning that individuals were not

---

45 Monika Mattes, "Krisenverliererinnen? Frauen, Arbeit und das Ende des Booms [Losers of the Crisis? Women, Work and the End of the Boom]," in *"Nach dem Strukturbruch"? Kontinuität und Wandel von Arbeitsbeziehungen und Arbeitswelt(en) seit den 1970er Jahren*, ed. Knut Andresen, Ursula Bitzegeio, and Jürgen Mittag (Bonn: Verlag J. H. W. Dietz Nachf. GmbH, 2011), 127–40.
46 Anselm Doering-Manteuffel and Lutz Raphael, "Nach dem Boom [after the Boom]," in *Vorgeschichte der Gegenwart. Dimensionen des Strukturbruchs nach dem Boom*, ed. Anselm Doering-Manteuffel, Lutz Raphael, and Thomas Schlemmer (Göttingen: Vandenhoeck & Ruprecht, 2016), 9–34; Dietmar Süß and Meik Woyke, "Schimanskis Jahrzehnt? Die 1980er Jahre in historischer Perspektive [Schimanski's Decade? The 1980s in a Historical Perspective]," *Archiv für Sozialgeschichte* 52 (2012), 3–20; Doering-Manteuffel and Raphael, *Perspektiven auf die Zeitgeschichte seit 1970*.
47 Axel Schildt, "Das letzte Jahrzehnt der Bonner Republik. Überlegungen zur Erforschung der 1980er Jahre [The Last Decade of the Bonner Republic: Considerations for the Investigation of the 1980s]," *Archiv für Sozialgeschichte* 52 (2012), 21–46; Nicole Kramer, "Neue soziale Bewegungen, Sozialwissenschaften und die Erweiterung des Sozialstaats. Familien- und Altenpolitik in den 1970er und 1980er Jahren [New Social Movements, Social Sciences and the Expansion of the Social State: Politics for Families and Elderly in the 1970s and 1980s]," *Archiv für Sozialgeschichte* 52 (2012), 211–30.
48 Süß and Woyke, "Schimanskis Jahrzehnt?," 3–20; Schildt, "Das letzte Jahrzehnt der Bonner Republik," 21–46.

free to withdraw money from their insurance when they believed they needed it.[49] Discussions ensued over the explosion of costs and how to contain them. Although increasing costs were mainly due to pension insurance, the cost explosion argument in the healthcare sector was used to restructure its financing and transform it into an enterprise.[50] Nevertheless, health insurance expenses continued to increase after the hospital law of 1972.[51] This law re-organized the financing of hospitals in Germany. Payment was retrospective and was calculated on the basis of beds in use per day, which likely encouraged hospitals to keep patients longer.[52] The responsibility of guaranteeing good healthcare was shifted to the federal level, where the provinces were obligated to develop hospital plans to register all capable healthcare institutions. Compensation for hospitals was based on their fiscal consciousness, with a focus on recovering costs and not making a profit. The costs of hospital care were split between the public sphere, meaning both the central and regional government budgets, and health insurance, meaning their paying members.[53]

According to nursing scientist Michael Simon, after the implementation of the law, the costs of the healthcare system increased for the following reasons: First, financial support from the state sector was decreased, leading to a higher financial burden on health insurance. Additionally, the system through which daily healthcare costs were paid changed as well. Before the hospital law, it was a three-class system in which first- and second-class patients were charged a higher part of costs than that paid by the health insurance for third-class patients. After the law, the three-class system was changed so that all patients were charged a uniform amount of daily healthcare costs. This, in consequence, led to a lower

---

49 Heddy Neumeister, "Autoritäre Sozialpolitik [Authoritarian Social Policy]," *ORDO Jahrbuch für die Ordnung von Wirtschaft und Gesellschaft* 12 (1961), 187–252; Hubertus Müller-Groeling, "Zur ökonomischen Problematik der gesetzlichen Krankenversicherung [About the Economic Problems of the Statutory Health Insurance]," *ORDO Jahrbuch für die Ordnung von Wirtschaft und Gesellschaft* 19 (1968), 485–98.
50 Wismar, *Gesundheitswesen im Übergang zum Postfordismus*; Michael Simon, *Krankenhauspolitik in der Bundesrepublik Deutschland. Historische Entwicklung und Probleme der politischen Steuerung stationärer Krankenversorgung [Hospital Policy in the Federal Republic of Germany: Historical Developments and Problems of the Political Control of Stationary Healthcare]*, Studien Zur Sozialwissenschaft Band 209 (Wiesbaden: Springer Fachmedien Wiesbaden GmbH, 2000).
51 Simon, *Krankenhauspolitik*.
52 Rolf Rosenbrock and Thomas Gerlinger, *Gesundheitspolitik. Eine systematische Einführung [Health Policy. A Systematic Introduction]*, 3rd. ed. (Bern: Verlag Hans Huber, 2014).
53 Simon, *Krankenhauspolitik*; Michael Simon, "Die ökonomischen und strukturellen Veränderungen des Krankenhausbereichs seit den 1970er Jahren [The Economic and Structural Changes in the Hospital Setting since the 1970s]," in *Mutationen des Krankenhauses: Soziologische Diagnosen in organisations- und gesellschaftstheoretischer Perspektive*, ed. Ingo Bode and Werner Vogd (Wiesbaden: Springer Fachmedien Wiesbaden, 2016), 29–45.

amount of money coming from private patients, which had to be made up by the health insurance.[54]

Second, the change in healthcare personnel, especially nurses, increased costs. Up until the 1950s nurses often worked more hours for less money than women in comparable vocations. This specific working model in nursing became increasingly unattractive to young women (see chapter 3.1). Additionally, the number of patients increased, exacerbating a nursing shortage. The countermeasures to make nursing more attractive such as increasing nurses' salaries and decreasing the number of hours worked in consequence to raise the costs for nursing personnel.[55]

Third, in the two decades after WWII, hospitals hardly had any money to rebuild and replace old and destroyed structures and equipment. Furthermore, inpatient care did not correspond with the modern needs of medicine anymore. One aim of the hospital law of 1972 was to modernize hospitals by investing in their rebuilding and restructuring. As Simon argues, it was these efforts at modernization, rather than uneconomic behaviour, that led to increasing hospital expenses in the first years after the law was introduced. After a few years of catching up, hospital expenses decreased.[56]

Hence, Simon argued that only the health insurance plan faced increasing costs and not the whole sector of hospital care. Furthermore, these costs did not occur because of uneconomic behavior but rather because of a modernization deficit that had to be solved, of a change in the organization of health personnel, and of the changes in the financial structure of hospital-based healthcare.

However, as Simon argued in retrospect, the term "cost explosion" was politically important to justify cost-containment policies thereafter. Here, he draws on the neoliberal argument and economic principle that reducing financial resources ("benefits") would lead to an increase in cost-effective behaviour. According to Simon, behind the officially declared cost-explosion in the healthcare system was the need to cover the financial deficits of pension insurance. In order to cover these state deficits the premise of covering all expenses was substituted for the premise of limiting resource consumption. Cost containment, therefore, became an important strategy to lower the financial deficits in other social insurance plans. Consequently, one cost containment act for health insurance [*Krankenversicherungs-Kostendämpfungsgesetz*] was released in 1977 and in 1981 the Hospital Cost Containment Act [*Krankenhaus-Kostendämpfungsgesetz*] was passed. Both were developed officially to ease the consequences of the hospital act of 1972. However, as Michael Simon argues, the acts actually pio-

---

54 Simon, *Krankenhauspolitik*.
55 Simon, *Krankenhauspolitik*.
56 Simon, *Krankenhauspolitik*.

neered a new mode of regulation in healthcare. Under the 1977 act, the financial support of healthcare by the public sector was decreased and the hospitals were urged to act according to the rules of the market by negotiating for themselves the cost of daily hospital care [*Pflegesätze*] with regional hospital societies. The 1981 act aimed at regulating costs in the healthcare system.[57] These transformations emerging in the hospital sector can also be found in the nursing field. Interestingly, several nursing scholars declare that this is the exact starting point of professionalization in nursing.

---

57 Simon, *Krankenhauspolitik*.

Chapter 3:
Studies on Developments in German Nursing and on the Nursing Process

To date, there is no publicized nursing study on the history of implementing the nursing process in Germany. However, discussions of the history of German nursing – its progress, evolution, and professionalization – as well as scientific papers on the nursing process, can be found. First, I will summarize the current state of research in regard to developments in German nursing. In several historical studies, an overarching narrative was developed from the 1980s on that explained nursing in Germany as evolving from a submissive and Christian female vocation into a professionalizing occupation based on rationality and science. Nursing activists reproduced and reused this narrative as they argued for a professionalization in nursing that was based on fostering scientific rationality, on academization, and on nursing research. Newer historical studies, however, have begun to critically reflect on this narrative to question this professionalization project.

In the second part, I present publications discussing the nature and reception of the nursing process. Here, the focus is especially on papers with a critical perspective, most of which can be found in the edited book, *The Nursing Process: A Global Concept*,[58] where authors with different critical perspectives discuss the concept of the nursing process. Other articles also view the situation regarding the nursing process critically, although much of their criticism is related more to the way the nursing process was implemented rather than to its inherent logic. The solutions these articles provide point towards a better implementation of the process through improving the education and training of nurses to show them how to use the nursing process, and through more profoundly understanding the theoretical considerations of the different elements of the nursing process in order to handle it in the "right" way.[59]

---

58 Monika Habermann and Leana R. Uys, *The Nursing Process: A Global Concept* (Edinburgh; New York: Elsevier/Churchill Livingstone, 2006).
59 E. g. Michael Isfort, "Prozessuale Pflege – Oder die nächste Fahrt geht rückwärts! [Processural Nursing Care: Or is the Next Turn Backwards]," *Die Schwester Der Pfleger* 44, no. 6 (Son-

3.1 Historiography

Nursing scientist Claudia Bischoff analyzes nursing as a female vocation, suggesting that femininity was commonly understood as an antidote to the "bad" characteristics of egoism, aggression, and competitiveness. She emphasizes that nursing was only constructed as a typical female vocation in the 19th century. According to Bischoff, equipping nursing with women benefits society because so-called typical female characteristics such as patience, friendliness, and a caring attitude are included automatically and gratuitously in nursing care. On the one hand, she sees this "female competence" as important in social vocations such as nursing or childcare to provide emotional and humanistic hospital care. However, she also emphasizes that it is exactly these "female" characteristics that put nurses in a subordinate position because they are only barely applicable to the "male" logic of vocational or professional work.[60] Bischoff accuses nurses of supporting the cost-saving politics of the 1970s and 1980s because of their female work ethos that centred on patient-oriented care, which helped to keep the image of humanity in hospitals at the same time as these institutions were implementing and "maintaining conditions and structures which actually [made] healthcare inhuman."[61] For her, progress in nursing draws on the changed societal values especially for women who now can choose work within a broader vocational and professional field; on the social and demographic changes which have led to new patient groups, such as older and/or chronically ill patients with multimorbidities; on medical and technical progress, which calls for better and scientifically educated nurses; and on the scientification of nursing, which has attempted to move nursing out of its formerly subordinate role, especially in regard to medicine.[62]

---

derdruck 7/05) (2005), 1–10; Peter Stratmeyer, "Ein historischer Irrtum der Pflege. Plädoyer für einen kritisch-distanzierten Umgang mit dem Pflegeprozess [A Historical Error in Nursing: A Plea for a Critical and Distanced Attitude Towards the Nursing Process]," *Dr. med. Mabuse* 106 (1997), 34–38.

60 Claudia Bischoff, *Frauen in der Krankenpflege: Zur Entwicklung von Frauenrolle und Frauenberufstätigkeit im 19. und 20. Jahrhundert [Women in Nursing: On the Development of the Female Role and Female Employment in the 19th and 20th Century]*, vol. 3rd (Frankfurt am Main; New York: Campus-Verlag, 1997); Claudia Bischoff, "Krankenpflege als Frauenberuf [Nursing as a Female Vocation]," *Das Argument/Sonderband* 86 (1982), 13–27.

61 "Unter den gegebenen Bedingungen ist zu vermuten, daß hinter der 'unzeitgemäßen' Forderung nach Patientenorientierter Pflege auch noch andere als humane, patientenbezogene Interessen stehen: daß nämlich Krankenhaus und Medizin die Patientenorientierte Pflege als humanes Alibi gegenüber Kritik von außen (miß)-brauchen, um alle diejenigen Bedingungen und Strukturen aufrechtzuerhalten, die die Krankenversorgung erst inhuman machen" (Bischoff, *Frauen in der Krankenpflege*, 11; my translation).

62 Bischoff, *Frauen in der Krankenpflege*.

In her arguments, Bischoff conceptualizes the nursing process as part of professional nursing. She explains that the nursing process is a supportive element in planning nursing care that connects two different logics. On the one hand, it carries the rational and organizational (male) component, opens nursing to managerial processes, and helps to foster effectivity and efficiency in nursing care. On the other hand, Bischoff states, it supports holism and the relational aspect between nurses and patients. This relational aspect, in turn, calls for emotional work and individuality, which she connects with typical female work capacity. Bischoff sees that the benefit of the nursing process lies in the integration of "female" logic with the gender-neutral vocabulary of this process-logic. However, she emphasizes that the problem-solving aspect of the nursing process (and hence, "male" logic) is more dominant than the relational aspect of the nursing process ("female" logic), but claims to value both equally in order to establish a true nursing professional that acknowledges not only the managerial necessities but also the emotional work required.[63] In my study, however, I question Bischoff's optimistic picture of the nursing process and its impact on the nursing profession. I will show that activities that cannot be verbalized in a rational way, such as emotional work, cannot be captured in the steps of the nursing process. These activities, hence, are in danger of becoming ignored in a newly constituted nursing vocation (see chapter 7.2.1).

Bischoff's narrative on the evolution of professionalization in nursing develops out of the positioning of nursing, as a female vocation, as subordinate to medicine (and hence, nurses to physicians) in the 18th and 19th century. It was taken further by German nursing scholars and historians and was used, along with the Christian foundation of nursing, as an explanation for the delay in and obstacles to professionalization. With re-orientation to nursing's "actual" activities (away from a medical focus), the development of academic nursing education courses, and a higher standardization of nursing activity, the next steps seem to have been taken towards professionalization in nursing.[64]

---

63 Bischoff, *Frauen in der Krankenpflege*.
64 Martin Albert, "Krankenpflege auf dem Weg zur Professionalisierung [Nursing on Its Way to Professionalization]," 1998, http://phfr.bsz-bw.de/files/12/93_1.pdf; Renate Fischer, *Berufliche Identität als Dimension beruflicher Kompetenz: Entwicklungsverlauf und Einflussfaktoren in der Gesundheits- und Krankenpflege [Vocational Identity as Dimension of Vocational Competence: Development and Influencing Factors in Nursing]* (Bielefeld: Bertelsmann, 2013); Hilde Steppe, "Das Selbstverständnis der Krankenpflege in ihrer historischen Entwicklung [The Self-Conception of Nursing in Its Historical Development]," *Pflege – Die wissenschaftliche Zeitschrift für Pflegeberufe* 13 (2000), 77–83; Johanna Taubert, *Pflege auf dem Weg zu einem neuen Selbstverständnis: Berufliche Entwicklung zwischen Diakonie und Patientenorientierung [Nursing on Its Way to a New Self-Concept: Occupational Development between Diaconry and Patient Orientation]*, 2nd ed. (Frankfurt am Main: Mabuse-Verlag, 1994); Horst-Peter Wolff and Jutta Wolff, *Geschichte der Krankenpflege: Mit 5 Tabellen*

This narrative, I argue, has to be viewed critically. It is based on a teleological understanding of the development of the German nursing vocation towards professionalism and ignores other potential outcomes. Moreover, the empirical findings of my study instead show tendencies of de-professionalization. Furthermore, I question that there are "actual" nursing activities that do not change over time and to which nurses only have to return. Rather, for example, in Germany in the 1970s and 1980s, the nursing vocation was re-constituted and a nurse's scope of practice expanded with new nursing activities. Sociologist Marianne Schmidbaur discusses the professionalization narrative by analyzing professionalization discourses and the vocational and professional developments in nursing throughout the whole 20th century. Drawing on aspects of power and gender, in her feminist work she asks about the relationship between professionalization and emancipation in nursing. For the 1970s and 1980s, she focuses particularly on developments in nursing education, on the attempts to academize, and on the perception of nursing. According to Schmidbaur, although finding less supportive political and economic conditions in the 1980s, German nursing achieved reasonable progress, which she ascribes to international developments in the nursing vocations of other states that positively affected what was happening in German nursing. In this regard, she values the medium-term program of the World Health Organization (WHO) for its introduction of research and study of the nursing process.[65] Other notions of holistic or patient-oriented/patient-centred care became absorbed by the theme of this nursing process.

However, Schmidbaur believes that the nursing process was introduced more because of pragmatic than philosophical or emancipatory concepts. She demonstrates the contradictory consequences that accompanied the legal recognition and institutionalization of the nursing process: an increase in control over and bureaucracy in nursing care but little regard for the idea that good nursing care is based on a holistic understanding of patients that was an underlying assumption of the nursing process. This led in the 1990s, according to Schmidbaur, even to the assumption that the emphasis on holistic care hinders or even precludes professionalization: "Purposeful action would always be directed to single problems, hence, holistic action, also in nursing, would not be possible. Between

---

[History of Nursing: With 5 Charts] (Basel [u.a.]: RECOM-Verlag, 1994); Claudia Bischoff-Wanner, "Pflege im historischen Vergleich [Nursing in Historical Comparison]," in *Handbuch Pflegewissenschaft*, ed. Doris Schaeffer and Klaus Wingenfeld (Weinheim und Basel: Beltz Juventa, 2014), 19–36.

65 Marianne Schmidbaur, *Vom "Lazaruskreuz" zu "Pflege Aktuell": Professionalisierungsdiskurse in der deutschen Krankenpflege 1903–2000 [From "Lazaruskreuz" to "Pflege Aktuell": Discourses on Professionalization in German Nursing Care 1903–2000]* (Königstein: Helmer, 2002).

the goals 'professionalization' and 'holism' there would be a contradiction that could not be solved."[66] Schmidbaur summarizes the attempts of professionalization in the 1970s and 1980s as being instrumental, that is, directed to a concrete utopia based on certain characteristics of professions, or as being emancipatory. These were based on the focus on holism.[67]

Schmidbaur analyzes the developments in German nursing that took place over a whole century based on the relations and interconnections between professionalization and emancipation. She shows the contradictions between attempts to professionalize and their consequences after application. She also carves out the tensions underlying the introduction of the nursing process as a tool of professionalization and provides a good starting point for this present study in which to analyze the two-fold image of the nursing process, in this case, in regard to professionalism and to accounting.

Nursing pedagogist Anne Kellner grounded her historical analysis about self-care in nursing on Foucault. She points to the influence of neoliberalism at the end of the 20th century but does not connect it with the specific role of professionalization in nursing. She argues rather for the professionality of nurses, for example, that empowered the patient to become an active and knowledgeable decision maker in healthcare. She focusses on the self-disciplining mechanisms and practices of nurses as attempts at self-management and self-optimization. She also analyzes the neoliberal patient-subject who becomes constructed as a consumer of nursing care and an entrepreneur of him-/herself. Patients are perceived and should perceive themselves as active and as responsible for their own health.[68]

Kellner outlines the following regarding professionalization: It was not until the 1970s that the professionalization project, which had actually begun in 1903 with the foundation of what is today the dominant professional nursing association, resumed. The female vocation began to integrate male nurses into its professionalization project. Emancipating itself from medicine, searching for a new identity with the help of the nursing process, and attempting to academize nursing education were steps of the professionalization project. Kellner puts a strong emphasis on the strategic actions of nurses. While reflecting on developments in German nursing in the 1990s, she does acknowledge that the pro-

---

66 "Zielgerichtetes Handeln sei immer auf Einzelprobleme gerichtet, 'ganzheitliches' Handeln somit – auch in der Pflege – gar nicht möglich. Zwischen den Zielen 'Professionalisierung' und 'Ganzheitlichkeit' bestehe ein nicht zu lösender Widerspruch" (Schmidbaur, *Vom "Lazaruskreuz" zu "Pflege Aktuell"*, 199; my translation).
67 Schmidbaur, *Vom "Lazaruskreuz" zu "Pflege Aktuell"*.
68 Anne Kellner, *Von der Selbstlosigkeit zur Selbstsorge. Eine Genealogie der Pflege [From Selflessness to Self-Care: A Genealogy of Nursing]*, ed. Regina Lorenz-Krause, vol. 4, Pflege und Gesundheit (Berlin: LIT Verlag Dr. W. Hopf, 2011).

fessionalization project became constrained or questioned, especially within the context of neoliberal ideology (tendencies of de-professionalization).[69] However, she does not explicitly connect professionalization in nursing with the introduction of neoliberal mechanisms.

Nursing scientist Eva-Maria Krampe analyzes the academization of the nursing vocation in Germany and asks whether nursing achieved autonomy with the introduction of academic study programs in nursing. She uses a Foucauldian critical analysis of discourses, focusing her analysis on the neoliberal transformations predominantly from the 1980s on. She argues that the severe economic pressure felt by the end of the 1970s fostered the addition of measurability and empirical provability as new dimensions of scientific nursing.

Krampe discusses a broad, superordinate discourse in nursing that consists of three streams. One stream is about the professionalization of the nursing vocation, which, if accomplished, would gain it more power and increase participation in the healthcare system as well as improve the actual practice of nursing. However, she asserts that no published agreement can be found on what exactly professionalization is and what it should look like for nursing in Germany. The second stream calls for nursing to develop its own knowledge base to be able to justify scientific and practical autonomy and to substantiate nursing activities and make them transparent. The third stream is the claim that nursing had adapted to the changing healthcare system, taking into account new market structures as well as quality management and standardization. Here, she emphasizes that "structural changes of the healthcare system were not only accepted without question but were even used as a vehicle for gaining importance and status."[70] Krampe concludes that nursing discourses at the end of the 1980s and in the 1990s verify and legitimate the neoliberal agenda in the healthcare system by using the same neoliberal arguments. She also criticizes the tendency to use professionalization and modernization synonymously. According to Krampe, modernization is simply an adaptation to new developments and hence, just guarantees the same except in changing circumstances. Professionalization, on the other hand, would be progress and is more than simply adapting.[71]

---

69 Kellner, *Von der Selbstlosigkeit zur Selbstsorge*, 4.
70 "Gleichzeitig wird aber auch offenbar, dass Strukturveränderungen des Gesundheitswesens nicht nur unhinterfragt akzeptiert werden, sondern dass sie sogar als Vehikel für den eigenen Bedeutungs- und Statusgewinn benutzt werden" (Eva-Maria Krampe, *Emanzipation durch Professionalisierung: Akademisierung des Frauenberufs Pflege in den 1990er Jahren; Erwartungen und Folgen [Emancipation through Professionalization: The Academization of a Female Vocation in the 1990s; Expectations and Consequences]* (Frankfurt am Main: Mabuse-Verlag, 2009), 104; my translation).
71 Krampe, *Emanzipation durch Professionalisierung*.

Krampe also shows that in regard to the relationship between nursing and medicine, the discourse contains different and apparently contradictory perspectives. While adapting to the medical paradigm was promoted as important in the case of specializations especially in acute and intensive care, those specialized streams in nursing were at the same time excluded from the "actual" nursing field to avoid nurses looking like medical assistants.

Krampe's results are interesting for my study because some of the discursive changes I will describe are no longer debated or questioned in her time frame, especially the now indisputable understanding that modern and even professional nursing care needs to be efficient, justified, and planned. Moreover, as Krampe emphasizes, modern or professional nursing is already being viewed through the frame of austerity. The pressure of economization has been argued as a chance to establish autonomy and independence from physicians, for example, by collaborating with managers or by producing higher educated nurses who can oversee activities in the healthcare system for less money.[72] However, I argue that many of these developments had already started one to two decades earlier than when Krampe dates them, like, for instance, the promise that patient-oriented care would help to save costs.[73] Moreover, I will focus on the nursing process in particular and its impact on perceptions of professional nursing.

Nursing historian Susanne Kreutzer centres her work especially on the rationalization in and transformation of the nursing vocation. She considers developments in nursing after WWII up until the 1980s and focusses on the upheavals or rapid changes in the perception of nursing, as well as the structures and organization in which nursing was carried out. Using archival material such as minutes of meetings, reports, and letters, as well as oral history interviews of nurses working in different nursing streams (Deaconesses, Hollywood Nurses of Heidelberg, Association of Free Sisters [*Bund freier Schwestern*] as part of the Union ÖTV (now *ver.di*)), Kreutzer shows how the traditional Christian-based nursing image declined from the 1960s on, how nursing, therefore, lost its former identity and became a medical assistant vocation, and how rationalization in the healthcare system affected nursing work.[74]

---

72 Krampe, *Emanzipation durch Professionalisierung*.
73 Krampe, *Emanzipation durch Professionalisierung*, 153.
74 Susanne Kreutzer, *Vom "Liebesdienst" zum modernen Frauenberuf: Die Reform der Krankenpflege nach 1945 [From "Labor of Love" to a Modern Female Profession: Nursing Reform after 1945]*, vol. 45, Reihe Geschichte und Geschlechter (Frankfurt am Main u. a.: Campus-Verlag, 2005); Susanne Kreutzer, *Arbeits- und Lebensalltag evangelischer Krankenpflege. Organisation, soziale Praxis und biographische Erfahrungen, 1945–1980 [Daily Work and Living in Protestant Nursing: Organization, Social Practice, and Biographical Experiences, 1945–1980]* (Göttingen: V&R unipress, 2014); Susanne Kreutzer, ""Before, We Were Always There – Now, Everything Is Separate": On Nursing Reforms in Western Germany," *Nursing History Review* 16 (2008), 180–200; Susanne Kreutzer, ""Hollywood Nurses" in West Ger-

According to Kreutzer, changes can be found in different realms. Societal changes fostered the decline of the motherhouse-based organization in German nursing. Motherhouses are confessional institutions in which unmarried women live and serve God as deaconesses and Catholic sisters. The organization of nursing service by the motherhouse system became dominant in the 19th century and remained relatively stable until the 1950s and early 1960s. Motherhouses either managed their own hospitals and healthcare institutions or concluded contracts with healthcare service institutions. Unmarried women lived in the motherhouse and were sent out to work as nursing personnel in hospitals, community care, and other social institutions. The motherhouse system provided an acceptable alternative way of life for single women besides being a wife and a mother. Women acquired a vocational education as well as lifelong support and a guarantee of care in sickness and old age. Nursing and medicine were perceived as complementary, with physicians treating the patient in regard to his/her illness and nurses caring for individuals holistically. Nurses had their own distinct area of competence and autonomy based on certain activities that belonged to nurses alone. Nurses worked 70 to 80 hours a week, making any private life impossible,[75] and nursing care was perceived as a charity service.[76]

Less attraction to this way of living coincided with an increasing societal acceptance that married women with a family could still be employed. Furthermore, possibilities of employment for women emerged outside of nursing, and women were less willing to live under a motherhouse regime. The Protestant and Catholic motherhouses in particular experienced a huge decline in members. As nursing shortages increased, nursing was restructured from a labor of love carried out by unmarried women to an occupation in which part-time work by married women was possible. Working hours were also reduced significantly – a process that had already happened in other vocations in German society. In the 1950s, a maximum of 54 working hours per week was slowly implemented, and in the 1960s the hours were again slowly reduced to 48 per week. By 1973, the 40-hour week was established.[77]

The decline of the motherhouse structure worsened the nursing shortage and led to a huge increase in costs for healthcare. "The crisis of the motherhouses

---

many: Biographies, Self-Images, and Experiences of Academically Trained Nurses after 1945," *Nursing History Review: Official Journal of the American Association for the History of Nursing* 21 (2013), 33–54.
75 Kreutzer, "On Nursing Reforms in Western Germany," 180–200.
76 Kreutzer, *Vom "Liebesdienst" zum modernen Frauenberuf.*
77 Axel Schildt, *Die Sozialgeschichte der Bundesrepublik Deutschland bis 1989/90 [The Social History of the Federal Republic of Germany until 1989/90]*, ed. Lothar Gall, vol. 80, Enzyklopädie deutscher Geschichte (München: R. Oldenbourg Verlag, 2007); Kreutzer, *Vom "Liebesdienst" zum modernen Frauenberuf.*

made it clear that the operation and the extension of hospitals had up to this point been based on a high degree on the poorly paid but highly qualified work of women. Now not only did the immense financial costs of professional nursing became obvious, but so did the importance of the emotional support of patients and their relatives."[78]

Changes were also made in regard to the content of nursing and nursing education. The nursing act of 1965 restructured nursing education fundamentally, laying a stronger focus on theoretical knowledge. Whereas formerly experiential knowledge and continuing patient observation was the basis upon which nurses carried out their work, this theoretical knowledge was disentangled from the individual patient and became the foundation of nursing decisions and actions. This diminished the implicit and tacit body of knowledge on which nursing in Germany was mainly based. For example, patient observation, according to Kreutzer, which was formerly a key competence in German nursing, became devalued with this increasing scientification, and it became complicated by strategies of rationalization such as the introduction of nursing aids and of functional care. Moreover, the processes of rationalization also led to an intensification of work.[79]

However, as Kreutzer argues, the nursing act of 1965 was established as an important step towards professionalization in nursing by increasing the theoretical hours as well as the general time of education and training to three years. Additionally, a shift in the very substance of nursing occurred by discussing and differentiating what belonged to nursing activity and what did not. Housekeeping activities came under criticism over the course of the 1950s with the increasing nursing shortage. However, nurses in 1955 insisted that differentiation between tasks belonging or not to the vocation could not be determined based on whether they were domestic/housekeeping or healthcare tasks but only in regard to the individual needs of the patient. "Whether a task belongs to the nursing vocation or not could not be decided upon the task itself but on the required proximity to the patient. A relief for nurses [...] could only be [decided in regard]

---

78 Kreutzer, "On Nursing Reforms in Western Germany," 193.
79 Susanne Kreutzer, "Krankenbeobachtung. Zur Entwertung einer pflegerischen Schlüsselkompetenz in der Bundesrepublik und Schweden nach 1945 [Patient Observation: On the Devaluation of a Key Competence in Nursing in the Federal Republic of Germany and Sweden after 1945]," in *Gesundheit/Krankheit. Kulturelle Differenzierungsprozesse um Körper, Geschlecht und Macht in Skandinavien*, ed. Lill-Ann Körber and Stefanie von Schnurbein, Berliner Beiträge zur Skandinavistik, Bd. 16 (Berlin: Nordeuropa-Institut, 2010), 167–88; Kreutzer, *Vom "Liebesdienst" zum modernen Frauenberuf*; Kreutzer, "On Nursing Reforms in Western Germany," 180–200; Kreutzer, *Arbeits- und Lebensalltag evangelischer Krankenpflege*.

to the activities outside of the patient room."[80] However, with the legislated introduction of nursing aides in 1965, a lower educated nurse type was established who could (and should) carry out the domestic or housekeeping tasks.[81]

The work of Kreutzer provides a critical perspective on the narrative of progress in nursing. Although it is argued that the Christian foundation of German nursing made it submissive to medicine, Kreutzer emphasizes that through its focus on the souls of patients and on emotional work, nurses held an elevated position and reputation even in relation to physicians. Only after the decline of this linkage between Christianity and nursing in the 1950s and 1960s was there no new image of autonomous nursing, and nurses came to be perceived (and perceived themselves) as mere assistants to physicians.[82]

My study builds on this critical perspective and questions whether the developments in German nursing in the second half of the 20th century, especially in the 1970s and 1980s, can be understood as professionalizing and gaining autonomy. Rather, as I argue in this study, those developments have to be seen in the context of a new governmental rationale, neoliberalism, in which the nursing vocation was obliged to become accountable in order to be accepted as a valuable part of society. In order to analyze and answer this complex question, I will use the nursing process as an example. The nursing process is based on a managerial structure to make nursing care transparent and was acknowledged by nurses as an instrument to provide professional nursing care. Therefore, on the following pages, I will describe the few scientific studies which discuss the nursing process from a critical perspective.

3.2 Critiques on the Nursing Process

Historical studies about the nursing process and its introduction to nursing are rare. Studies critically reflecting on the nature of the nursing process, its underlying rationale, and its positivist and reductive character are also rather difficult to find. It is interesting that critical analyses concerning the nursing process focus mostly on the poor implementation and take up of the nursing process in

---

80 "Ob eine Aufgabe berufsspezifisch oder berufsfremd war, entschied sich damit nicht an den auszuführenden Tätigkeiten, sondern an der erforderlichen Nähe zum Patienten. Eine Entlastung der Schwestern konnte sich nach den Vorgaben der Arbeitsgemeinschaft demnach nur auf Tätigkeiten jenseits des Krankenzimmers beziehen." (Kreutzer, Vom "Liebesdienst" zum modernen Frauenberuf, 257; my translation).
81 Kreutzer, Vom "Liebesdienst" zum modernen Frauenberuf.
82 Susanne Kreutzer, "Conflicting Christian and Scientific Nursing Concepts in West Germany, 1945–1970," in Routledge Handbook on the Global History of Nursing, ed. Patricia D'Antonio, Julie A. Fairman, and Jean C. Whelan (London, New York: Routledge, 2016), 151–64.

nursing care. Additionally, criticism is raised that despite the fact that the nursing process is not evidence-based, it is acknowledged globally. The following section contains critical analyses of the nursing process with a focus on different countries but also with a focus on its nature. One major editorial work has been published by nursing scientists Monika Habermann and Leana Uys, who sampled international contributions and put critical analyses of the nursing process in a historical perspective.[83] The cybernetic logic of the nursing process is the focus of critique by all of the authors.

Issues Regarding the Implementation of the Nursing Process in Nursing Care

In different countries, nurses at the bedside struggled with implementing the nursing process. While the official implementation of the nursing process into formulas, regulations, and legislations happened rather quickly, it seems that in actual nursing practice the reception was slower and is still not complete. Nursing scientist Daniel Kelly analyzed the implementation of the nursing process in the UK and asserts that the nursing process was integrated into nursing care within just a few years, suggesting "that the Nursing Process was highly significant to nurses and policymakers of the time. It is unusual for a nursing philosophy to be adopted so rapidly and on such a grand scale. The nursing elite clearly must have believed it offered more than a systematic approach for delivering nursing care."[84] This rapidity in implementing the nursing process is also the case for Germany, as my study shows. It took about ten years from the first official calls to apply the nursing process to nursing care to its statutory enactment.

However, despite its fast official adoption in British nursing, the nursing process is still not fully accepted and implemented in general nursing practice in the UK.[85] Analyzing the reception of the nursing process in German nursing, Monika Habermann points to the difficulties in considering and acknowledging non-physical aspects – the spiritual, cultural, social, and communicative aspects – within the nursing process. Furthermore, she argues, the nursing process is hardly followed in its complete circle by bedside nurses. Only some steps are utilized. Steps like goal-setting or evaluation are often forgotten.[86] The poor

---

83 Habermann and Uys, *The Nursing Process: A Global Concept*.
84 Daniel Kelly, "Opening New Discourses in Nursing: The History of the Nursing Process in the UK," in *The Nursing Process: A Global Concept*, ed. Monika Habermann, Leana R. Uys, and Barbara Parfitt (Edinburgh; New York: Elsevier/Churchill Livingstone, 2006), 24.
85 Kelly, "Opening New Discourses in Nursing," 15–29.
86 Monika Habermann, "The Nursing Process: Developments and Issues in Germany," in *The Nursing Process: A Global Concept*, ed. Monika Habermann, Leana R. Uys, and Barbara Parfitt (Edinburgh; New York: Elsevier/Churchill Livingstone, 2006), 95–105.

reception of the nursing process by nurses at the bedside themselves might be a sign of resistance against the official program.

Nursing scientist Barbara Stevens Barnum clearly articulated the contradictions between the political propagation of the nursing process and its low appreciation in bedside care: "Never was a system of nursing more politicized than the Nursing Process. Advocates pushed the system until it was adopted worldwide by nations and health organizations as well. There was just one problem: nurses who actually had to work with the system were seldom happy."[87] The bad reception of the nursing process by nurses themselves shows the flaws of this concept. According to Barnum, those flaws can be found in the inefficient use of resources because the nursing process is time-consuming; in the theoretical work that has to be done by filling out documents, which was perceived contrary to nurses' work; and in the misfit with the cultural demands of the respective environments. She also doubts that holistic care can be provided with the nursing process since the nursing process values steps and pieces of nursing care. The wholeness of nursing, then, is rather the understanding that every task has been completed. But the importance of nursing care to be with the patient, rather than completing a task, is not acknowledged in the nursing process.[88]

Professionalization as Illusion?

While critical analyses question whether the nursing process brought the positive result that has been ascribed to the process, they do not clearly and extensively discuss whether it helped to professionalize nursing. Definitely, the nursing process was pushed and appreciated as an instrument to improve nursing care and to professionalize the nursing vocation in anglophone countries[89] as well as in Germany.[90] Reasons for this hope of professionalization in nursing with the implementation of the nursing process were found in its promise to improve quality in nursing care as well as to its potential for research and management. Instruments of managerialism such as the nursing process seem to have been appreciated and fostered by nurses because they enhanced their confidence and promised professional status.

---

87 Barbara Stevens Barnum, "The Nursing Process Worldwide: What Is Its Future?" in *The Nursing Process: A Global Concept*, ed. Monika Habermann, Leana R. Uys, and Barbara Parfitt (Edinburgh; New York: Elsevier/Churchill Livingstone, 2006), 163.
88 Barnum, "The Nursing Process Worldwide," 155–67.
89 Kelly, "Opening New Discourses in Nursing," 15–29; Niels Buus and Michael Traynor, "The Nursing Process: Nursing Discourse and Managerial Technologies," in *The Nursing Process: A Global Concept*, ed. Monika Habermann, Leana R. Uys, and Barbara Parfitt (Edinburgh; New York: Elsevier/Churchill Livingstone, 2006), 31–46.
90 Habermann, "The Nursing Process: Developments and Issues in Germany," 95–105.

Barnum, for example, argues that the nursing process constantly integrates new developments such as nursing diagnoses and evidence-based practices and grows with this integration. In consequence, the nursing process not only became larger and added more steps but was also more and more introduced into nursing research. Ultimately, so Barnum believes, the nursing process became associated with progress and professionalization in nursing.[91]

According to Kelly, the nursing process was welcomed in the UK first as a tool to push the "rather disgruntled profession during the 1970s", and second, as a political tool which allowed "each item of expenditure [in healthcare] to be accounted for and, more importantly, justified."[92] Here, however, Kelly criticizes that the reconstitution of nursing care to an administrative activity seems to have turned against this understanding of professional nursing practice by valuing management values over values of individual nursing care.[93]

Nursing scientists Niels Buus and Michael Traynor argue that the nursing process with its managerial logic reconstituted nursing care and nurses themselves. This not only made nurses participate in implementing the nursing process but also opened them up to control. Hence, by establishing the nursing process as the norm in nursing care, disciplinary mechanisms are introduced that are also directed against the nurses themselves.[94] The appreciation of nurses regarding the nursing process and its backlash to nurses themselves, Buus and Traynor ascribe to the two different logics underlying the nursing process. One is the logic of the nursing process as understood by Ida Orlando and one as understood by Yura and Walsh.

The first emergence of the nursing process can be dated to the late 1950s at the Yale School of Nursing and to Ida Orlando. Nursing care was seen as "communication and interpersonal relations [...and] the collaborative striving of the patient and the nurse towards healing in terms of a process."[95] In the 1970s, Yura and Walsh from The Catholic University seem to have reconceptualized the process in nursing to a more science- and research-based process, similar to biomedical thinking. In this logic of the nursing process, problems are linked with concrete planning to solve those problems. That means the focus is more on plans than on actions. They argue that today both logics still exist with one focus on the relational aspect in the healing of and the caring for a patient and the other on a rather biomedical and problem-solving cycle. While with the first logic the emphasis is on two people (a patient and a nurse) who are acting through the process, the nurse is removed in the second logic due to a passive sentence

---

91 Barnum, "The Nursing Process Worldwide," 155–67.
92 Kelly, "Opening New Discourses in Nursing," 24.
93 Kelly, "Opening New Discourses in Nursing," 15–29.
94 Buus and Traynor, "The Nursing Process," 31–46.
95 Buus and Traynor, "The Nursing Process," 36.

structure in the planning of nursing care. Only the patient is focused on. But the plans can be evaluated regarding their effectiveness.[96] It seems, the authors emphasize, that the differences in the conceptualization of the nursing process became blurred (and ignored) over time, leading to a "doublethinking" regarding the nursing process. Doublethinking they define as "the power of holding two contradictory beliefs in one's mind simultaneously and accepting both of them."[97] These two logics are carried further and so is the contradiction, as they state.[98] This doublethinking, as well as its negative impact on the nursing vocation and on nursing care, can also be found in German nursing, as I will show in my study.

For Germany, the implementation of the nursing process seems to have had an even stronger value. Habermann constructs the nursing vocation in Germany as behind in comparison to the nursing vocations of the neighboring states of Germany, and finds this lower status historically in the religious foundation of German nursing. After WWII, the nursing vocation in Germany suffered from a "continuing fragmented and controversial representation […] in the public and political field."[99] According to Habermann, throughout the 1980s the nursing process was seen as an answer for difficulties in the nursing vocation regarding the definition of its scope of practice and its contribution to society. It was also perceived as a valid instrument for quality assurance in hospitals and by nurse managers of healthcare organizations as well as by organizations that judged the quality of healthcare organizations.[100] However, as Habermann criticized, using the nursing process accompanies a reduction in the complexity in nursing care by translating this complexity into a means-end language and squeezing highly various information into a simplified problem-solving cycle. Patient orientation and holistic and individual nursing care, according to Habermann, cannot be rightly acknowledged in the reductive structure. By fragmenting nursing care, Habermann emphasizes, the nursing process is close to the medical logic of the patient and does not provide a unique nursing perspective.[101] This criticism is interesting because it stands against the hope of nurses to move away from medicine and establish their own scope and logic of practice with the implementation of the nursing process (see chapter 8.1.1).

Moreover, as Barnum emphasizes, the logic of the nursing process is not unique to nursing. Hence, neither does the nursing process originate in nursing

---

96 Buus and Traynor, "The Nursing Process," 31–46.
97 Buus and Traynor, "The Nursing Process," 40.
98 Buus and Traynor, "The Nursing Process," 31–46.
99 Habermann, "The Nursing Process: Developments and Issues in Germany," 100.
100 Habermann, "The Nursing Process: Developments and Issues in Germany," 95–105.
101 Habermann, "The Nursing Process: Developments and Issues in Germany," 95–105.

nor has the nursing process potential to function as a core instrument of a unique profession:

> One could just as easily have created the plumbing process. First, the plumber *assesses* the situation (e.g. water is not going down the sink). Then he *diagnoses* the problem (e.g. clogged drain). Then he creates a *plan* (get out the snake), and then he *intervenes* (e.g. use the snake). Finally he *evaluates* (e.g. the water is running through the pipes again). In other words, the only thing that makes the Nursing Process *nursing* is that the process is applied to nursing content. The process is not unique to our profession.[102]

Criticism of the Cybernetic Logic of the Nursing Process

In a non-historical study, I found a critical analysis emphasizing the (scientific) underpinnings of the nursing process – especially its cybernetic logic. German nursing scientist Manfred Hülsken-Giesler argues that the nursing process developed in the scientific logic of pragmatism.[103] Science within the understanding of pragmatism would be based on "universal calculability" [*universaler Berechenbarkeit*][104] with functionality or usefulness as the premise of this pragmatism, contrary to a continuous (self-)critical premise.[105] Hülsken-Giesler analyzes the nursing process as a non-trivial machine or system. Those machines or systems are based on the cybernetic logic, that is, the input-output procedure. This logic opens non-trivial machines to past events and to "time." Non-trivial systems are not predictable; however, with cybernetic logic within a normative frame the predictability can be increased.[106] Hence, restructuring nursing according to the nursing process is the attempt to make nursing with its uncertain realities predictable. Moreover, a distinction between relevant and irrelevant information is established with the tendency to standardize these procedures. The translation of these standardized processes into digitalized computing

---

102 Barnum, "The Nursing Process Worldwide," 155–67 161; italics in original.
103 Manfred Hülsken-Giesler, *Der Zugang zum Anderen. Zur theoretischen Rekonstruktion von Professionalisierungsstrategien pflegerischen Handelns im Spannungsfeld von Mimesis und Maschinenlogik [Access to and Approach of the Other: For a Theoretical Reconstruction of Professionalization Strategies of Nursing Care in the Tension between Mimesis and Machine Logic]*, ed. Hartmut Remmers, vol. 3, Pflegewissenschaft und Pflegebildung (Göttingen: V&R unipress, 2008).
104 Hartmut Remmers, *Pflegerisches Handeln. Wissenschafts- und Ethikdiskurse zur Konturierung der Pflegewissenschaft [Nursing Action: Scientific and Ethical Discourses to Outline Nursing Science]*, Reihe Pflegewissenschaft (Bern: Verlag Hans Huber, 2000), 126.
105 This might have given German nursing a new foundation after the loss of its traditional Christian foundation. However, the integration of foreign nursing theories and nursing concepts always comes along with an adaption and transformation process into the German nursing culture and with the development of German nursing theories and concepts (Hülsken-Giesler, *Der Zugang Zum Anderen*; Remmers, *Pflegerisches Handeln*).
106 Hülsken-Giesler, *Der Zugang Zum Anderen*.

programs perpetuates the already established logic of accounting in nursing and reaffirms the new nursing perception.[107] As Hülsken-Giesler explains, this new nursing perception acknowledges the need for formalized, controllable, and rational nursing care. The digitalization of nursing planning and of the nursing process, in particular, is strengthened with the reduction of complexity by enabling and producing prefabricated phrases and a standardized structure. Hence, the nursing documentation programs based on the nursing process do not call for a nurse to write the nursing care plan for a specific patient but to create the nursing care plan with nursing goals and interventions by themselves. Nurses only have to do simple mouse clicks and the algorithm of the digitalized documentation program does the rest, even comparing the target and real situation of the patient and evaluating nursing care apart from the nurse.[108] Hülsken-Giesler concludes that the nursing process likely removes documented nursing care and professional nursing logic from the bedside by pushing nurses, in their attempts to professionalize, to the managerial area with the danger of the mechanization of nursing.[109]

Drawing on these critical discussions about the nursing process, I will analyze this concept and its meaning for German nursing from a Foucauldian perspective. The historical lens of the discussions surrounding the implementation of the nursing process helps to understand why and from which sites the nursing process was appreciated and pushed in the 1970s and 1980s. I will trace the discursive structures and conditions of that time and discuss how the nursing process can be understood as an accounting tool to enforce a neoliberal agenda.

---

107 Hülsken-Giesler, *Der Zugang Zum Anderen*.
108 Hülsken-Giesler, *Der Zugang Zum Anderen*.
109 Hülsken-Giesler, *Der Zugang Zum Anderen*.

Chapter 4:
Methodological Considerations

In this chapter, I present the epistemic and methodological underpinnings that will guide my analysis of the developments in German nursing in the 1970s and 1980s. In order to follow the theoretical framework, I need to introduce some of the concepts that are necessary to understand Foucault's theoretical considerations about the governing of our societies. By presenting more information about the historical approach of my study, I will also briefly summarize Foucault's notions of discourses and how he understood them, and the interplay between power and knowledge, events, genealogy, and problematizations. In the next part of this chapter, I introduce the method of historical discourse analyses and in the last part, I present the empirical data I used in this study and how I analyzed them discursively.

4.1 The History of the Present

Before I discuss some of Foucault's theoretical concepts that are important for my research, I want to describe the epistemic stance of my thesis. To analyze the transformations of (nursing) expertise and professionalism through the implementation of accounting tools I will use what Foucault calls the history of the present. According to Foucault, the approach of the history of the present starts by questioning existent taken-for-granted concepts or knowledges considered to be true by confronting them with their own history.[110] Using history in this way enables us to critically question the present and to ask what the discursive conditions of the present are. Thus, the starting point of this study is the recognition that healthcare systems all over the Western world, including Germany, are currently "restructured" through cost containment interventions. These particularly target nurses and their work by transforming nursing actions into

---

110 Michel Foucault, "Nietzsche, Genealogy, History," in *The Foucault Reader*, ed. Paul Rabinow (New York: Pantheon Books, 1984), 76–100.

standardized, evidence-based interventions that can hardly be seen as professionalized.[111] However, at the same time, German nursing considers itself well on the way in its professionalization project. Throughout the last two decades, more and more academic nursing programs have been established, academic nursing education is now possible for entry level nurses, and the newest nursing act defines exclusive tasks for professional nurses, including most of the steps of the nursing process except for intervening and documenting.[112] Thus, for my study, I will analyze the discourses around the perceived need to professionalize nursing in Germany that became particularly powerful in the second half of the 20th century. As I will highlight in my project, the nursing process was perceived by many nurses, nursing scholars, and managers as a central tool to advance the process of professionalization. My study will critically question this assumption and demonstrate that the nursing process was a first step in rendering nurses' actions (and healthcare in general) calculable, increasing control over nursing actions and implementing a foundation to increase the financial pressure on hospitals and other healthcare providers.

Discourses

Probably one of the most important concepts, particularly in Foucault's earlier work, is what he called discourses, understood as overarching entities or "as practices that systematically form the objects of which they speak."[113] Discourses not only determine what can be said, what is thought to be true and how to act, but they also create and restructure the elements and aspects that are talked about. Discourses, therefore, are repressive and productive at the same time. Discourses are repressive in the way that they constrain the possibilities of speaking, thinking, and acting by reducing them to the reality they organize. By limiting what can be said they also produce or create the reality people live in and determine the knowledge those people have of this reality. Discourses produce truth and with this truth comes a specific societal power personified in the expert who is "in the truth." Statements can only be heard and acknowledged as true or credible when they are made by using and obeying the rules of the discourse.

---

111 See for example Dave Holmes, Amélie Perron, and Patrick O'Byrne, "Evidence, Virulence, and the Disappearance of Nursing Knowledge: A Critique of the Evidence-Based Dogma," *Worldviews on Evidence-Based Nursing* 3, no. 3 (2006), 95–102.
112 PflBRefG, "Gesetz zur Reform der Pflegeberufe (Pflegeberufereformgesetz) vom 17. Juli 2017 [Law for the Reformation of the Occupations in Nursing from July 17th, 2017]," in *Teil I Nr. 49,*, ed. Bundesgesetzblatt (ausgegeben zu Bonn am 24. Juli 2017).
113 Michel Foucault, *The Archaeology of Knowledge and the Discourse of Language*, ed. Michel Foucault, Vintage Books Edition, January 2010 ed. (New York: Vintage Books, 2010), 49.

Power and discourse are interdependent: power is a foundation of discourse but discourses, in turn, produce power relations.[114]

Hence, it is only possible to think, experience, act, and speak inside of the discourses we never chose. Only in these discursive systems is the real accessible. Also, the subject is the result of these discursive regimes. They establish the frame and norms to make individuals recognizable, to make them subjects. Therefore, there is no way to apprehend a reality outside of language or discourse and despite the fact that material objects exist, the meaning that is attributed to these objects will always be within discourse and language. This means also that objects pre-existing to language, such as accidents or natural catastrophes that happen without our intention, are not in doubt in Foucault's notion of discourse. But the interpretation of these events depends on the discourses that are at work. Therefore, our perception is already structured in a certain way, based on the discourse, and even our experiences and thoughts depend on the discourses around us.[115] However, discourses are not static but change over time and a genealogical perspective aims to trace discursive changes that often occur in sudden ruptures and shifts.

Power/Knowledge

Power, in a Foucauldian understanding, is relational and must be analyzed "in action." It is not an entity or thing that someone possesses and others do not – as scholars in the Weberian tradition would have it.[116] Power circulates within networks and it is not solely exclusionary or repressive but rather productive, in the sense that it produces desires and knowledge, for example, and incites certain conducts or behaviours.[117] Thus, power "exists only when it is put into action" and it acts indirectly by influencing the context of possible action, making certain actions more likely than others, or, in Foucault's words, power is "an action upon

---

114 Achim Landwehr, *Historische Diskursanalyse [Historical Discourse Analysis]*, 2nd. ed. (Frankfurt am Main: Campus-Verlag, 2009).
115 Philipp Sarasin, *Geschichtswissenschaft und Diskursanalyse [History and Discourse Analysis]*, 4 ed. (Frankfurt am Main: Suhrkamp Verlag, 2014).
116 Steven Lukes, *Power: A Radical View*, 2nd ed. (Hampshire, New York: Palgrave Macmillan, 2005); Michel Foucault, "Afterword: The Subject and Power," in *Michel Foucault: Beyond Structuralism and Hermeneutics. With an Afterword by and an Interview with Michel Foucault*, ed. Hubert L. Dreyfus and Paul Rabinow (Chicago: The University of Chicago Press, 1983), 208–26.
117 Michel Foucault, "Body/Power," in *Power/Knowledge: Selected Interviews and Other Writings 1972-1977*, ed. Colin Gordon (New York: Harvester Press, 1980), 55–62; Foucault, "Two Lectures," 78–108.

an action, on existing actions or on those which may arise in the present or the future."[118]

Foucault demonstrated in his work on the birth of the prison, the psychiatric asylum, and the hospital how power produced subjects through disciplinary power.[119] By separating the mad, the criminal, or the sick in special institutions, a particular knowledge developed like criminology, psychiatry, or medicine that became possible through the disciplinary regime in these institutions. Only certain experts are authorized to decide who must be excluded and kept in these institutions, and mutually these institutions produce the "true" knowledge (discourses) that justifies the power of the expert.[120] Hence, "there is no power relation without the correlative constitution of a field of knowledge, nor any knowledge that does not presuppose and constitute at the same time power relations."[121] The notion of power/knowledge describes this interdependence of power and knowledge and its "correlative" relationship.[122] "[P]ower regularly promotes and utilizes a 'true' knowledge of subjects and indeed in a certain manner constitutes the very field of that truth."[123]

Events

As already mentioned earlier, Foucault's genealogical approach aims to identify ruptures or shifts – moments when discourses changed and knowledge until then considered true suddenly became obsolete. Thus, Foucault criticizes the way historical research had been conducted in his time. This form of historical research took the exact opposite approach of what Foucault proposed – always looking for connections and continuity, trying to ground an event within structures and systems that have always been there, and not valuing the random character of events.[124] According to Foucault's definition, events are sudden changes or shifts or "the reversal of a relationship of forces, the usurpation of power, the appropriation of a vocabulary turned against those who had once used it, a feeble domination that poisons itself as it grows lax, the entry of a masked

---

118 Foucault, "The Subject and Power," 219–20.
119 Michel Foucault, *The Birth of Biopolitics: Lectures at the Collège De France, 1978-79* (Basingstoke, New York: Palgrave Macmillan, 2008).
120 Michel Foucault, *Discipline and Punish: The Birth of the Prison*, vol. 2nd Vintage books (New York: Vintage Books, 1995).
121 Foucault, *Discipline and Punish*, 27.
122 Hubert L. Dreyfus and Paul Rabniow, *Beyond Structuralism and Hermeneutics: With an Afterword by and an Interview with Michel Foucault*, 2nd ed. (Chicago: The University of Chicago Press, 1983), 203.
123 Colin Gordon, "Afterword," in *Power/Knowledge: Selected Interviews and Other Writings 1972-1977*, ed. Colin Gordon (London, New York: Harvester Press, 1980), 229–59: 239.
124 Michel Foucault, "Orders of Discourse," *Social Science Information* 10, no. 2 (1971), 7–30.

'other'.[125] To focus on events or eventalization implies that the historian must abstain from searching for historical constants or extra-historical structures as a foundation for their historical analysis, such as an "economic mechanism, an anthropological structure or a demographic process."[126] Instead, historians should analyze processes and discourses that led to the formation of singularities. The question to be asked is "how is it that one particular statement appeared rather than another?"[127]

Studying history from a Foucauldian perspective leads to a history of the present. That is, "to link the present to the past not as its inevitable outcome, but as the contingent product of changes in relationships of power and in the ideas through which such relationships are conceived."[128]

Genealogy

As already discussed, studying history from a genealogical perspective is an analysis of the present through a historical critique in order to reveal and analyze the emergence of practices and concepts that are today taken for granted. In relation to traditional approaches, the perspective on historic material is different. The attempt is not so much to discover the past but rather to obtain more knowledge about the present and the function of contemporary practices.[129]

In my research project, I will not use Foucault's other more "structural" approach that he called archaeology and that focused more on structural differences between the past and the present.[130] My intention is to analyze the emergence and changes of discursive processes or events in German nursing that led to and enabled current transformations, practices, and concepts in nursing. Thus, my project is the study of the discontinuous and unsteady production and formation of discourses around professionalization and accountability in nursing.[131] For Foucault, "it is to discover that truth or being does not lie at the root of what we know and what we are, but the exteriority of accidents."[132]

---

125 Foucault, "Nietzsche, Genealogy, History," 88.
126 Michel Foucault, "Questions of Method," in *The Foucault Effect: Studies in Governmentality. With Two Lectures by and an Interview with Michel Foucault*, ed. Graham Burchill, Colin Gordon, and Peter Miller (Chicago: University of Chicago Press, 1991), 78.
127 Foucault, *The Archaeology of Knowledge*, 27.
128 Editors of the History of the Present, "Introducing History of the Present," *History of the Present: A Journal of Critical History* 1, no. 1 (2011), 1-4: 1.
129 Robert Castel, ""Problematization" as a Mode of Reading History," in *Foucault and the Writing of History*, ed. Jan Goldstein (Cambridge, Massachusetts: Basil Blackwell Ltd, 1994), 237-52: 303-04.
130 E.g. Foucault, *The Archaeology of Knowledge*.
131 Foucault, "Orders of Discourse," 7-30.
132 Foucault, "Nietzsche, Genealogy, History," 81.

Therefore, from a genealogical perspective, it is interesting to analyze how power/ knowledge through practices produce reality and how this reality became fixed in legislations and rituals.[133] In the sense of critique and prevention of a teleological understanding of history, genealogy should not establish a new 'truth' but should disturb or "destabilize"[134] the existing thinking of the past and question the already written history especially in regard to images of consistencies and evolution. It is both a criticism of the produced historical narrative as well as of the perception of the present, opening them to new interpretations.[135]

In order to write a genealogy, the contemporary practice or concept has to be identified, the discursive condition in which this practice or concept emerged has to be described, and the problematization the practice or concept became an answer for has to be identified.[136] In my study, I look at the nursing process as a contemporary practice in German nursing. The discursive condition is the discourses around the cost explosion of healthcare and the societal and economic conditions in the 1970s and 1980s, which led to a reconstitution of organizations and individuals, for example, the responsibilization of citizens. In this discursive condition, it was problematized that the healthcare services provided were controllable and nursing services ineffective and inefficient.

But even the narratives produced in history are limited by discursive conditions that allow only certain meanings to be ascribed to past events. According to historian Elizabeth Deeds Ermarth, the history of the present

> requires acknowledgement of that limit and, in so doing, opens a new and productive gap between discursive system and enunciation: not a gap between 'past and present' to be filled with emergent causalities and the data that confirm them; but a gap between potential and enunciation that invites creativity and remains always open. A creative opportunity appears in that gap which is literally the space of choice: closed, limited and personal, yet respectful of the collective intelligence, the social memory, contained in the semiological systems available to individuals every moment of every day.[137]

---

133 Dreyfus and Rabniow, *Beyond Structuralism and Hermeneutics*; Foucault, "Nietzsche, Genealogy, History," 76–100.
134 Andrew Barry, Thomas Osborne, and Nikolas Rose, "Introduction," in *Foucault and Political Reason. Liberalism, Neo-Liberalism and Rationalities of Government*, ed. Andrew Barry, Thomas Osborne, and Nikolas Rose (Chicago: The University of Chicago Press, 1996), 1–17: 5.
135 Foucault, "Nietzsche, Genealogy, History," 76–100; Achim Landwehr, "Die Kunst, sich nicht allzu sicher zu sein: Möglichkeiten kritischer Geschichtsschreibung [The Art of Being Uncertain: Options in Writing Critical History]," *Werkstatt Geschichte* Sonderdruck Esseypreis 2012 (2012), 3–12.
136 David Garland, "What Is a "History of the Present"? On Foucault's Genealogies and Their Critical Preconditions," *Punishment & Society* 16, no. 4 (2014), 365–84.
137 Elizabeth Deeds Ermarth, "The Closed Space of Choice: A Manifesto on the Future of History," in *Manifestos for History*, ed. Keith Jenkings, Sue Morgan, and Alun Munslow (London, New York: Routledge Taylor & Francis Group, 2007), 50–66: 64.

Problematization

The transformation of discourses and practices or the emergence of new ones are not the result of the intentions of specific historical actors. "Rather, the transformations are seen as the outcome of the interplay of various socially and historically situated discourses and practices which may have had, and may continue to have, unforeseen and unintended consequences."[138] Discourses change because practices were perceived as problematic in specific historical constellations and these problematizations will lead to what I, following Foucault, characterize as events – the sudden change or disruption of discourses and discursive formations. It might even be the case that the unintended consequences of the transformations become themselves problematized and a solution must be found leading to another discursive event. Critically analyzing current taken-for-granted discourses and practices means to go back in time and to find the point when these discourses and practices emerged as a response to specific problematizations. This means, in turn, that the transformed discourses or practices are already predetermined by the way the issue has been problematized in the first place.[139] Problematization "develops the conditions in which possible responses can be given; it defines the elements that will constitute what the different solutions attempt to respond to."[140]

Therefore, in this study I focus on the way healthcare in general and nursing service, in particular, became problematized in the second half of the 20th century. I will show that healthcare became criticized in economic terms, which in turn was followed by the establishment of processes and concepts to restructure nursing service (as an example for healthcare) into an economic good. Accounting tools such as the nursing process especially in its materialized forms of documentation systems have not only transformed discourses and practices in nursing but have also shifted the logic of nursing actions and the way nursing is understood today.[141]

---

138 Alistar M. Preston, "The Birth of Clinical Accounting: A Study of the Emergence and Transformations of Discourses on Costs and Practices of Accounting in U.S. Hospitals," *Accounting Organizations and Society* 17, no. 1 (1992), 63–100: 65.
139 Foucault, "Polemics, Politics and Problematizations," 381–90; Peter Miller, "The Margins of Accounting," *The Sociological Review* 46, no. 1_suppl (1998), 174–93.
140 Foucault, "Polemics, Politics and Problematizations," 389.
141 Kirsten Beedholm, Kirsten Lomborg, and Kirsten Frederiksen, "Ruptured Thought: Rupture as a Critical Attitude to Nursing Research," *Nursing Philosophy* 15, no. 2 (2014), 102–11.

4.2 Historical Discourse Analysis

The overall purposes of discourse analysis in historical research are to identify the point of time at which certain discourses emerged or have been transformed; to answer the question of how discourses changed in the course of their history; to visualize the interconnectedness of discourses; and to clarify the historical formations of knowledge and the reality that this knowledge produced.[142] From a Foucauldian perspective, discourse analysis does not try to reconstruct the reality of the author who produced the documents used in the analysis or to discover the real intentions of the author in the written words, nor does a discourse analysis try to prove or refute the credibility of the author or the truth or falsity of the statements made in the documents. Discourse analysis does not try to interpret the real meaning of the text. Instead, Foucault argues, what the analysis should reveal are the conditions that made the production of the documents possible or how they come to exist in the form in which they exist.[143] It is not the matter of analyzing the "formal structure and laws of construction [of a statement], but that of its existence and the rules that govern its appearance."[144]

Thus, discourse analysis is not interested in the individual author's perspective but rather analyzes the discourses that made "the conditions under which certain statements will be considered true and appropriate."[145] Those underlying discourses emerged accidentally in history and studying those means to "focus[…] on gaps, ruptures, and shifts of meaning."[146]

Furthermore, texts – whether they are historical or not – must be understood as belonging to a certain linguistic system that determines the structure and grammar of the language in which the text is written. By using the concepts that language provides, reality can only be described in a way that is predetermined by the language. Thus, language is the key element constructing reality. And the concepts that language provide are determined by the discourses. There is no reality outside of language and outside of discourse because only through language is reality accessible. Furthermore, a gap exists between what people perceive (the world they experience) and what they can articulate (the words used to describe the world). Therefore (historical) texts carry and recreate a certain (past) reality that is narrower or a more restricted version of the one a subject actually

---

142 Landwehr, *Historische Diskursanalyse*.
143 Foucault, *The Archaeology of Knowledge*; Landwehr, *Historische Diskursanalyse*.
144 Foucault, *The Archaeology of Knowledge*, 30.
145 Sara Mills, *Michel Foucault* (London; New York: Routledge, 2003), 66.
146 Elizabeth A. Clark, *History, Theory, Text. Historians and the Linguistic Turn* (Cambridge, Mass.: Harvard University Press, 2004), 116.

perceived and experienced.[147] "[P]ast reality that can be found in texts is an already discursively communicated reality."[148]

Therefore, a reconstruction of the past is not the purpose of my genealogical study but the analysis of the contemporary discourses in the second half of the 20th century that problematized the provision of healthcare in general and nursing in particular that led to a new understanding of nursing care, creating a new image of what it meant to be a nurse. My aim is to answer the question of how a certain understanding of and reality in nursing care came into being. Following discursive discontinuities and ruptures, I will analyze which "truth" and "reality" become constructed and established and what became silent at a certain point in time.

Foucault proposed a completely anti-hermeneutic analysis of discourses. Not the meaning behind the statements but the statements themselves, their pure existence, are the objects of analysis. Statements, here, should be understood as constitutive elements of the discourse. Statements can be determined with two different characteristics: First, statements are not free in space but connected or integrated into different relations such as their social and institutional environments, the structures of statements, and discursive strategies. Therefore, statements are only important because of their function. Second, statements do not appear only once but are characterized by their repetition. Hence, he defines discourse as a mass of statements that belong to the same discursive formation.[149]

Therefore, discourses have to be analyzed by focusing on how they are limited and cut off (mechanisms of rarification). The discontinuity of discourses needs to be acknowledged as well as their variety of manifestations. Discourses become obvious in practices "as a violence that we do to things, or [...] as a practice we impose upon them."[150]

4.3 Data Collection and Data Analysis

In order to reveal the discursive transformation of nursing and the establishment of a new nursing discourse, I retrieved my empirical data predominantly from articles published in healthcare journals. Those articles were mostly written by

---

147 Beverley Southgate, "Postmodernism," in *A Companion to the Philosophy of History and Historiography*, ed. Aviezer Tucker (Chichester: Blackwell Publishing Ltd., 2009), 540–49; Landwehr, *Historische Diskursanalyse*; Sarasin, *Geschichtswissenschaft Und Diskursanalyse*.
148 "... dass die in den Texten repräsentierte Wirklichkeit immer bereits diskursiv kommunizierte Wirklichkeit ist" (Landwehr, *Historische Diskursanalyse*, 52; my translation).
149 Landwehr, *Historische Diskursanalyse*.
150 Foucault, "Orders of Discourse," 22.

the nurses themselves, but ministers of health, hospital managers, and physicians can also be found as authors.

To follow the discussions in the German nursing vocation, I selected two nursing journals that were published by the most influential nursing organizations in the 1970s and 1980s. Furthermore, I also used a journal of hospital management in order to integrate the discussions from the nursing journals into the managerial context of the hospital setting. Additionally, I used published documents of the WHO because the nursing process was introduced into German nursing based on a medium-term program of the WHO.

Documents of the WHO

The documents I used from the WHO are both on the global as well as on the European level. On the global level, the reports concerning 10 years of WHO's work are especially interesting because they reflect overall strategies of the WHO in restructuring national healthcare systems and reorganizing healthcare personnel. The WHO started to evaluate its work in ten-year reports starting in 1958 with a report on *The First Ten Years of the World Health Organization*.[151] The report of the second decade from 1958 to 1967 was published in 1968.[152] However, the reports of the third and the fourth decade were published many years later and need to be considered recent and not historic documents.[153] Of special interest in regard to the WHO strategies is a report about the organizational study on *Methods of Promoting the Development of Basic Health Services*.[154] Here, the background of WHO strategies is described in more detail.

Furthermore, as a main secondary source, I used the work of historians Marcos Cueto, Theodore M. Brown, and Elizabeth Fee, who provided comprehensive historical insights into the work of the WHO with their book, *The World Health Organization: A History*.[155]

For the European level, the work of the WHO, as well as its strategies, are recorded in session and annual reports. Moreover, the study, *People's Needs for*

---

151 WHO, "The First Ten Years of the World Health Organization," (Geneva: World Health Organization, 1958).
152 WHO, "The Second Ten Years of the World Health Organization 1958–1967," (Geneva: World Health Organization, 1968).
153 WHO, "The Third Ten Years of the World Health Organization 1968–1977," (Geneva: World Health Organization, 2008); WHO, "The Fourth Ten Years of the World Health Organization 1978–1987," (Geneva: World Health Organization, 2011).
154 WHO, "Organizational Study on "Methods of Promoting Development of Basic Health Services". Report of the Working Group, 16 January 1973," (World Health Organization, 1973).
155 Marcos Cueto, Theodore M. Brown, and Elizabeth Fee, *The World Health Organization: A History* (Cambridge: Cambridge University Press, 2019).

Data Collection and Data Analysis 63

Nursing Care: A European Study, which is one of the main results of the medium-term program for the introduction of the nursing process, gives insights into how the program was carried out.[156]

Krankenpflege – the Publication of the DBfK

The first nursing journal is the publication of the largest nursing association in Germany, the Deutscher Berufsverband für Pflegeberufe (DBfK) [the German Professional Association for Nursing Vocations], and is the main empirical source for this study. The DBfK is the successor of the German nursing association Berufsorganisation der Krankenpflegerinnen Deutschlands (B.O.K.D.) [Vocational Organization of the Female Nurses of Germany] which was founded in 1903 by Agnes Karll, who was also a co-founder of the International Council of Nurses (ICN). The B.O.K.D. was a nursing association for "free" nurses, meaning nurses who were not associated with a religious association. However, the B.O.K.D. and its successors did ground their work on Protestant thinking. The association was closed down in the Third Reich. After WWII, a new nursing association was founded in the memory of the B.O.K.D and named itself Agnes-Karll-Verband (AKV) [Agnes-Karll-Association]. In 1974 and with the integration of several smaller nursing associations, the AKV was re-named the DBfK. The DBfK is the main German nursing association and is highly politically active. For example, it represents the nursing vocation in political issues with the aim of obtaining a higher recognition for nurses and better working conditions. The journal of the DBfK and its predecessors also have been renamed several times. It was published until the beginning of the Third Reich, and then resumed publication after World War II in 1946 as *Die Agnes-Karll-Schwester* [*The Agnes-Karll Sister*]. In 1967, it was renamed *Die Agnes-Karll-Schwester, der Krankenpfleger* [*The Agnes-Karll Sister, the Male Nurse*]; in 1972, *Krankenpflege* [*Nursing*)] in 1993, *Pflege Aktuell* [*Current Nursing Care*]; and became integrated into the new nursing journal *Die Schwester, der Pfleger* [*The Sister, the Male Nurse*] in 2006.

I scanned this journal, which is published monthly, from 1960 to 1993, using the keywords "*Pflegeprozess*" [nursing process], "*Pflegeplan*" [nursing plan], and "*Pflegeplanung*" [nursing care plan]. I found the first mention of the nursing process in 1969. In this article, the nursing process was introduced as an answer to the increase in scientific knowledge in nursing, to a shorter hospitalization time, to the need for new nursing techniques in rehabilitation, and to the shift to

---

156 Pat Ashworth et al., *People's Needs for Nursing Care: A European Study*, ed. World Health Organization (Copenhagen: World Health Organization, 1987).

patient-oriented care.[157] Chronologically earlier and more often, however, I could find the term nursing plan instead of process. In these descriptions, nursing care was constituted as a process. From the middle of the 1970s on, and especially after 1976 when the medium-term program of the WHO began, nursing process appeared more often. However, both nursing process and nursing care plan coexisted throughout the following decades. Sometimes nursing care plan was correctly defined as one step of the nursing process, sometimes the two terms (nursing care plan and nursing process) were used synonymously. The nursing care plan was then described as the sum of the serial steps of the nursing process: "nursing anamnesis," "nursing goals," "nursing plan" and "nursing report" (or 'nursing documentation').[158] In 1961, an exchange nurse who wrote about her experiences in the USA mentioned a *"Schwesternfürsorgeplan"* [sister caring plan], which was discussed in a team meeting of healthcare personnel.[159]

In general, I found 147 articles discussing the nursing process or the nursing care plan. Between 1961 to 1975 only 12 of those articles were published, while from 1976 to 1983 – during the time of the medium-term program of the WHO – 88 articles could be found. From 1984 to 1986 – surrounding the new nursing act in 1985 and the integration of the nursing process into the new regulations on nursing education – I found 38 published articles.

The early articles mentioning the nursing process or similar terms talk about rehabilitation and health education, which is connected in these articles with the goal to re-integrate the individual as a useful member of society. Later on, the articles are focused more on individual nursing care as well as control of and transparency in nursing care. From 1976 on, the nursing process became clearly linked to the WHO and to an improvement in both nursing care and recognition of nurses. The issues of constraints in nursing such as having less time and fewer financial resources were already connected to the nursing process in the late 1960s and continued to be an issue (directly or indirectly) throughout the decades. From 1974 on, the articles increasingly contained the call for more pro-

---

157 Liselotte Hölzel-Seipp, "Der praktische Krankenpflegeprozeß [The Practical Nursing Process]," *Die Agnes-Karll-Schwester, der Krankenpfleger* 23, no. 5 (1969), 201–03.
158 E. g. Cornelia Send, "Mittel für die Durchführung der individuellen Pflege (I) [Instruments for Providing Individual Nursing Care I]," *Krankenpflege* 29, no. 7 (1975), 274; Cornelia Send, "Mittel für die Durchführung der individuellen Pflege (II) [Instruments for Providing Individual Nursing Care II]," *Krankenpflege* 29, no. 8 (1975), 324; Cornelia Send, "Mittel für die Durchführung der individuellen Pflege (III) [Instruments for Providing Individual Nursing Care III]," *Krankenpflege* 29, no. 9 (1975), 368; Cornelia Send, "Mittel für die Durchführung der individuellen Pflege (IV) [Instruments for Providing Individual Nursing Care IV]," *Krankenpflege* 29, no. 10 (1975), 409.
159 Barbara Schattat, "Bericht über meine ersten Monate in USA im Rahmen des Schwestern-Austauschprogramms [Report About My First Months During a Nurse Exchange in the USA]," *Die Agnes-Karll-Schwester* 15, no. 8 (1961), 263–64: 264.

ductivity, effectiveness, and efficiency.[160] At the same time, and in connection with the medium-term program of the WHO, the nursing process became increasingly the foundation for autonomy in nursing.[161] Over the course of the 1980s, computerization and electronic documentation became an important part of the discussions around the nursing process. The potential to build electronic programs for nursing based on the nursing process was a particular focus and the articles presented attempts and projects.[162]

Deutsche Krankenpflegezeitschrift – The Publication of the Deutsche Schwesterngemeinschaft

Another journal of interest for this study was the publication of the Deutsche Schwesterngemeinschaft [The German Nursing Sister Association]. This association was founded in 1948 with the aim of federating the different German nursing associations in order to establish an international association with the ICN. Besides the Agnes-Karll-Verband (later DBfK), the motherhouses of the Red Cross as well as the association of free sisters, Bund freier Schwestern, it also became members of this national nursing confederation.[163] Although the confederation was dissolved in 1972, the nursing journal continued to be published on a monthly basis by the publisher Kohlhammer Verlag. It was founded in 1948 as the *Deutsche Schwesternzeitung* [*German Sisters' Journal*]. In 1971, it was

---

160 E.g. Hölzel-Seipp, "Der praktische Krankenpflegeprozeß," 201–03; Bayern, "Mitgliederversammlung am 9.11.1974 [General Meeting on November 9th, 1974]," *Krankenpflege* 28, no. 12 (1974), 521; Detlef Hohlin, "Notwendigkeit der Adaption der Krankenhäuser an Strukturänderungen aus pflegerischer Sicht [A Nursing Perspective on the Necessity of Hospitals Adapting to Structural Changes]," *Krankenpflege* 31, no. 9 (1977), 287–90; Renate Reimann, "Information im Dienst des Kranken [Information at Patient's Service]," *Krankenpflege* 33, no. 7/8 (1979), 249–53.
161 E.g. Rosemarie Weinrich, "Gedanken zum Berufsbild Krankenpflege [Thoughts on the Vocation of Nursing]," *Krankenpflege* 36, no. 1 (1982), 2–3; Margit Schellenberg, "Die Bedeutung einer patientenorientierten Pflegeplanung [The Importance of a Patient-Oriented Nursing Care Plan]," *Krankenpflege* 31, no. 9 (1977), 291–93; Reimann, "Information im Dienst des Kranken," 249–53.
162 E.g. Friederike Dittrich, "Der Terminal auf der Station [The Computer on the Ward]," *Krankenpflege* 38, no. 9 (1984), 278–79; Friederike Dittrich, "Pflege ist Leistung – Dokumentation ist Beweis [Nursing Is a Service: Documentation Is the Proof]," *Krankenpflege* 38, no. 4 (1984), 142–44; Rupert Ringelhann, "Eindrücke von der Interhospital '85 in Düsseldorf [Impression from the Interhospital '85 in Düsseldorf]," *Krankenpflege* 39, no. 7–9 (1985), 236–38; Roland Trill, "Anforderungen an ein EDV-Gestütztes Kommunikationssystem für den Pflegebereich [Requirements for a Computing-Based Communication System in Nursing]," *Krankenpflege* 40, no. 9 (1986), 342–44.
163 Susanne Kreutzer, *Vom "Liebesdienst" zum modernen Frauenberuf: Die Reform der Krankenpflege nach 1945 [From "Labor of Love" to a Modern Female Profession: Nursing Reform after 1945]*, vol. 45, Reihe Geschichte und Geschlechter (Frankfurt am Main u.a.: Campus-Verlag, 2005).

renamed the *Deutsche Krankenpflegezeitschrift* [*German Nursing Journal*] and in 1994, the *Pflegezeitschrift* [*Nursing Journal*]. The journal was understood as a publication medium for different nursing associations where authors, who were academic and more science-oriented scholars, could publish peer-reviewed papers. Hence, this journal had a more theoretical and scientific approach to nursing and was less influenced by any agenda of a specific nursing association, such as happened with the journal of the DBfK.

Although this journal contains more articles related to the scientification of nursing it interestingly did not participate in the discussions surrounding the introduction of the nursing process in the 1970s and 1980s. It was not until later on in the 1980s, when the implementation of the nursing process into the nursing vocation was already completed, that I found examples of the nursing care plan and how it could be used in nursing practice. In 1984, a section called *Pflegeplanung/Pflegeprozess* was added to the content of the journal; however, it contained only descriptions of patient cases under the structure of the nursing care plan or process.

Das Krankenhaus – the Journal of the Deutsche Krankenhausgesellschaft

The Deutsche Krankenhausgesellschaft (DKG) [The German Hospital Society] was founded in 1949 as an association for hospital operators [*Krankenhausträger*]. Its objective was to establish a new hospital system in Germany after WWII and maintain its financial stability. It worked at the federal level of Germany and negotiated healthcare services and costs with federal representatives of the social insurances. The DKG is an influential association in the politics underlying the healthcare system, for example, collaborating in the development and adoption of laws concerning the healthcare sector in general and the hospital sector in particular.[164] The journal of the Deutsche Krankenhausgesellschaft, *Das Krankenhaus* [*The Hospital*], provides insight into hospital management and offers a managerial perspective for this study. It includes articles on legislative decisions and their impact on the healthcare system and on the providers and organization of healthcare. In the 1960s and 1970s especially, it discussed the architecture of hospital buildings as well as possibilities for rationalization in hospital processes. Discussions about nursing care services during that time were rarely found. By the middle of the 1970s, discussions began to be raised about outsourcing hospital processes such as cleaning and cooking.

---

164 Falk Illig, *Gesundheitspolitik in Deutschland. Eine Chronologie der Gesundheitsreformen der Bundesrepublik* [*Health Politics in Germany: A Chronology of the Health Reforms of the Federal Republic*] (Wiesbaden: Springer VS, 2017); DKG, "Wir stellen vor: Die Deutsche Krankenhausgesellschaft [We Present: The German Hospital Society]," *Krankenpflege* 37, no. 3 (1983), 106–07.

Data Collection and Data Analysis   67

From 1983 on, however, I found articles in which the nursing vocation became constituted as an important component of hospitals. They discussed nursing service and its relevance for technical and electronic processes such as digital documentation systems, or the potential for nurses to be responsible for administrative hospital work.[165] In 1984, the nursing process was mentioned for the first time and declared as central to quality nursing care.[166] Two years later, the nursing process was again constituted as a foundation for nursing quality by Roland Trill, health manager and expert in computing.[167] Trill published articles on electronic data processing in nursing in both *Das Krankenhaus* as well as in *Die Schwester, der Pfleger* of the DBfK. Especially interesting in *Das Krankenhaus* is that the increasing relevance of the nursing process for hospitals coincided with discussions on the computerization of hospital work. In 1990, one article examined the nursing process as a central component of a computer program for the administration of nursing service within a hospital.[168]

Analysis of the Empirical Data

Although discourse analysis can be seen as more of an attitude than a concrete method,[169] certain steps can be followed. First, the focus is on the place the statements are produced, that is, the historical, social, and/or cultural starting point where a series of similar statements can be found. This is what is meant by the location of power.[170] The primary time frame for my study is the 1960s to the late 1980s because the discussions around the nursing process began in the 1960s, strengthened in the late 1970s and early 1980s, and reached a peak when the nursing process was legally accepted in the nursing act of 1985. At that time, it became officially accepted as a part of German nursing, and afterwards, journal discussions focused more on the concrete introduction of the nursing process in

---

165 Josefia Schulte, "Betriebliche Steuerung Aufgabe des Krankenpflegepersonals? Modelle zur Stellenbeschreibung – 1. Teil [Operational Administration Tasks of Nursing Personnel? Models for a Job Description – 1st. Part]," *Das Krankenhaus* 75, no. 1 (1983), 23–26; Manfred Ellrich, "Kommunikationsbeziehungen im Pflegebereich und ihre Auswirkungen auf technische Rufsysteme [Communication Relations in Nursing Service and Their Impact on Technical Call Systems]," *Das Krankenhaus* 75, no. 1 (1983), 8–10.
166 Edith Büchner and Wilhelm Thiele, "Untersuchungen über Patientenversorgung und Pflegequalität [Research on Patient Care and Nursing Quality]," *Das Krankenhaus* 76, no. 9 (1984), 401–03.
167 Roland Trill, "Qualitätssicherung in der Krankenpflege [Quality Assurance in Nursing]," *Das Krankenhaus* 78, no. 9 (1986), 380–84.
168 Jörg Lanig and Günther Hanke, "PIK – Ein Bund-Länder EDV-Verfahren für den Pflegedienst im Krankenhaus [PIK – A Federal-'Länder' Computing Procedure for Nursing Service in the Hospital]," *Das Krankenhaus* 82, no. 3 (1990), 131–34.
169 Sarasin, *Geschichtswissenschaft und Diskursanalyse*; Landwehr, *Historische Diskursanalyse*.
170 Sarasin, *Geschichtswissenschaft und Diskursanalyse*.

clinical nursing care and its application and utility as German nursing care became more digitalized. With the fall of the Berlin wall and the reunification of Germany in 1989/1990 journal topics shifted further, more to healthcare and nursing care in East Germany.

The actions of people were not relevant to my study but more important was the analysis of the documents – the topics, discussions, arguments, and future projections for nursing which the articles transmitted. The reports and documents of the WHO, as well as the articles of the hospital journal *Das Krankenhaus* in the 1960s and first half of the 1970s, provided the framework to understand the conditions within which the new nursing discourse emerged. From the middle of the 1970s on, I analyzed the articles of the journal *Das Krankenhaus* with regard to the respective topics that emerged alongside articles in the nursing journals at the same time. Interestingly, by the middle of the 1980s, the articles in the hospital journal appeared to be responding to the discursive shift that happened in the nursing journal: The newly reconstituted nursing vocation was presented as compatible with (digitalized) administrative processes in the hospital setting. Articles in the DBfK journal constitute the main source for data analysis, where the debate on the nursing process broadened and deepened during the 1970s when the WHO's middle-term program was first announced.

Second, the focus should be put on its inscription: Statements are repetitions of similar statements, generating schemes or patterns of orders or discursive regularities.[171] The articles contained discussions I analyzed around the nursing process in regard to the way nursing was constituted and in regard to themes and other topics that were connected to this construction of nursing. Moreover, I focused on the explanation given as to why the nursing process was important for the nursing vocation. Especially during the years of the medium-term program of the WHO, I could see how statements from the introductory articles were captured and developed further. The nursing process became an entity very quickly: the steps of the nursing process were translated into image form and their visualization helped to further spread the concept. Several articles provided forms and examples of patient charts in which the nursing process could be found. This inscription of the nursing process on paper forms or later in digital structures (see chapter 7.3) supported the persistence of the nursing process.

Third, limitations and the inter-discourse should also be recognized. Limitations are prohibitions on what can be said. The inter-discourse establishes connections and elements of connections to other discourses.[172] Themes and explanations connected to the nursing process were observed from the late 1960s to the late 1980s, with a focus on their dominance, continuity or discontinuity,

---

171 Sarasin, *Geschichtswissenschaft und Diskursanalyse*.
172 Sarasin, *Geschichtswissenschaft und Diskursanalyse*.

and interconnections. During discussions of the medium-term program of the WHO especially, the themes of autonomy, transparency, control, and administration in nursing care became so closely connected that it became increasingly difficult to differentiate between them. As I will show in my empirical chapters, the discourse of professionalization that emerged throughout the discussions on the nursing process became interrelated with an economic discourse. With the particular rational, objective, transparent language and the mode of documentation of the nursing process, the value placed on rationality led to the devaluation and gradual ignoring of emotionality, especially of nurses.

Fourth, as the analysis develops, the discourse becomes visible in more detail.[173] The empirical structure I have used differentiates between the importance of accountability of this newly constituted nursing and the argument for professionalization that was connected to the nursing process. As I mentioned in the third step, the different aspects connected to the nursing process increasingly grouped together in such a way that a clear differentiation was barely possible. Thus, dividing the chapters into issues of accounting and professionalization is rather artificial. However, this structure is necessary to show the apparent contradictions and interdependence between accountability and professionalization in order to constitute a new nursing vocation based on the neoliberal rationale.

---

173 Sarasin, *Geschichtswissenschaft und Diskursanalyse*.

Chapter 5:
Theoretical Framework

In this chapter, I present the theoretical underpinnings of my study, which contain an interdisciplinary perspective drawing on Foucauldian approaches of power and governmentality, as well as different theoretical insights from scholars who adopted some concepts from Foucault. I combine these with a critical perspective on accounting in order to demonstrate how calculation became an integral part of strategies aimed at indirectly influencing the behaviour of subjects. This interdisciplinary perspective will help me to analyze the contradictory discussions in German nursing regarding the introduction of the nursing process, which valued accountability and professionalism in nursing at the same time.

I will use the concept of governmentality in order to analyze developments in German nursing in the 1970s and 1980s. From the perspective of governmentality, government cannot be reduced to "the state" or to the bureaucratic, administrative institutions that often are imagined as government. Governing consists rather of practices understood as a complex interplay between apparatuses of tactics, calculations, procedures, strategies, analyses, etc. to govern the population.[174] From the perspective of studies of governmentality, neoliberalism is a particular rationale of governmentality rather than merely an ideology or economization of societies. This neoliberal rationale became the leading form of governmentality at the time the nursing process was implemented and the state of nursing professionalization in Germany was problematized.

Understanding the nursing process as an accounting tool draws on the approach of critical accounting. Using this approach, I will analyze the transformation of how nursing has been understood and how nursing actions have been analyzed. The work of some scholars from the field of critical accounting provides the theoretical instruments to analyze the way organizations and in-

---

174 Thomas Lemke, *Eine Kritik der politischen Vernunft: Foucaults Analyse der modernen Gouvernementalität* [*A Critique of Political Reason: Foucault's Analysis of Modern Governmentality*], vol. 6. (Berlin: Argument Verlag, 2014).

dividuals can be transformed through accounting techniques and processes. These scholars also highlight the decisive role accounting plays in the operationalization of the neoliberal rationale.

5.1 Biopower and the Development of Expertise in Healthcare

First, I introduce the concept of biopower in order to trace the establishment of physicians as experts in the area of the health of a population. In his later work, Foucault increasingly focused on another dimension of power, a power that was not only directed toward singularities but increasingly trained on the phenomena of the mass. With the emergence of big administrative states, the wealth of the population was acknowledged as the wealth of the state and a new power, directed at the population in order to govern its society, began to dominate.[175] Before the 17th and 18th century, monarchs had perceived their territory as the true wealth of their kingdom and as the foundation of their power, disregarding the lives of their subjects whenever they deemed it appropriate – Foucault summarizes this power as the "the right to take life or let live."[176] Sovereign power at that time could only demonstrate its power by taking life – it was the power of the sword.

But from the 18th century on, a decisive shift occurred and a new form of power complemented this old sovereign power. This new form of power, which Foucault called biopower, focused on living beings. Perceiving the population, the mass, as a resource of the state, the health of the population became a major preoccupation of governments. With the emergence of disciplinary institutions a second form of power materialized. Disciplinary power addressed the individual body and used direct forms of surveillance and correction.[177] Consequently, Foucault called this dimension the anatomo-politics of the human body.[178]

Biopower focuses not on individuals or society, as a totality of individuals, but on the population as one whole body. It tries to control this body with its strategies and mechanisms directed at the health of the population, fostering well-being and trying to improve sanitary conditions. This dimension of biopolitics tries to modify phenomena that cannot directly be altered – for example, it tries to decrease the mortality rate or increase the fertility rate, etc. Mass phenomena can only indirectly be influenced or controlled – biopower is a power

---

175 Michel Foucault, *"Society Must Be Defended:" Lectures at the College De France 1975–76* (New York: Picador, 2003).
176 Foucault, *Society Must Be Defended*, 241.
177 Michel Foucault, *Discipline and Punish: The Birth of the Prison*, vol. 2nd Vintage books (New York: Vintage Books, 1995).
178 Foucault, *Society Must Be Defended*.

of control and regulation that tries to establish regularities at the level of populations.[179]

Demographics, statistics, and accounting thus became major preoccupations for the administration and managing of populations. These biopolitical societies are societies of normalization because statistically established norms become the defining instances of how to behave in society. These norms, however, are not static. Rather, subjects are encouraged to constantly adjust to flexible norms calculated though the statistical normal distribution of populations. Everybody knows where he/she stands compared to his/her neighbour in the statistical normal curve and accordingly tries to adjust.[180]

Medical Expertise as Component of Government

It was in the context of this new emerging biopower in the 18th century that medical expertise became established as a key component of governing a population. Affecting economics and politics, a growing population in Western Europe made new ways of governing this population necessary; for example, new ways and techniques in the surveillance, control and co-ordination of the population were developed with the goal of increasing its productivity.[181] The health and wealth status of the population became a main political objective; the concerns of political authority were less focused on the individual and more on the issue of "how to raise the level of health of the social body as a whole."[182]

The different variables that were retrieved from both the population as a whole, as well as individual bodies, connected medicine and statistics, and biological characteristics came to be understood as relevant for economics. Furthermore, this understanding suggested that those biological factors could be manipulated to govern individuals and the population body, with the possibility of improving the economy and the wealth of the population.

Subsequently, the individual became medicalized; health and hygiene became important. The structure and organization of space around the population, such as the structure of cities, came under surveillance regarding hygienic aspects and was restructured to improve the health of the population.[183] During these

---

179 Foucault, *Society Must Be Defended*.
180 Michel Foucault, ""Society Must Be Defended," Lectures at the Collège De France, March 17, 1976," in *Biopolitics: A Reader*, ed. Timothy C. Campbell and Adam Sitze (Durham: Duke University Press, 2013), 61–81; Ian Hacking, "Biopower and the Avalanche of Printed Numbers," *Humanities in Society*, no. 5 (1982), 279–95.
181 Michel Foucault, "The Politics of Health in the Eighteenth Century," in *Power/Knowledge: Selected Interviews and Other Writings 1972–1977*, ed. Colin Gordon (New York: Harvester Press, 1980), 166–82.
182 Foucault, "The Politics of Health 1980," 170.
183 Foucault, "The Politics of Health 1980," 166–82.

changes, a politics of health merged with medicine in a new role, with an important administrative function to develop techniques to improve and sustain the health of the population. Medical tasks shifted to teach individuals the rules of hygiene, to design or re-design areas of poor hygiene, and to set up surveys of the status of the population regarding its health and wealth. In this way, doctors, as hygienists, gained social power since they, besides their therapeutic work, took on the task of urban restructuring and influencing the behaviour of people. In other words, disease became connected with amoral behaviour and bad government.[184] "The doctor [became] the great advisor and expert, if not in the art of governing, at least in that of observing, correcting and improving the social 'body' and maintaining it in a permanent state of health."[185] Since the population was perceived as a social *body*, medicine perceived this same body as its central focus. By medicalizing the social body, medicine needs to be understood as a "profoundly 'social' science."[186]

The medical profession developed itself as an apparatus of administration and government, claiming the right to produce truth and developing its knowledge into expertise. Hence, medicine can be defined as a form of power/knowledge because it can, based on its scientific knowledge and its ability to work on different levels and in different ways in society, operate upon the individual body within the modus of disciplinary power and upon the population, as the social body, within the modus of regulatory or biopolitical power.[187] Physicians, as well as other experts, established themselves "as those who can speak and enact truth"[188] and in consequence, received power and authority to directly govern people in accordance to norms that were established by the very same experts.[189]

---

184 Foucault, "The Politics of Health 1980," 166–82; Michel Foucault, "The Politics of Health in the Eighteenth Century," *Foucault Studies* 18 (2014), 113–27; Nikolas Rose, "Medicine, History and the Present," in *Reassessing Foucault: Power, Medicine and the Body. Studies in the Social History of Medicine*, ed. Colin Jones and Roy Porter (London, New York: Routledge, 1994), 48–72.
185 Foucault, "The Politics of Health 1980," 177.
186 Rose, "Medicine, History and the Present," 54.
187 Foucault, "'Society Must Be Defended," Lectures at the Collège De France, March 17, 1976," 61–81; Foucault, "The Politics of Health 1980," 166–82; Foucault, "The Politics of Health in the Eighteenth Century," 113–27; Rose, "Medicine, History and the Present," 48–72.
188 Nikolas Rose, "Government, Authority and Expertise in Advanced Liberalism," *Economy and Society* 22, no. 3 (1993), 283–99: 293.
189 Interesting historical analyses about how physicians successfully asserted themselves against other (medical) healthcare providers such as (barber-)surgeons, midwives, or so-called white women in 19th century Germany can be found in the following studies: Claudia Huerkamp, *Der Aufstieg der Ärzte im 19. Jahrhundert vom gelehrten Stand zum professionellen Experten: Das Beispiel Preußens [The Rise of Physicians in the 19th Century from the Intellectual's Rank to the Professional Expert: The Example of Prussia]*, ed. Helmut Berding, Jürgen Kocka, and Hans-Ulrich Wehler, vol. 68, Kritische Studien zur Geschichtswissenschaft (Göttingen: Vandenhoeck & Ruprecht, 1985); Peter Lundgreen, "Wissen und

As long as governments functioned in a mode of welfarism, the emphasis was laid on distributing the risks that came with industrialized societies more collectively by introducing mechanisms like accident insurance, social security, and pension plans. But welfare came at a price because these societies were what Foucault called disciplinary societies, in which citizens had to follow a strict regime and a pre-determined lifepath. Social workers became the privileged experts who could intervene in the everyday lives of those considered non-compliant with the societal order. Throughout the welfare state, expertise necessary for the maintenance of these disciplinary societies became more and more institutionalised in the form of professions, which would later form enclosures. Those enclosed professions professed to act in the name of neutral knowledge. The organization of expertise in these enclosures was acknowledged to guarantee value-free judgments and interventions made by experts who had no other interest than intervening in the best interest of society.[190]

Sociology of Professions

The study of the sociology of professions is a domain which contains different theoretical approaches on professions. These theoretical approaches provide different explanations on the development, role, importance and organization of professions. They use for their analysis primarily the classic professions such as medicine, law, or the clergy. I argue that these approaches derive their assumptions from these images of professions under welfarism. Since these are the theories on which arguments for professionalization are based, I will provide a rough overview of these theories. Although these sociological theories of pro-

---

Bürgertum. Skizze eines historischen Vergleichs zwischen Preußen/Deutschland, Frankreich, England und den USA, 18.–20. Jahrhundert [Knowledge and Bourgeoisie. Outline of a Historical Comparision between Prussia/Germany, France, England, and the USA, 18th-20th Century]," in *Bürgerliche Berufe. Zur Sozialgeschichte der freien und akademischen Berufe im internationalen Vergleich*, ed. Hannes Siegrist (Göttingen: Vandenhoeck & Ruprecht, 1988), 106–24; Annette Drees, *Die Ärzte auf dem Weg zu Prestige und Wohlstand. Sozialgeschichte der Württembergischen Ärzte im 19. Jahrhundert [Physicians on Their Way to Prestige and Prosperity. A Social History About the Physicians of Württemberg in the 19th Century]*, ed. Hans J. Teuteberg and Peter Borscheid, vol. 9, Studien zur Geschichte des Alltags (Münster: F. Coppenrath Verlag, 1988); Michael Stolberg, "Heilkundige: Professionalisierung und Medikalisierung [Healers: Professionalization and Medicalization]," in *Medizingeschichte: Aufgaben, Probleme, Perspektiven*, ed. Norbert Paul and Thomas Schlich (Frankfurt am Main, New York: Campus-Verlag, 1998), 69–86.

190 Foucault, ""Society Must Be Defended," Lectures at the Collège De France, March 17, 1976," 61–81; Rose, "Government, Authority and Expertise," 283–99; Peter Miller and Nikolas Rose, "Governing Economic Life," *Economy and Society* 19, no. 1 (1990), 1–31; Peter Miller and Nikolas Rose, "Political Power Beyond the State: Problematics of Government," in *Governing the Present: Administering Economic, Social and Personal Life*, ed. Peter Miller and Nikolas Rose (Cambridge, Malden: Polity Press, 2008), 53–83.

fessions ascribe different characteristics, functions, positions, or meanings to professions, they have in common a perception that professions have a distinct and troublesome relationship to the "state" instead of acknowledging that they are part of government. These theories can be sorted into different perspectives explaining professional status based on certain indicators, specific functions, powerful positions in society, or on practical action in uncertain circumstances.[191] Indicator theories ascribe certain characteristics to professions such as autonomy and self-control, professional knowledge and high educational requirements, ideals of service and a code of ethics, high income, prestige and influence, as well as monopoly over professional activity.[192] In a functional perspective, professions are described as overseeing central tasks in a modern society and therefore have certain rights and responsibilities: Priests are responsible for the spiritual welfare of members of society, lawyers build and maintain social consensus, physicians work with conditions of health and illness, and engineers regulate the physical environment.[193]

---

191 Alexander M. Carr-Saunders and Paul A. Wilson, *The Profession* (London: Frank Cass & Co. Ltd., 1964); Talcott Parsons, "Professions," in *International Encyclopedia of the Social Sciences.*, ed. David L. Sills (London: Crowell Collier and McMillan, Inc., 1968), 536–47; Talcott Parsons, "The Professions and Social Structure," *Social Forces* 17, no. 4 (1939), 457–67; Harold L. Wilensky, "The Professionalization of Everyone?," *American Journal of Sociology* 70, no. 2 (1964), 137–58; Amitai Etzioni, *The Semi-Professions and Their Organization: Teachers, Nurses, Social Workers* (New York: Free Press, 1969); William J. Goode, "The Theoretical Limits of Professionalization," in *The Semi-Professions and Their Organization: Teachers, Nurses, Social Workers*, ed. Amitai Etzioni (New York: Free Press, 1969), 266–313; Rudolf Stichweh, "Professionen in einer funktional differenzierten Gesellschaft [Professions in a Functional Differentiated Society]," in *Pädagogische Professionalität: Untersuchungen zum Typus pädagogischen Handelns*, ed. Arno Combe and Werner Helsper (Frankfurt am Main: Suhrkamp Verlag, 1996), 49–69; Eliot Freidson, *Professionalism: The Third Logic* (Chicago: University of Chicago Press, 2001); Anne Witz, *Professions and Patriarchy* (London, New York: Routledge, 1992); Ulrich Oevermann, "Theoretische Skizze einer revidierten Theorie professionalisierten Handelns [Theoretical Outline of a Revised Theory of Professional Action]," in *Pädagogische Professionalität: Untersuchungen zum Typus pädagogischen Handelns*, ed. Arno Combe and Werner Helsper (Frankfurt am Main: Suhrkamp Verlag, 1996), 70–182; Andrew Delano Abbott, *The System of Professions: An Essay on the Division of Expert Labor* (Chicago: University of Chicago Press, 1988); Magali Sarfatti Larson, *The Rise of Professionalism: A Sociological Analysis* (Berkeley: University of California Press, 1977); Angelika Wetterer, *Arbeitsteilung und Geschlechterkonstruktion. "Gender at Work" in theoretischer und historischer Perspektive [Division of Labor and Gender Construction. "Gender at Work" in a Theoretical and Historical Perspective]*, vol. 19, Theorie und Methode (Köln: Herbert von Halem Verlag, 2002/2017).
192 William J. Goode, "Encroachment, Charlatanism, and the Emerging Profession: Psychology, Sociology, and Medicine," *American Sociological Review* 25, no. 6 (1960), 902–65; Wilensky, "Professionalization of Everyone?," 137–58; Etzioni, *The Semi-Professions and Their Organization*; Carr-Saunders and Wilson, *The Profession*.
193 Parsons, "Professions," 536–47; Stichweh, "Professionen in einer funktional differenzierten Gesellschaft," 49–69.

Criticizing, but also building on the functional perspective on professions, some approaches acknowledge professions as powerful organizations in a society. Professions gain specialized knowledge about issues and increasingly attain control over their work. Their specialized body of knowledge and specialized tasks exclude those who are not members, making it difficult to understand and evaluate their service.[194] Feminist approaches on professions analyze exactly this enclosure, criticizing that it leads to the structural exclusion of women. Several feminist studies have examined the relationship between the medical (male) profession and the nursing (female) vocation.[195]

Those sociological theories of professions, however, do not acknowledge that the change of political rationale (from welfarism to neoliberalism) created fundamental changes for professions as institutionalized expertise. Nurses, when arguing for a professionalization in nursing, are also not providing an exact definition of a profession, but are rather drawing on certain characteristics they want to achieve. For example, they call for nursing to be recognized for its autonomy through the establishment of certain structures and accomplishments such as nursing research, nursing standards, or a professional nursing language (see especially chapter 8). Their arguments are derived from an understanding of profession that is closely related to sociological approaches towards the concept of professions. Here is where I believe the contradiction of the professionalization attempts of German nurses has its origin. In the next sub-chapter, I will present this conflict by introducing the concept of governmentality.

5.2 Governmentality and the Issue of Professionalism

Studies of governmentality have developed into an academic field on their own in North America and elsewhere. For over three decades, governmentality studies have entered the scientific systems of many different countries such as France and Germany.[196] It is difficult to provide a uniform definition of what studies of governmentality comprise, because since the 1970s/80 s it has developed a wide range of themes, directions, and research projects but lacks a homogeneous research program and school of thought.

From the perspective of governmentality, the focus on the state as the actor of government is shifted to encompass a broader understanding of governing as a strategic way to indirectly influence the conduct of people through different

---

194 Freidson, *Professionalism*; Larson, *The Rise of Professionalism*; Abbott, *The System of Professions*.
195 Witz, *Professions and Patriarchy*; Wetterer, *Arbeitsteilung und Geschlechterkonstruktion*.
196 Thomas Lemke, *Gouvernementalität und Biopolitik [Governmentality and Biopolitics]*, vol. 2. (Wiesbaden: VS Verlag für Sozialwissenschaften, 2008).

technologies, mechanisms, and strategies.[197] In contrast to disciplinary or monarchist societies that forced their subjects to behave in the way the government wanted them to behave, necessitating huge apparatuses of surveillance and correction, governmentality is about how to govern in the most efficient and economical way, meaning how to govern not too much. Michel Foucault explains the notion of governmentality as the art of governing a population, a question which, according to him, was raised in the 16th century.[198]

The act of governing changed into the art of how best to govern and the acknowledgement that the population, as the real wealth of the nation, needs to prosper. The art of governing became trying "to know and regulate the wealth, health, [and] happiness of populations through an ensemble of institutions, procedures, analyses, reflection, calculations and tactics."[199] This touches on the concept of bio-power or bio-politics.[200] The most crucial point is that governmentality is about influencing the context or milieu in which citizens live in order to direct their behaviour toward a desired conduct. It is a combination of a specific form of self-government, often linked to moral imperatives and a scientific way to govern a state. In this way, governing becomes decentralized and interwoven within a web of power and knowledge.[201] Particularly important in this regard became a form of power that Foucault traced back to the beginning of the Christian faith. What he called pastoral power is based upon the knowledge of the souls of people, a knowledge that was meant to help the faithful to find redemption in the other world. One technique used by Christian pastors was the practice of confession through which individuals would open up to the authority of the pastor and display their innermost secrets, enabling the pastor to function as a guide. In order for it to function, the very insights of the individual had to be known. This pastoral power was later secularized and integrated into the governing of Western societies. Pastoral power "is salvation oriented (as opposed to political power). It is oblative (as opposed to the principle of sovereignty); it is individualizing (as opposed to legal power); it is coextensive and continuous with

---

197 Miller and Rose, "Political Power Beyond the State," 53–83.
198 Michel Foucault, "Governmentality," in *The Foucault Effect: Studies in Governmentality: With Two Lectures by and an Interview with Michel Foucault*, ed. Graham Burchell, Colin Gordon, and Peter Miller (Chicago: University of Chicago Press, 1991), 87–104.
199 Nikolas Rose, "Expertise and the Government of Conduct," *Studies in Law, Politics, and Society* 14 (1994), 359–97: 363.
200 Sven-Olov Wallenstein, "Introduction: Foucault, Biopolitics, and Governmentality," in *Foucault, Biopolitics, and Governmentality*, ed. Jakob Nilsson and Sven-Olov Wallenstein (Stockholm: Södertörn Philosophical Studies, 2013), 7–34.
201 Marianne Pieper and Encarnación Gutiérrez Rodríguez, "Einleitung [Introduction]," in *Gouvernementalität: Ein sozialwissenschaftliches Konzept in Anschluss an Foucault*, ed. Marianne Pieper and Encarnación Gutiérrez Rodríguez (Frankfurt am Main [u. a.]: Campus-Verlag, 2003), 7–21.

life; it is linked with a production of truth – the truth of the individual himself."[202] In its secularized form it was no longer about the salvation of the individual after death but rather about achieving one's potential in the here and now on earth. The motor of pastoral power in the second half of the 20th century is the hope for wealth, security, well-being, and protection.[203] In nursing, pastoral power is found in the professional call to be a self-reflective practitioner[204] and also in the concept of holism.

Thus, governmentality is about strategies and tactics employed to direct individuals and populations in a certain way that require another form of specific knowledge based on the ancient "science of 'police.'" This police science produced detailed knowledge about individuals who live in a national territory, helping to make them calculable.[205] Knowledge or expertise have to be understood as an integral part of government, but any transformation of governmental rationale and its objectives and policies also changes the shape and form of expertise. Therefore, professions as an institutionalized form of expertise have to be understood historically.[206]

5.2.1 The Neoliberal Rationale and Professions

Neoliberalism emerged in the Global North as a result of the problematization of the welfare state. According to political scientist Wendy Brown, the neoliberal shift did not encounter sharp resistance.[207] Rather, by influencing the context of actions in order to make certain actions and behaviours of individuals more likely than others, as in the sense of the "conduct of conduct,"[208] neoliberalism became integrated more deeply into the language and consciousness of individuals and in their everyday life. Hence, subjects became reconstituted and perceived themselves differently. Neoliberalism cannot be understood as a single consistent concept but rather as a constellation of conceptions that developed

---

202 Michel Foucault, "Afterword. The Subject and Power," in *Michel Foucault: Beyond Structuralism and Hermeneutics. With an Afterword by and an Interview with Michel Foucault*, ed. Hubert L. Dreyfus and Paul Rabinow (Chicago: The University of Chicago Press, 1983), 208–26: 214.
203 Foucault, "The Subject and Power," 208–26.
204 Andreas Fejes, "Governing Nursing through Reflection: A Discourse Analysis of Reflective Practices," *Journal of Advanced Nursing* 64, no. 3 (2008), 243–50.
205 Miller and Rose, "Governing Economic Life," 3.
206 Terry Johnson, "Governmentality and the Institutionalization of Expertise," in *Health Professions and the State in Europe*, ed. Terry Johnson, Gerald Larkin, and Mike Saks (London, New York: Routledge, 1995), 7–24.
207 Wendy Brown, *Undoing the Demos: Neoliberalism's Stealth Revolution* (New York: Zone Books, 2015).
208 Foucault, "The Subject and Power," 208–26.

into very different, sometimes even contradictory, directions. Thus, some authors use the notion of neoliberalism as a "thought collective."[209] "Neoliberalism is a specific and normative mode of reason, of the production of the subject, 'conduct of conduct,' and scheme of valuation [...]," but in different cultures and political perspectives "[...] it takes diverse shapes and spawns diverse content and normative details, even different idioms."[210]

However, one basic assumption shared by different neoliberalists is that a really "free" society can only exist if limitless competition prevails. "Freedom" in the neoliberal understanding means the ability to make choices and act freely from constraints and dictation of the state, based only on the rules of economy. Economic behaviour, striving to maximize its own interests and competition are, according to neoliberals, natural characteristics of individuals.[211] Hence, a "free" society has to be based on the principles of the market. Proponents argue that markets imply or possess a specific, complex knowledge that cannot be apprehended by governments. For this reason, governments/states should not intermingle with markets because they would only distort their rational development.[212]

Ordoliberalism

In the German variant of neoliberalism, however, the state was conceptualized as strong in order to control the rules of the market (for example, by preventing monopolies because these would disturb the free competition of the different players in the market) and to mitigate some of the harsh consequences of the market economy through a social system.[213] The idea of a strong state should not only maintain a stable framework for a competitive economy but also guarantee

---

209 Philip Mirowski and Dieter Plehwe, *The Road from Mont Pe`Lerin: The Making of the Neoliberal Thought Collective* (Cambridge, Mass.: Cambridge, Mass.: Harvard University Press, 2009).
210 Brown, *Undoing the Demos*, 48.
211 Franz Böhm, "Die Idee des Ordo im Denken Walter Euckens [The Idea of Ordo in the Mindset of Walter Eucken]," *ORDO Jahrbuch für die Ordnung von Wirtschaft und Gesellschaft* 3 (1950), XV–LXIV; Heddy Neumeister, "Autoritäre Sozialpolitik [Authoritarian Social Policy]," *ORDO Jahrbuch für die Ordnung von Wirtschaft und Gesellschaft* 12 (1961), 187–252; Walter Hamm, "Programmierte Unfreiheit und Verschwendung: Zur überfälligen Reform der gesetzlichen Krankenversicherung [Programmed Bondage and Dissipation: On the Overdue Reform of the Statutory Health Insurance]," *ORDO Jahrbuch für die Ordnung von Wirtschaft und Gesellschaft* 35 (1984), 21–42.
212 Miller and Rose, "Political Power Beyond the State," 53–83.
213 Michel Foucault, *The Birth of Biopolitics: Lectures at the Collège De France, 1978–79* (Basingstoke, New York: Palgrave Macmillan, 2008).

social security.²¹⁴ As German economist Ralf Ptak states, the emphasis on the strong state and its responsibility to provide minimal social security and the emphasis on a free market which the state would abstain from directly intervening in, may have blurred the line between the welfare state and the ordoliberal economic perspective.²¹⁵

This German neoliberal variant is called *Ordoliberalism* after the journal *Ordo* ('Ordnung' [order])²¹⁶, which has been published since the 1920s. In this journal especially, discussions occurred during WWII regarding how Germany should be rebuilt after the war. Prominent authors were, for example, Walter Eucken,²¹⁷ Friedrich von Hayek,²¹⁸ Ludwig Erhard,²¹⁹ and Alfred Müller-Armack.²²⁰ Throughout the decades following the war, articles were published concerning issues of economy, the social system, and healthcare.²²¹ By the 1960s, the Ordoliberals were already criticizing the social security and healthcare system for its high costs and authoritarian style in governing the population, meaning that individuals were not given the freedom to withdraw money at will from their insurance.²²² The construction of the social pension fund was criticized as a non-transparent organization for saving money, in which the saving process was anonymous and uncontrollable for the individual. It had been set up in a way that believed the logical reaction of the individual as a rational acting subject would be to misuse this fund and demand as many resources as possible from it. Due to

---

214 Rudolf Morsey, *Die Bundesrepublik Deutschland, Entstehung und Entwicklung bis 1969 [The Federal Republic of Germany, Its Formation and Development until the Year 1969]* (München: De Gruyter Oldenbourg, 2007).
215 Ralf Ptak, *Vom Ordoliberalismus zur sozialen Marktwirtschaft [From Ordoliberalism to Social Market Economy]* (Wiesbaden: VS Verlag für Sozialwissenschaften, 2004).
216 Walter Eucken, "Das ordnungspolitische Problem [The Regulative Problem]," *ORDO Jahrbuch für die Ordnung von Wirtschaft und Gesellschaft* 1 (1948), 56–90.
217 Walter Eucken taught economics at the University of Freiburg/Germany in the 1930s and 1940s. He ranks as a founder of the German social market economy.
218 Friedrich von Hayek was a scientist in law and political economics. He taught economics at the University of Freiburg/Germany in the 1960s and 1980s and won the Nobel Prize in economics.
219 Ludwig Erhard was Minister of Economic Affairs from the beginning of the Federal Republic of Germany on until 1963 and subsequently became the second German Chancellor.
220 Alfred Müller-Armack was a professor of economy and sociology, and worked in the Federal Ministry of Economics when Ludwig Erhard was Minister of Economic Affairs.
221 Hamm, "Programmierte Unfreiheit und Verschwendung" 21–42; Neumeister, "Autoritäre Sozialpolitik," 187–252; Roland Vaubel, "Die deutschen Staatsausgaben: Wende oder Anstieg ohne Ende? [The German Government Expenditures: Turning Point or Recession without Ending?]," *ORDO Jahrbuch für die Ordnung von Wirtschaft und Gesellschaft* 35 (1984), 3–19; Eucken, "Das ordnungspolitische Problem," 56–90.
222 Neumeister, "Autoritäre Sozialpolitik," 187–252; Hubertus Müller-Groeling, "Zur ökonomischen Problematik der gesetzlichen Krankenversicherung [About the Economic Problems of the Statutory Health Insurance]," *ORDO Jahrbuch für die Ordnung von Wirtschaft und Gesellschaft* 19 (1968), 485–98.

this misconstruction, the social pension fund would need to act in an authoritarian fashion towards the individual, similar to the care of paupers rather than as a real insurance scheme, and would treat the individual as a suppliant rather than a creditor.

Ordoliberals wanted the establishment of a controllable and democratic saving system with clear and documented amounts of savings for each individual in order to urge individuals to continue saving and prevent the wasting of money and resources. Social insurance should be transformed into saving deposits and only a few people in need should receive social insurance, which would pay only in cases of catastrophe for which they were not responsible.[223] They also blamed the health insurance system for providing hospitals with the incentive to use resources excessively. Ordoliberals proposed establishing incentives for economic and cost-conscious behaviour and stipulated that everybody in the healthcare system, including patients, physicians, and the health insurance system, were to become profit-oriented.[224]

One example of this shift to base healthcare services on an economic rationale in a neoliberal sense can be found in the hospital journal *Das Krankenhaus* (see chapter 4.3). Siegfried Eichhorn, an economist and board member of the German Hospital Institute (DKI),[225] called for adapting hospital structures to those of the economy. In 1966, Eichhorn compared adapting to the economy an "internal secularization of hospital work."[226] In 1974, he called for the participation of physicians and nurses in the management of the hospital and its economic constraints to transform hospital processes economically. Thus, Eichhorn recommended introducing benefits for good economic behaviour and penalizing bad economic behaviour to induce or foster rational and self-responsible behaviour of the hospital personnel. By showing such a self-responsible behaviour, and by understanding their actions in economic terms, nurses and physicians could help the hospital achieve its economic goals. Hence, acting economically was presented as moral behaviour. As part of the internal secularization of

---

223 Neumeister, "Autoritäre Sozialpolitik," 187–252.
224 Walter Hamm, "Verschwendung in Krankenhäusern durch falsche Anreize [Wastefulness in Hospitals Because of False Incentives]," *ORDO Jahrbuch für die Ordnung von Wirtschaft und Gesellschaft* 33 (1982), 363–68.
225 The German Hospital Institution was founded in 1953 with the task to improve hospital work in regard to its medical, nursing, and economical effectivity (Peter Ossen and Anja Wunsch, "Am Puls der Zeit. Interview: Perspektiven des DKI 60 Jahre nach seiner Gründung [In Pace with the Times. Interview: Perspectives of the German Hospital Institute (DKI) 60 Years after Its Foundation]," *Das Krankenhaus*, no. 2 (2014), 110–14).
226 "[D]ie Anpassung der Arbeitsbedingungen im Krankenhaus an die der Wirtschaft ... [als] eminent wichtige[n] Prozeß der 'inneren Säkularisierung' der Krankenhausarbeit." (Siegfried Eichhorn, "Die betriebswirtschaftlichen Aspekte der Leistungssteigerung durch Zusammenarbeit [Economic Aspects to Increase Performance through Collaboration]," *Das Krankenhaus* 58, no. 8 (1966), 315–23: 315; my translation).

hospital work, Eichhorn hoped to achieve a "demystification of the healing and nursing vocations."[227] The call for de-mystification is important for this study because it is a central element in the question of whether or not developments in German nursing can be understood as professionalization.

From the late 1970s on, criticisms of the German social system increased. A growing number of critics believed that the social and healthcare systems needed to be transformed economically by the introduction of managerial and accounting mechanisms and should even be privatized.[228] Economist Walter Hamm criticized statutory health insurance as being "alien to the free economic and social order" and as treating the insured as "an incapable citizen."[229] Additionally, he complained that the state assumed it had all the information to evaluate and calculate every local event in healthcare, whereas, in reality, only individuals had the necessary information and awareness of local conditions that enabled them to make the best decisions, based on their economic interests. He also argued that the state was trying to control ever-broader areas of the healthcare system, leading to more and more state intervention; that hospitals were funded independent of their efficiency, leading to the wasteful use of healthcare services, to prescribing more services than necessary, to choosing the most expensive therapies, and to keeping uneconomic processes in place, etc.[230]

According to Hamm's understanding, the patient constantly and naturally strove for personal advancement, and this had to be considered in the construction (or transformation) of the healthcare system. The way the system was, as Hamm argued, selfishness produced behaviour that violated the principle of solidarity and jeopardized the community. Hamm called this the "moral hazard" of the healthcare system.[231] In his opinion, the state needed to provide a framework that enabled "everybody by pursuing his/her own advantage to

---

227 "'Entmystifizierung' der Heil- und Pflegeberufe." (Siegfried Eichhorn, "Zielkonflikte zwischen Leistungsfähigkeit, Wirtschaftlichkeit und Finanzierung der Krankenversorgung [Conflicts of Objectives between Performance, Efficiency and Financing of Healthcare]," *Das Krankenhaus* 66, no. 5 (1974), 186–96: 192; my translation.
228 E.g. Hamm, "Programmierte Unfreiheit und Verschwendung," 21–42; Hamm, "Verschwendung in Krankenhäusern," 363–68; Joachim Wiemeyer, "Die konzertierte Aktion im Gesundheitswesen nach dem Krankenversicherungs-Kostendämpfungsgesetz [Concerted Action in the Healthcare System after the Cost-Containment Act for Health Insurance]," *Jahrbuch für Christliche Sozialwissenschaften* 20 (1979), 251–88; Vaubel, "Die deutschen Staatsausgaben," 3–19.
229 "Die soziale Krankenversicherung bildet in ihrer heutigen Gestalt unzweifelhaft einen Fremdkörper in der freiheitlichen Wirtschafts- und Gesellschaftsordnung der Bundesrepublik Deutschland. [...] Die Versicherten werden als unmündige Bürger behandelt." (Hamm, "Programmierte Unfreiheit und Verschwendung," 21; my translation).
230 Hamm, "Programmierte Unfreiheit und Verschwendung," 21–42.
231 Hamm, "Programmierte Unfreiheit und Verschwendung," 23.

contribute to the attainment of macroeconomic goals and goals of the society."[232] His conclusion was to introduce competition in healthcare so that hospitals needed to compete against each other and behave as economic entities with the possibility of generating profits. Competition, according to Hamm, helped to guarantee both good quality and fewer costs in healthcare services.[233]

Hamm's argument clearly includes a moral dimension. Neoliberalism is not only about the economization of the social sphere or the introduction of management techniques. It is as much a moral project that aims to "produce" new subjects – both healthcare workers and patients. It was in this context that the nursing process was implemented in Germany. The discourse of self-responsibility was essential to efficiency technologies and was exemplified by the introduction of accounting techniques to the nursing process.

To realize a neoliberal agenda in healthcare, it was first of all necessary to transform hospitals and healthcare services into economic entities. One precondition was that nursing services could be calculated (and I argue that the nursing process had a decisive function in this transformation). All these technologies were not invented by nurses but derived from business and management accounting and the private economy.

The Economic Individual in the German Context

Neoliberalism emerged by weakening the formerly close relationship between political authority and the social field, and by putting the focus on markets, economy, efficiency, competition, and autonomous subjects with free choice. The aim of government became the fostering of self-responsibility and autonomy of subjects in a way that the goals of the state become integrated into the personal goals of individuals.[234] This trend of individualization is focused on the economization of the subject and requires accounting strategies.[235] Moreover, in the area of organization management and human resources, an appreciation of hierarchies shifted to calls for a non-hierarchical organization and creative, independently thinking, and actively acting employees. The striving for self-fulfilment as characteristic of individuals became an acknowledged and fostered

---

232 "Diese Vorschriften müssen jedoch so ausgestaltet sein, daß alle Beteiligten mit ihrem Streben nach eigenem Vorteil zugleich einen Beitrag zu Erreichung gesamtwirtschaftlicher und gesamtgesellschaftlicher Ziele leisten." (Hamm, "Programmierte Unfreiheit und Verschwendung," 22; my translation.
233 Hamm, "Programmierte Unfreiheit und Verschwendung," 21–42.
234 Miller and Rose, "Governing Economic Life," 1–31; Foucault, *The Birth of Biopolitics*.
235 Peter Miller and Michael Power, "Accounting, Organizing, and Economizing: Connecting Accounting Research and Organization Theory," *Academy of Management Annals* 7, no. 1 (2013), 557–605.

rationale, which was used to establish an efficient and non-hierarchical order of corporate management. Slogans such as the "humanization of working lives" cover this change in the administration and management of enterprises.[236] They were used to create motivation and incentives to make the individual employee feel part of the production process. Employees "should fulfil their needs of recognition and self-fulfilment within the enterprise and not outside it."[237] Here individual freedom became framed by the logic of a market-oriented organization which ultimately should lead to an "entrepreneurial self."[238]

Related to this is the notion of *homo œconomicus*, where social conduct must be understood as a calculative action based on economic principles. Contained within *homo œconomicus* is the idea that we consider ourselves as a form of capital – *human capital*, meaning that investments in ourselves are investments in our enterprise of the self and our human capital will pay out in the future (e.g. the education we undergo will give us better job opportunities). The individual, perceived as *homo œconomicus*, becomes an entrepreneurial subject, seeking to constantly increase its competitive potential by improving its value in every part of its life and by acting and deciding in a strategic manner.[239]

This new conception of the individual as creative and productive promised a higher autonomy in decisions and actions than before. However, this expected

---

236 Brigitta Bernet, "Vom "Berufsautomaten" zum "Flexiblen Mitarbeiter.". Die Krise der Organisation und der Umbau der Personallehren um 1970 [From the "Occupational Machine" to the "Flexible Employee"]," in *Wertewandel in der Wirtschaft und Arbeitsweltarbeit, Leistung und Führung in den 1970er und 1980er Jahren in der Bundesrepublik Deutschland*, ed. Bernhard v. Dietz and Jörg Neuheiser, Wertewandel im 20. Jahrhundert (Berlin: De Gruyter Oldenbourg, 2016), 31–54.
237 "…um ihnen Anreize zu bieten, sich selbst in den Arbeitsprozess einzubringen und ihre Bedürfnisse nach Anerkennung und Selbsterfüllung im Rahmen des Betriebs – und nicht außerhalb desselben – zu befriedigen" (Bernet, "Vom 'Berufsautomaten' zum 'Flexiblen Mitarbeiter'," 35; my translation).
238 Anselm Doering-Manteuffel and Lutz Raphael, *Nach dem Boom. Perspektiven auf die Zeitgeschichte seit 1970 [After the Boom: Perspectives on Contemporary History since 1970]*, 3rd ed. (Göttingen: Vandenhoeck & Ruprecht, 2012), 9; see also Gabriele Metzler, "Staatsversagen und Unregierbarkeit in den siebziger Jahren? [Government Failure and Ungovernability in the 1970s?]," in *Das Ende der Zuversicht? Die siebziger Jahre als Geschichte*, ed. Konrad H. Jarausch (Göttingen: Vandenhoeck & Ruprecht, 2008), 243–60; Metzler, "Staatsversagen und Unregierbarkeit," 243–60; Dieter Sauer, "Permanente Reorganisation [Permanent Re-Organization]," in *Vorgeschichte der Gegenwart. Dimensionen des Strukturbruchs nach dem Boom*, ed. Anselm Doering-Manteuffel, Lutz Raphael, and Thomas Schlemmer (Göttingen: Vandenhoeck & Ruprecht, 2016), 37–56; Anne Seibring, "Die Humanisierung des Arbeitslebens in den 1970er-Jahren: Forschungsstand und Forschungsperspektiven [Humanization of the Work Life in the 1970s: State of and Perspectives in Research]," in *"Nach dem Strukturbruch"? Kontinuität und Wandel von Arbeitsbeziehungen und Arbeitswelt(en) seit den 1970er Jahren*, ed. Knut Andresen, Ursula Bitzegeio, and Jürgen Mittag (Bonn: Verlag J. H. W. Dietz Nachf. GmbH, 2011), 107–26.
239 Brown, *Undoing the Demos*; Foucault, *The Birth of Biopolitics*.

autonomy also comes with responsibility. One example from the context of public health is the movement for working on an individual's health fitness. Sports events, active holidays, and, prominently in Germany, the exercise trail Trimm-Dich-Pfad became popular for many people.[240] "The proper modern agentic individual, for instance, manages a life, carrying a responsibility not only to reflect self-interest but also to the wider rationalized rules conferring agency. Helplessness, ignorance, and passivity may be very natural human properties, but they are not the properties of the proper effective agent."[241] Hence, following the economic rationale became a moral obligation. In turn, citizens who stayed healthy decreased the financial burdens of all and would thus behave in an economically responsible way regarding society as a whole. Rational behaviour to stay healthy was thus conceptualized as economic behaviour.

Within neoliberalism then, all areas of human relations are understood and conceptualized as following an economic rationale and are part of a market economy. If people follow *only* their own interests, wealth for society will increase. Hence, from the perspective of studies of governmentality, economic conduct is conceptualized as a moral obligation for citizens and a particular mode of governing individuals in neoliberalism. The most important task for governments is to secure competition in a free market.

In comparison to welfarism, a neoliberal rationale propagated the strength of the market instead of a planned and state-regulated economy; the encouragement of individuals to become active citizens in determining their life and quality of life, and to be entrepreneurs of their selves with the freedom to make rational decisions; the privatization of former public services and economization of the private sphere; efficiency based on economic competition between organizations instead of depending on the expertise of enclosed and uncontrollable professions; and transparency by enhancing visibility through monetarization and calculations through the systematic implementation of accounting technologies.[242] The introduction of techniques such as "monetarization, marketization, enhancement of the powers of the consumer, financial accountability and [the] audit" were meant to increase the operability and transparency of the workplace.[243]

---

240 Lemke, *Eine Kritik der politischen Vernunft*, 6; Anselm Doering-Manteuffel, "Langfristige Ursprünge und dauerhafte Auswirkungen [Long-Term Origins and Lasting Effects]," in *Das Ende der Zuversicht?* (Vandenhoeck & Ruprecht, 2008) *Die siebziger Jahre als Geschichte*, ed. Konrad H. Jarausch (Göttingen: Vandenhoeck & Ruprecht, 2008), 313–29; Thomas Foth and Dave Holmes, "Governing through Lifestyle: Lalonde and the Biopolitical Managemnt of Public Health in Canada," *Nursing Philosophy* 19, no. 4 (2018), 1–11.
241 John W. Meyer and Ronald L. Jepperson, "The 'Actors' of Modern Society: The Cultural Construction of Social Agency," *Sociological Theory* 18, no. 1 (2000), 100–20: 107.
242 Miller and Rose, "Political Power Beyond the State," 53–83.
243 Rose, "Government, Authority and Expertise," 294.

Expertise in Neoliberalism

The role of expertise thus has become the translation and alignment of political principles, industrial aims, and the goals of individuals: the economic objective of a firm becomes linked with the personal goals of a worker within this firm under the general political aim of economic growth.[244] Professions in the welfare state tended to form what Rose called "enclosures."[245] These enclosures of expertise made it difficult to directly intervene in professional matters. In neoliberalism, professions are perceived as hindrances and against the realization of competition. To break up these enclosed professions, mechanisms of competition such as audits, accounting strategies, and management processes were increasingly introduced. In consequence, the power of professions became less connected to their trusted ability to claim truth and to define reality. In the neoliberal rationale, even professions must compete with each other or with other vocations. The economic and autonomous subject, then, chooses the experts that promise the most efficient solutions for the subject's problems. It was no longer the absolute claim of true knowledge that was important, which had characterized the relationship between experts and subjects in the welfare state, but the decision of free subjects based on principles like accountability and transparency. Hence, economy came to function as a new body of knowledge and the new truth within the nexus of knowledge and power.[246]

In this way, professions have lost the traditional status they had enjoyed in the welfare state and that was due to their respective fields of recognized expertise. In neoliberalism, professions have increasingly been transformed into service institutions attempting to meet customers' demands. Financial and market mechanisms have reduced the control that the formerly enclosed professions had, for example, in the area of self-regulation, because of the demands of market orientation and work transparency.[247] In other words, for experts, the right to speak based upon a positive knowledge of human conduct vanishes within neoliberalism and is replaced by a right to speak upon principles of efficacy, accountability, economics, and self-management. Rose provides two examples of this transformation: First, the trust people had in professional work has been replaced by the necessity of the audit in professional practice. Second, the importance of "true" knowledge of human conduct based on the social and human

---

244 Miller and Rose, "Governing Economic Life," 1–31.
245 Rose, "Government, Authority and Expertise," 259.
246 Wallenstein, "Foucault, Biopolitics, and Governmentality," 7–34; Rose, "Government, Authority and Expertise," 283–99.
247 Rose, "Government, Authority and Expertise," 283–99.

sciences has been replaced by an emphasis on accounting and financial management.[248]

In summary, while in the welfare state expertise became institutionalized in professions in which professionals established autonomy and formed enclosures that protected them from competing knowledges, in neoliberalism this monopolized structure of professions has increasingly been opened up. Expertise in neoliberalism is not acknowledged anymore as an absolute, especially if it is contained within a closed system of professions. In neoliberalism, experts must demonstrate that the expertise they provide is effective and efficient. For traditional professions that stabilized their status during the welfare state, this change in governmental rationale threatens their autonomy to claim truth "just" because of their expert status. And newly (in the neoliberal rationale) awakening professions such as nursing will never reach the status and shape of traditional professions but can only become recognized as important societal vocations when they can make the positive impact of their work transparent and help to further establish strategies of the market. It seems, however, that nurses hardly acknowledge the understanding of neoliberal expertise and what it means for their eagerness to professionalize. Instead, they still believe in and promote the image of the traditional profession.

5.2.2 De-professionalization or the Concept of New Professionalism

As I discussed in the last section, professions have been the preferred target of criticism by neoliberals and thus, it seems to be contradictory to talk about professionalization in neoliberal times. Expertise in neoliberalism can only be acknowledged as such when it can show its effectivity and efficiency. A precondition is that experts need to be transparent, controllable, and accountable to the customer who purchases their services. Therefore, the traditional understanding of professions is replaced by the claim that experts have to compete in the market like everybody else and to constantly show that they deliver what they promise. This comes along with the decline of traditional professional core values such as closure, authority, and autonomy. Moreover, managerial strategies seem to be ethically superior because they break up the professional enclosure and produce through techniques of control (which are based on distrust) more trust than a traditional discourse of professionalism based on "paternalism, arrogance and self-interest."[249]

---

248 Rose, "Government, Authority and Expertise," 283–99.
249 Tony P. Gilbert, "Trust and Managerialism: Exploring Discourses of Care," *Journal of Advanced Nursing* 52, no. 4 (2005), 454–63: 455.

Why, then, did discussions around the professionalization of several vocations occur with the transformation of the welfare state to neoliberalism? Discussions around the so-called professionalization of nursing, for example, began predominantly in the 1970s and 1980s, which was exactly the time neoliberalism became the leading global governmental rationale. Interestingly, at exactly that time, the first articles were published discussing the issue of de-professionalization. For example, a British nursing activist stated in 1988: "The true professions' monopolies are under threat and nursing leaders are undoubtedly sufficiently aware of this to make it a factor in forming their policies. They know that full professional status for nursing cannot be achieved, and they are facing an unprecedented combination of threats to their already limited autonomy."[250]

Authors predicting the de-professionalization (partly called "proletarianization") especially of physicians but also other healthcare vocations based their argument on the ongoing introduction of managerial and bureaucratic mechanisms, the emphasis on entrepreneurialism (such as the logic of efficiency and for-profit or cost-effectiveness), and the increasing introduction of accounting and control systems in former professions. The implementation of an economic logic as the dominant logic of professions threatened the former taken-for-granted idea of what professions should be and must, thus, be read as a trend to de-professionalize.[251] The process of substituting the importance of scientific

---

250 Jane Salvage, "Professionalization or Struggle for Survival? A Consideration of Current Proposals for the Reform of Nursing in the United Kingdom," *Journal of Advanced Nursing* 13, no. 4 (1988), 515–19: 519; see also Goode, "Theoretical Limits of Professionalization," 266–313.
251 George Ritzer and David Walczak, "Rationalization and the Deprofessionalization of Physicians," *Social Forces* 67, no. 1 (1988), 1–22; John B. McKinlay and Joan Arches, "Towards the Proletarianization of Physicians," *International Journal of Health Services* 15, no. 2 (1985), 161–95; Maximiliane Wilkesmann, Birgit Apitzsch, and Caroline Ruiner, "Von der Deprofessionalisierung zur Reprofessionalisierung im Krankenhaus? Honorarärzte zwischen Markt, Organisation und Profession [From De-Professionalization to Re-Professionalization in the Hospital? Fee-Based Physicians between the Market, Organization, and Profession]," *Soziale Welt* 66, no. 3 (2015), 327–46; Paul A. C. Parkin, "Nursing the Future: A Re-Examination of the Professionalization Thesis in the Light of Some Recent Developments," *Journal of Advanced Nursing* 21, no. 3 (1995), 561–67; Julian Wolf and Werner Vogd, "Professionalisierung der Pflege, Deprofessionalisierung der Ärzte oder vice versa? [Professionalization of Nursing, Deprofessionalization of Physicians, or Vice Versa?]," in *Professsionskulturen – Charakteristika unterschiedlicher professioneller Praxen*, ed. Silke Müller-Hermann, et al. (Wiesbaden: Springer Fachmedien, 2018), 151–73. A more positive understanding of this introduction of managerial thinking into medicine can be found in an article about the transformation of Finnish hospital care. Liisa Kurunmäki, professor of accounting, refers to Andrew Abbotts' theory of professions, arguing that the medical profession in Finland became hybridized by integrating knowledge and techniques of accounting into their scope of practice (Liisa Kurunmaki, "A Hybrid Profession: The

progress in medicine with questions of costs of medical treatment and healthcare were already happening in the 1970s and 1980s in the US, especially with the introduction of the DRG system. DRGs are Diagnostic Related Groups that sort patients in hospitals. This DRG-based financing system was implemented in the German hospital sector from 2003 on. It contains a patient classification system that categorizes patients according to their main and secondary diagnoses and rates the heaviness of individual cases. Based on this the costs of healthcare for each patient are calculated. This categorization and calculation happens not by physicians or healthcare teams but is chosen by a standardized and registered software program.[252] In the DRG-based financing system, medical and economic aspects are merged and physicians become economically accountable for the use of resources in treating patients.[253] Here, medical knowledge becomes linked to cost-benefit approaches leading to the governing of physicians based on economy. This is based on the call to de-mystify professional medical knowledge and the tendency to value objective and standardized mechanisms of diagnosis and treatment over subjective and experiential knowledge of the professionals because it can more easily be linked to cost-benefit approaches. This coincides with decreasing trust in professional knowledge and leads, in consequence, to a decline of medicine as an organized profession. The introduction of a standardized, objective and measurable language threatens physicians with losing the exclusiveness (in content and value) of their knowledge. Rather, the rationale of economy become implemented as the foundation upon which to act. This becomes even more intensified with the increasing use of computers making formerly enclosed knowledge more and more accessible in a way that is rational, economic, and applicable to the increased call for multi-professional collaboration.[254]

Acquisition of Management Accounting Expertise by Medical Professionals," *Accounting, Organizations and Society* 29, no. 3 4 (2004), 327–47).

252 Michael Simon, *Das Gesundheitssystem in Deutschland. Eine Einführung in Struktur und Funktionsweise [The Healthcare System in Germany: An Introduction in Structure and Functionality]*, 4th ed. (Bern: Verlag Hans Huber, 2013); Rolf Rosenbrock and Thomas Gerlinger, *Gesundheitspolitik. Eine systematische Einführung [Health Policy: A Systematic Introduction]*, 3rd. ed. (Bern: Verlag Hans Huber, 2014).

253 Alistar M. Preston, "The Birth of Clinical Accounting: A Study of the Emergence and Transformations of Discourses on Costs and Practices of Accounting in U.S. Hospitals," *Accounting Organizations and Society* 17, no. 1 (1992), 63–100. For the introduction of DRGs in Australia in the 1990s see Wai Fong Chua, "Experts, Networks and Inscriptions in the Fabrication of Accounting Images: A Story of the Representation of Three Public Hospitals," *Accounting, Organizations and Society* 20, no. 2 (1995), 111–45.

254 Marie R. Haug, "The Deprofessionalization of Everyone?," *Sociological Focus* 8, no. 3 (1975), 197–213; Ritzer and Walczak, "Rationalization and the Deprofessionalization of Physicians," 1–22; Maren Siepmann and David A. Groneberg, "Der Arztberuf als Profession – Deprofessionalisierung [The Medical Vocation as Profession: Deprofessionalization],"

Perceiving the introduction of scientific management strategies as a threat to the professional development of nursing can also be found quite early in the literature. Here as well, the de-mystification of nursing knowledge is emphasized as a de-professionalizing development.[255] This trend of de-professionalization strengthened with the introduction of computers in nursing and with the obligation of nurses to adapt their actions and thinking to the "thinking" and procedures of the computer, leading to a de-individualization of patients and to a de-expertizing of nurses.[256]

Another reason for de-professionalization in healthcare vocations or professions can be seen in the downsizing knowledge gap between experts and the public because of an "increased education and knowledge development [...] and the democratization of knowledge and skills"[257] that leads to a loss of expert authority over the patient, of trust in the public, and of professional monopoly over knowledge and skills. This needs to be understood as a consequence of the neoliberal rationale that encourages patients to become informed consumers and who take responsibility for their decisions regarding their health. Nurses in particular enhanced this development in their field with nursing models and theories that encouraged perspectives on partnership and participation in nursing care. This can be understood as a positive outcome or even desired result of de-professionalization.[258]

These arguments concerning the increasing de-professionalization of professions through the implementation of managerial strategies can be found from the 1970s on. Nonetheless, nursing scholars, nursing associations, and nurses in Germany have pushed for the professionalization in nursing in Germany since the 1970s. It is even more surprising that nurses saw the introduction of managerial strategies as a driver for professionalism in nursing. This contradiction between professionalization and de-professionalization was discussed by Mirko

---

Zentralblatt für Arbeitsmedizin, Arbeitsschutz und Ergonomie 62 (2012), 288–92; Heinrich Bollinger and Joachim Hohl, "Auf dem Weg von der Profession zum Beruf: Zur Deprofessionalisierung des Ärzte-Standes [On the Way from a Profession to a Vocation: On the Deprofessionalization of the Physicians]," *Soziale Welt* 32, no. 4 (1981), 440–64; Preston, "The Birth of Clinical Accounting," 63–100; Chua, "Experts, Networks and Inscriptions," 111–45.

255 Janet L. Storch and Shirley M. Stinson, "Concepts of Deprofessionalization with Application to Nursing," in *Political Issues in Nursing: Past, Present, and Future*, ed. Rosemary White (Chichester: John Wiley & Sons Ltd, 1988), 33–44; Parkin, "Nursing the Future," 561–67; Salvage, "Professionalization," 515–19.

256 L. Barbara Harris, "Becoming Deprofessionalized: One Aspect of the Staff Nurse's Perspective on Computer-Mediated Nursing Care Plans," *Advances in Nursing Science* 13, no. 2 (1990), 63–74.

257 Parkin, "Nursing the Future," 565.

258 Parkin, "Nursing the Future," 561–67; Storch and Stinson, "Concepts of Deprofessionalization," 33–44.

Noordegraaf, a Dutch professor of Public Management. He explains that the loss of autonomy and a loss of a monopoly of knowledge in professions "often happens in the name of professionalization and by introducing new professional methods (e. g., measurement and monitoring)."[259] De-professionalization takes place in the name of professionalization. These new professional methods are based on a managerial logic, for example, cybernetic problem-solving processes, and promise to enhance professionality.[260] Noordegraaf uses the term of "Hybridized professionalism [which] offers new opportunities for maintaining the notion of professionalism in times that weaken the notion of professionalism."[261] Calling it "new professionalism," sociologist Julia Evetts also emphasizes that "managerial demands for quality control and audit, target setting and performance review become reinterpreted as the promotion of professionalism."[262] She connects this change and the introduction of output measures with the discourse of enterprise, the discourse of competition, or the trend of individualization, making it a neoliberal agenda. The understanding of professionalism changes with the integration of market mechanisms, commodifying professional service and constraining it financially. Additionally, the relationship between the professional and the client or patient is "being converted into customer relations through the establishment of quasi-markets, customer satisfaction surveys and evaluations as well as quality measures and payment, results."[263]

However, the connection of professionalism with managerial logic enables, as Evetts states, other vocations to call themselves "professional,"[264] meaning that managerial logic opens up the enclosures of traditional professions leading to a "professionalization of everyone."[265] One example is the introduction of evidence-based practice into different societal fields. With the introduction of evidence-based practice, actions and interventions are evaluated based on the best available (quantifiable and measurable) evidence. Actions are conceptualized as following a

---

259 Mirko Noordegraaf, "From "Pure" to "Hybrid" Professionalism: Present-Day Professionalism in Ambiguous Public Domains," *Administration & Society* 39, no. 6 (2007), 761–85: 762.
260 Noordegraaf, "From "Pure" to "Hybrid" Professionalism," 761–85; Reimer Gronemeyer and Charlotte Jurk, "Entprofessionalisieren wir uns! Über die Sprache der Versorgungsindustrie: Wie Plastikwörter die Sorge um andere infizieren und warum wir uns davon befreien müssen [We Should De-Professionalize! On the Language of the Supply Industry: How Plastic Words Contaminate the Care for the Other and Why We Need to Free Ourselves from It]," in *Entprofessionalisieren wir uns! Ein kritisches Wörterbuch über die Sprache in Pflege und Sozialer Arbeit*, ed. Reimer Gronemeyer and Charlotte Jurk (Bielefeld: transcript Verlag, 2017), 9–12.
261 Noordegraaf, "From "Pure" to "Hybrid" Professionalism," 775.
262 Julia Evetts, "A New Professionalism? Challenges and Opportunities," *Current Sociology* 59, no. 4 (2011), 406–22: 412.
263 Evetts, "A New Professionalism?," 416.
264 Evetts, "A New Professionalism?," 406–22.
265 Wilensky, "Professionalization of Everyone?," 137–58.

purely instrumental logic, meaning all actions can be construed as based on means-end analyses. In consequence, activities within the rationale of evidence-based practice have to be transparent, rational, objective, and controllable. It was first implemented in medicine, where it was believed to avoid wasting resources with ineffective or less effective medical intervention.

The introduction of evidence-based medicine transformed the way and the space in which the medical profession could act. The highest value of evidence in evidence-based practise (e.g. evidence-based medicine or evidence-based nursing) is ascribed to quantitative and statistical research designs, especially randomized controlled trials (RCTs), and meta-studies. These are research studies conducted in a rather post-positivistic manner, meaning they purport to objectively discover *the* reality by developing hypotheses about this reality and to prove the validity of these hypotheses with falsifications. Scientific work in this understanding needs to be transparent, rational, and repeatable, and the language used has to be transparent, definite, and possibly numeric. However, with evidence-based practice comes the real danger of knowledge disappearing, in this case knowledge in medicine or nursing that is derived from other perspectives.[266]

It seems that the nursing vocation is welcoming this transformation, subordinating itself under managerial logic because it appears to provide nurses with the means to be free from subordination under a medical logic and to allow this female vocation to gain recognition in the understanding of a new or hybrid professionalism.

5.3 Critical Accounting and its Application in Healthcare

In what follows, I will use some insights from scholars who work in accounting and who developed some of Foucault's concepts further in order to analyze how accounting technologies became decisive technologies in the governing of our societies. I am not an accountant and my knowledge of accounting is more than limited, but some of the ideas developed in critical accounting are very helpful to better understand how the nursing process contributed to the transformations in nursing.

Accounting and how it is understood varies historically. The understanding of and research about accounting has differed throughout the decades, especially since the start of the second half of the 20th century. Besides scientific accounting,

---

266 Dave Holmes, Amélie Perron, and Patrick O'Byrne, "Evidence, Virulence, and the Disappearance of Nursing Knowledge: A Critique of the Evidence-Based Dogma," *Worldviews on Evidence-Based Nursing* 3, no. 3 (2006), 95–102; Rosenbrock and Gerlinger, *Gesundheitspolitik*.

cost accounting, and accounting with the focus on behaviour of members of organizations, critical accounting can also be found as a scientific strand. Scholars using Foucault's concepts in their work began to publish in the 1970s and 80s.[267] While the scientific literature of critical accounting is broad, I will focus only on some theorists of critical accounting like Peter Miller and Christopher S. Chapman, since they will help me to show how the neoliberal rationale has been implemented into the everyday context of nurses and how nurses adopted the approach as part of broader societal transformations.

Critical accounting does not view accounting as a neutral non-intervening activity that is concerned simply with the calculation of budgets and the representation of the economic situation of an enterprise or organization. Rather, it is understood as "spatially and historically varying calculative practices – ranging from budgeting to fair value accounting – that allows accountants and others to describe and act on entities, processes, and persons."[268] Accounting scholar Peter Miller ascribes to accounting "a low epistemological threshold"[269] and, together with his colleagues Christopher S. Chapman and David J. Cooper, even declares it to be a "craft without essence."[270] In more positive terms, the permeability of accounting should be considered, enabling it to oversee practices and rationales from other fields (such as engineering) and to establish itself in different contexts and localities.[271]

Four different characteristics can be related to accounting. These are territorializing, mediating, adjudicating, and responsibilizing. Accounting is territorializing in the sense that it demarks a territory and constitutes it as a calculable entity. "Territorializing is achieved by linking ideas of the market with the instruments of accounting, so as to allow households, hospitals, schools, retired persons, or whatever to be constituted as accounting subjects obligated to calculate or be calculated."[272] With its mediating activity, accounting moves between rationales. The processes and results of accounting become more likely accepted by individuals and organizations who orient their actions upon accounting practices. Hence, accounting has an adjudicating role, meaning that its practice is powerful and becomes the legitimized form of knowledge of the setting in which

---

267 Peter Miller, "The Margins of Accounting," *The Sociological Review* 46, no. 1_suppl (1998), 174–93; Peter Miller, "Calculating Economic Life," *Journal of Cultural Economy* 1, no. 1 (2008), 51–64; Miller and Power, "Accounting, Organizing, and Economizing," 557–605.
268 Christopher S. Chapman, David J. Cooper, and Peter B. Miller, "Linking Accounting, Organizations, and Institutions," in *Accounting, Organizations, and Institutions: Essays in Honour of Anthony Hopwood*, ed. Christopher S. Chapman, David J. Cooper, and Peter B. Miller (New York: Oxford University Press, 2009), 1–29: 1.
269 Miller, "The Margins of Accounting," 190.
270 Chapman, Cooper, and Miller, "Accounting, Organizations, and Institutions," 2.
271 Miller, "The Margins of Accounting," 174–93.
272 Miller and Power, "Accounting, Organizing, and Economizing," 579–80.

it is implemented. "In many cases, this role in adjudicating performance has acquired such legitimacy that it is now more or less binding on both organizations and societies if they are to be considered appropriate and modern. [...] From this point of view, accounting is fundamentally a responsibilizing practice even as its functionality in achieving desired outcomes is to be doubted."[273] This subjectivizing and responsibilizing characteristic installs accounting practices not only in organizational structures but also on the individual. By incorporating those accounting practices, such as audits, the individual becomes constituted as a calculable and calculative subject that is able to and has to make choices. Accounting constitutes individuals who acknowledge accounting practices and their representations as facts and perform according to the rules of the accounting practices. Equipped with knowledge and techniques, the calculable, and hence, economic subject, becomes an agent of itself and acknowledges its responsibility for the rational choices it made and their output.[274]

Accounting, by making entities accountable, constitutes these entities in the first place and, as Miller emphasizes, contains a moral dimension. Instead of the neutrality that is normally ascribed to accounting and calculations, accounting practices are based on particular visions and ideas of what efficient and effective management should look like – accounting comprises a particular rationale. With the introduction of an accounting logic into organizations, these organizations become restructured and reorganized based on this underlying rationale through the implementation of control mechanisms, such as monitoring, auditing, and the introduction of "a language with which to define and delineate organizational goals, procedures, and policies."[275] Calculations make practices operable in certain terms by giving it a structure, language, and hence, visibility:

> "[W]hile management or regulators may be concerned with issues of efficiency or value for money, it is accounting practices that enable such ideas to be operationalized and made real. In making visible and calculable the objects and activities that are at the heart of management, accounting creates a facticity that appears objective and unchallengeable, beyond the fray of politics or mere opinion."[276]

Miller argues that it is this capacity of calculative practices that makes them so important for analyses of governmentality because it is through calculation that programs for governing are made operable.[277] For example, management nowadays is closely connected to accounting, hence, accounting shapes the practices

---

273 Miller and Power, "Accounting, Organizing, and Economizing," 562.
274 Miller and Power, "Accounting, Organizing, and Economizing," 557–605.
275 Chapman, Cooper, and Miller, "Accounting, Organizations, and Institutions," 13.
276 Miller and Power, "Accounting, Organizing, and Economizing," 558–59.
277 Miller, "Calculating Economic Life," 57.

and perceptions of management.²⁷⁸ Moreover, accounting techniques have also successfully been implemented in all spheres of the market and have incorporated market practices in its repertoire. Thus, accounting established itself as a dominant discourse in the market setting. Through this, the accounting rationale of the market becomes not only implemented in various settings and organizations that were formerly governed by different rationales, but also into society in general. Therefore, practices of accounting have to be critically reflected on regarding their constitutive character and underlying rationales. For example, practices of calculations likely are based on the concept of efficiency, benchmarking, or competitiveness.²⁷⁹

In the case of the healthcare setting, accounting strategies were praised because they fostered a higher efficiency in the use of resources, better measurability in a complex setting, and more consistency and accuracy in management control. With a standardized language, nurses' work should be disentangled from the situatedness of nursing care and made measurable and calculable:

> Just as all music can be analyzed according to seven whole tones, elements of patient care may be expressed in about ten categories. One has only to look at one of the most basic categories – medication – to see that while medication is definable and quantifiable, each patient's requirement falls within a range of medication complexity. There is no element of patient care without this abstraction.²⁸⁰

Transforming individuals and organizations into calculating entities is a precondition to make them open to economic logic and economic procedures. This is important in the ordoliberal rationale which requires a restructuring of society based on economic thinking, meaning that competition and market orientation were introduced into societal practices in order to transform society into the shape of a market.²⁸¹ With certain concepts belonging to the idea of economy, such as efficiency, sustainability, and accountability, accounting practices "do not simply inform economic decision-making, but in many cases constitute the domain of economic activity itself, a process we refer to as *economization*."²⁸² Hence, economization is the practices which constitute individuals as economic subjects and organizations as economic entities.²⁸³

---

278 Miller and Power, "Accounting, Organizing, and Economizing," 557–605.
279 Miller, "Calculating Economic Life," 51–64.
280 Jenny K. Jarrard, "Engineered Standards in Hospital Nursing: Management Engineers Can Give Reinforcement and Correction to Problem Solving," *Nursing Management* 14, no. 4 (1983), 29–32: 31.
281 Foucault, *The Birth of Biopolitics*.
282 Miller and Power, "Accounting, Organizing, and Economizing," 579; italics in original.
283 Miller and Power, "Accounting, Organizing, and Economizing," 557–605.

5.4 Summary

In the second half of the 20th century, accountants, economists, hospital managers, and politicians became increasingly interested in nursing practices and in the multiple ways in which nurses and patients apparently wasted valuable resources. New policies were implemented that transformed healthcare practices. Processes of economization can be found in order to establish the rationale of economy upon which individuals and organizations should be governed. In the time of the neoliberal rationale, the nursing process was implemented.

Using nursing articles as well as articles of hospital management, I will analyze the discourse in nursing. In order to describe this discourse, it is necessary to reveal contradictions as well as silences and power relations. While the economization of nursing can be viewed as contradictory and inhibitory to nursing professionalization,[284] in this study, I will use the example of the nursing process to analyze the interdependencies between professionalizing in nursing and the call for accountable and economic nursing. I will use the perspective of critical accounting to analyze the nursing process as a managerial tool and its impact on German nursing, which came to perceive its introduction important for the professionalization process. This perspective helps to understand how managerial-based nursing became accepted as the "right" way of doing nursing care, as professional nursing.

---

284 Gilbert, "Trust and Managerialism," 454–63.

Chapter 6:
The Nursing Process and Its Way into German Nursing

6.1 Introductory Explanation

In the following chapters, I will present a complex discourse that emerged in German nursing in the 1970s and 1980s and that remains dominant today. In order to make this discourse understandable, I have to artificially separate it into different components, which explain the emergence of accounting and economic thinking in nursing on the one hand, and the concurrent movement toward the idea of professionalization on the other. The nursing process is a central part of this nursing discourse, as I will show in this empirical section, since it connects the development of accountability in nursing with the attempts and arguments of German nurses to professionalize the nursing vocation. In order to introduce this complex discourse I will first give an overview of the background and the discussions from which this discourse emerged. This chapter thus describes the movement of the nursing process into German nursing.

The Structure of the Discourse in Nursing

This discourse in German nursing contains mechanisms, knowledges, procedures, and strategies from accounting as well as from nursing. In this hybrid discourse, nursing and accounting become intermingled and the differences between them become blurred. This is what makes this discourse so complex and sometimes even contradictory. It seems that this discourse that developed in German nursing care in the 1970s and 1980s included all strategies and perspectives – even those that appeared contradictory – for the professionalization of the nursing vocation as long as the nursing process was included as a central component. Therefore, arguments for the professionalization of the nursing vocation were various and comprised technical and scientific progress, a needed change of thinking (about health) in patients and nurses.

One example is the nature of the nursing process, which has been described as "a revolutionary way to think about the patient"[285] or a "qualitative change"[286] in nursing. But some have thought the opposite: that the steps of the nursing process are just normal procedure in daily nursing practice and the nursing process only provides a distinctive language for this practice.[287] The following quote, for example, is from a report about a presentation of the nursing process provided by nursing scholars Antje Grauhan and Charlotte Katz. Reflecting on this presentation, the writer of the report concluded: "One perceived – however – that one always had done nursing care in this way [this the nursing process], but matron Antje Grauhan, Berlin, and Dr Charlotte Katz, nurse, Manchester, could analyze what nurses always do clearly and understandably."[288] This quote shows that the nursing process was not perceived as a totally new way of thinking in nursing but as a possibility to verbalize routines in daily nursing care in clear and understandable words.

The relationship of the nursing process to nursing research is also understood differently in the nursing journal *Krankenpflege*. One nurse active in scientific research valued the nursing process as an instrument to introduce research and science into nursing care.[289] On the contrary, another argued that it is the task of nursing research to develop the nursing process as a scientific instrument to prove the effectiveness of nursing care.[290]

A third example questions whether empathy or rationality is more desired in nursing. One nurse argued that as the healthcare system changed, nurses would need a higher level of empathy in order to provide the best care possible for the

---

285 "…eine revolutionäre Art des Denkens über den Patienten" (J. N. Thompson, "Der Krankenpflegeprozeß – Mit Vorsicht zu Behandeln! [The Nursing Process:Treat Carefully!]," *Krankenpflege* 34, no. 7/8 (1980), 243–44: 244; my translation).
286 "… der Pflegeprozess als qualitative Veränderung" (Sabine Bartholomeyczik, "Arbeitsplatz Krankenbett [Workplace Bedside]," *Krankenpflege* 41, no. 5 (1987), 158–61: 160; my translation).
287 Renate Reimann, "Pflegeplanung – Was bedeutet geplante Pflege in der Berufspraxis [Nursing Care Plan:The Meaning of Planned Nursing Care in Daily Professional Practice]," *Krankenplege* 33, no. 5 (1979), 154–57; Rosemarie Weinrich, "Ausblick auf die Arbeit des DBfD in den 80er Jahren [Outlook on the Work of the DBfK in the 80s]," *Krankenpflege* 35, no. 1 (1981), 16–18.
288 "Man fand zwar, daß man ja eigentlich immer schon so gearbeitet habe, aber Oberin Antje Grauhan, Berlin, und Dr. Charlotte Katz, Krankenschwester, Manchester, konnten das 'Immer-schon-so klar' und verständlich analysieren" (Wilma Jansen, "Überblick über die wesentlichen Referate [Overview of Essential Presentations]," *Krankenpflege* 32, no. 6 (1978), 197–200: 200; my translation).
289 Monika Krohwinkel, "Wie kann Krankenpflegeforschung uns helfen, besser zu pflegen? [How Can Nursing Research Help Us to Provide Better Nursing Care?]," *Krankenpflege* 34, no. 1 (1980), 14–15.
290 Reimann, "Pflegeplanung," 154–57.

patient.²⁹¹ But another nurse dismissed the family model of nursing calling for nurses to empathize with patients' needs, and instead called for rationality in the nurse-patient relationship. Instead of feeling with the patient, nurses should rather think themselves into the situation of the patient.²⁹²

As this nursing discourse became established, the need for modernization or professionalization was not always explained. Rather it seemed to be enough to state without explanation that the nursing vocation had to progress towards professionalization in order to strategize. As I will show in the following chapters (especially in chapter 8), with this unquestioning call for professionalization based on the nursing process, nurses did not realize that they were being led by the neoliberal discourse.

In the following discussion on the nursing process, the central component of the newly emerged discourse in German nursing, I will examine the role of the WHO in the establishment of this discourse. The medium-term program of nursing and midwifery of the WHO, which ran from 1976 to 1983, is of special importance because it introduced the nursing process into European, and thus German, nursing. The chapter concludes with an overview of how German nursing received this program.

6.2 The Nursing Process

The nursing process was developed in the USA over the course of changes in the healthcare payment system. In the mid-1960s, the government-sponsored health insurance systems – Medicare (for the financing of healthcare for elderly people) and Medicaid (for the financing of healthcare for poor people) – were introduced. With their introduction and the ongoing discussions about rising costs for healthcare, from the 1970s on hospitals were reimbursed for care provided prospectively rather than retrospectively, meaning that structures and procedures of healthcare planning were needed in order to calculate costs in advance.²⁹³ The nursing process developed within this climate of steadily increasing costs and changes in practices of hospital accounting and cost control. Besides the nursing process, other examples of approaches for managing patient care and treatment were developing, such as the Problem-Oriented System of Medical

---

291 Rosemarie Weinrich, "Der Wandel im bisher üblichen Verständnis von Krankenpflege [Change in the Common Perception of Nursing]," *Krankenpflege* 35, no. 4 (1981), 156–58.
292 Antje Grauhan, "Berufsethische Normen in der Krankenpflege [Ethical Norms in Nursing]," *Krankenpflege* 39, no. 7–8 (1985), 231–33.
293 Alistar M. Preston, "The Birth of Clinical Accounting: A Study of the Emergence and Transformations of Discourses on Costs and Practices of Accounting in U.S. Hospitals," *Accounting Organizations and Society* 17, no. 1 (1992), 63–100.

Care by Lawrence Weed in the early 1970s for both physicians and nurses. Other nursing care approaches were also being developed by nursing scholars like Virginia Henderson or Faye G. Abdellah in the 1950s and 1960s.[294]

Two originating strands can be found for the concept of the nursing process, and these carry different logics. The first emergence of the concept of nursing process can be dated to the late 1950s at the Yale School of Nursing by Ida Orlando.[295] In 1961, she published her considerations on how to integrate principles of psychiatric care into the curriculum for general nursing education. Her nursing process focused on the relationship and communication between the nurse and the patient. The "steps" of this nursing process are "The Patient's Behavior," "The Nurse's Reaction," and "the nursing actions which are designed for the patient's benefit."[296] While Orlando's nursing process was based on emphasizing nurse-patient communication, in the late 1960s another nursing process was developed that was more based on a cybernetic structure. Helen Yura and Mary B. Walsh, two US nursing scholars who worked at the Catholic University of America in Washington, DC, reconceptualized the process in nursing as a more natural science- and research-based process, similar to biomedical thinking.[297] They structured their study program for further education for nurses according to a number of steps they called the "nursing process." They defined this process as "the core process for the practice of nursing."[298] The first part of the process contained information on assessing patients' needs. The second part focused on the planning of nursing care based on these needs. In the third part of the program, nurses learned how to implement this planned care and in the fourth part, they evaluated the nursing care provided. The authors integrated the concept of problem-solving into the nursing process,[299] which in turn constituted the nursing process as a problem-solving process with a cybernetic structure.[300]

---

294 Virginia Henderson, *Principles and Practice of Nursing*, ed. Gladys Nite and Bertha Harmer, 6th ed. (New York: New York: Macmillan, c1978); Virginia Henderson, "The Concept of Nursing," *Journal of Advanced Nursing* 3, no. 2 (1978), 113–30.
295 Niels Buus and Michael Traynor, "The Nursing Process: Nursing Discourse and Managerial Technologies," in *The Nursing Process: A Global Concept*, ed. Monika Habermann, Leana R. Uys, and Barbara Parfitt (Edinburgh; New York: Elsevier/Churchill Livingstone, 2006), 31–46.
296 Ida Jean Orlando, *The Dynamic Nurse-Patient Relationship: Function, Process, and Principles* (New York: New York, Putnam 1961, 1961), xi, 31.
297 Helen Yura and Mary B. Walsh, *The Nursing Process: Assessing, Planning, Implementing, and Evaluating; the Proceedings of the Continuing Education Series Conducted at the Catholic University of America, March 2 through April 27, 1967* (Washington: Catholic University of America Press, 1968); Buus and Traynor, "The Nursing Process," 31–46.
298 Mary B. Walsh and Helen Yura, *Human Needs and the Nursing Process* (New York: Appleton-Century-Crofts, c1978., 1978), xi.
299 Frances H. Harpine, "Assessing the Needs of the Patient," in *The Nursing Process; Assessing, Planning, Implementing, and Evaluating; the Proceedings of the Continuing Education Series*

Cybernetics developed in the US,[301] and emerged as a science in the 1940s out of questions of communication and control being raised in different scientific and political fields, such as the US military and the neurosciences.[302] When dealing with complex issues, the regulatory cycle provided a standardized language of input, process, output, and feedback, allowing structural control. Increasingly issues and processes from various areas became described in those terms, and cybernetic language was eventually introduced into such diverse fields as biology, management, engineering, etc. As a simple solution to the question of how to process information it functioned as a first step in the development and running of computerized systems.[303] In the 1970s, cybernetic language and thinking gave an answer to societal questions such as rising societal plurality, economic and technologic renewals by providing unifying terms to diverse social and political demands.[304] The cybernetic logic "abstracts generally from the essence and correctness of the observed phenomenon and recognizes the behavior and organization based only on systematic aspects of communication. This procedure, thus, allows describing material and immaterial objects and processes as a circular algorithm."[305]

Conducted at the Catholic University of America, March 2 through April 27, 1967, ed. Helen Yura and Mary B. Walsh (Washington: Catholic University of America Press, 1968), 21–43.

300 Helen Yura, Mary B. Walsh, and Dorothy Ozimek, *Nursing Leadership: Theory and Process*, 2nd ed. (New York: Appleton-Century-Crofts, 1981).

301 Norbert Wiener, *Cybernetics or Control and Communication in the Animal and the Machine*, vol. 2nd edition, Fourth Printing (Cambridge, Massachusetts: The M.I.T. Press, 1985); Virginia Henderson, "Nursing Process – a Critique," *Holistic nursing practice* 1, no. 3 (1987), 7–18.

302 Arie C. Drogendijk, "Gesundheit, Krankheit und Kybernetik [Health, Illness, and Cybernetic]," *Elektromedizin* 7, no. 3 (1962), 160–71; Martin Lengwiler and Jeannette Madarász, "Präventionsgeschichte als Kulturgeschichte der Gesundheitspolitik [Prevention History as Cultural History]," in *Das präventive Selbst. Eine Kulturgeschichte moderner Gesundheitspolitik*, ed. Martin Lengwiler and Jeannette Madarász (Bielefeld: transcript Verlag, 2010), 11–28; Wiener, *Cybernetics or Control*, 2nd edition, Fourth Printing.

303 Stafford Beer, "Cybernetics: A Systems Approach to Management," *Personnel Review* 1, no. 2 (1972), 28–39; Wiener, *Cybernetics or Control*, 2nd edition, Fourth Printing.

304 Vincent August, *Technologisches Regieren. Der Aufstieg des Netzwerk-Denkens in der Krise der Moderne. Foucault, Luhmann und die Kybernetik [Technological Governing. The Rise of Network-Thinking During the Crisis of Modernity. Foucault, Luhmann, and Cybernetics]* (Bielefeld: transcript Verlag, 2021); Michael Hagner, "Vom Aufstieg und Fall der Kybernetik als Universalwissenschaft [On the Rise and Fall of Cybernetics as a Universal Science]," in *Die Transformation des Humanen. Beiträge zur Kulturgeschichte der Kybernetik*, ed. Michael Hagner and Erich Hörl, 2nd ed. (Frankfurt am Main: Suhrkamp, 2018), 38–71.

305 "Die Kybernetik abstrahiert dabei […] grundsätzlich von der Beschaffenheit und Gegenständlichkeit des betrachteten Phänomens und nimmt ausschließlich das Verhalten und die Organisation unter systematischen Aspekten der Kommunikation in den Blick. Durch diese Vorgehensweise gelingt die Beschreibung von materiellen und immateriellen Objekten und Prozessen als zirkuläre, algorithmische Schrittfolge" (Manfred Hülsken-Giesler, *Der Zugang zum Anderen. Zur theoretischen Rekonstruktion von Professionalisierungsstrategien pfle-*

As Virginia Henderson reflected, Yura and Walsh's understanding of the nursing process as a cybernetic process was more successful for its further replication in nursing than the understanding of a nursing process emphasizing nurse-patient communication as proposed several years earlier by Orlando.[306] Hence, cybernetic logic with input, output, and the feedback loop is inherent to the understanding of the nursing process today.

Depending on the nursing setting, the number of steps in the nursing process – usually between four and six – varies historically as well as contextually. However, they always contain assessing the problem, setting nursing goals and planning nursing care based upon the information derived from the earlier assessment, performing nursing care based on a nursing care plan, and documenting as well as evaluating the success or failure of the interventions in comparison with the proposed nursing goals. Sometimes the setting of nursing goals is defined as a separate step in the process and located between the assessment and the nursing care plan. To enhance the nursing process, in the late 1980s and in the 1990s, the classification systems "Nursing Outcomes Classification" (NOC) and "Nursing Interventions Classification" (NIC) were developed at the University of Iowa College of Nursing. Both contain a classification of either (proposed) nursing outcomes or nursing interventions in a standardized language. In the NOC, every outcome has a list of indicators describing and framing the outcome. A measurement scale from 1 to 5 is included to rate the indicators in regard to the patient, and these range from 1 as "never positive" to 5 as "consistently positive." But it is not only the actual status of the patient that can be evaluated; the proposed outcome for the patient has to be set out by planning the numbers the patient should achieve in the indicators. Comparing the numbers of the proposed outcome with the numbers that were ascribed to the patient during the assessment means that the progress of the patient in healthcare can be evaluated based on distinct numbers. The NIC contains lists of standardized nursing interventions for different domains concerning not only the individual patient but also a community or population.[307]

It was possible to implement these classification systems because the nursing process had already structured nursing care into different steps and defined

---

gerischen Handelns im Spannungsfeld von Mimesis und Maschinenlogik [Access to and Approach of the Other: For a Theoretical Reconstruction of Professionalization Strategies of Nursing Care in the Tension between Mimesis and Machine Logic], ed. Hartmut Remmers, vol. 3, Pflegewissenschaft und Pflegebildung (Göttingen: V&R unipress, 2008), 321; my translation).

306 Henderson, "Nursing Process," 7–18; Orlando, *The Dynamic Nurse-Patient Relationship*.
307 Sue Moorhead, *Nursing Outcomes Classification (NOC)*, 4th ed. (St. Louis, Mo.: Mosby Elsevier, 2008); Gloria M. Bulechek, Howard Karl Butcher, and Joanne McCloskey Dochterman, *Nursing Interventions Classification (NIC)*, 5th ed. (St. Louis, Mo: Mosby/Elsevier, 2008).

practices and parts of nursing care as nursing outcomes and interventions. As these systems were implemented in a nursing care setting, they simultaneously became part of the nursing process.[308] Regardless of the changes and adaptations the central concept of the nursing process is to solve problems in a goal-oriented, step-by-step manner based on rational decision-making and acting, and on cybernetic logic.

This rationale and the cybernetic structure of the nursing process, as I will show in this study, is a powerful technology that enabled significant changes in German nursing. The structure allows linking certain single nursing tasks to specific nursing problems as well as planned nursing goals to the actual outcome. This visualization of nursing care and the standardized language used that is based on input, process, and output enables it to act upon nursing action. That means nursing action becomes visible not only to nurses themselves but also to others external to the nursing vocation like managers and accountants. Furthermore, nursing actions become constituted in calculative terms via the nursing process, and hence, open to manipulation, for example, by installing management systems into nursing or calculating the quantity and quality of nursing personnel on the nursing process (see chapter 7).

The nursing process based on this cybernetic understanding was promoted by the WHO and was officially introduced into German nursing in the context of a medium-term program of the organization that ran from 1976 until 1983. This program declared as its central aim the establishment of nursing research and the strengthening of the status of nursing in European states. It also contained the largest European nursing study, *People's Needs for Nursing Care*, at that time with eleven countries participating in this study.[309] The aim of the study was to research the steps of the nursing process. From every participating centre in the eleven countries data were retrieved concerning each single step. For example, all the care needs from people were collected and compared, leaving a total of 24 identified care needs. Other steps were observed and data collected outlining how many nursing goals were set, how many and which nursing interventions were executed, and how the outcome was judged. This last step of the nursing process, the evaluation, was discovered to be the weakest part of nursing practice. Hence, the study identified areas in which nurses, using the nursing process, could improve. Moreover, as the authors stated, this study strengthened international collaboration in nursing research and practice. Participating nurses gained knowledge about the organization of their nursing setting and practice in

---

308 Heiner Friesacher, "Segen oder Fluch für die Pflege? Pflegediagnosen und Pflegeklassifikationssysteme [Boon and Bane for Nursing? Nursing Diagnoses and Nursing Classification Systems]," *Padua* 2, no. 4 (2007), 43–47.
309 Pat Ashworth et al., *People's Needs for Nursing Care: A European Study*, ed. World Health Organization (Copenhagen: World Health Organization, 1987).

the structure of the nursing process. The use of the nursing process was made legitimate by the results of the study that showed, on the one hand, that data could be retrieved from research on the nursing process, and on the other hand, that flaws in nursing practice could be identified when this nursing practice was based on the nursing process.[310]

Although Germany did not participate in this European study, the research that came out of this WHO program was published regularly.[311] German nursing scholars clearly recognized its value and spread the research. Nurses welcomed the nursing process quite enthusiastically as a chance to make their work visible, valuable, and to demonstrate their professionalism. The nursing process was developed further in German-speaking countries most prominently by Verena Fiechter and Martha Meier, two Swiss nursing pioneers and educators. Their 1981 book, *Pflegeplanung [Nursing Care Plan]*, which was an instruction manual on the use of the nursing process in nursing,[312] was very well received. It was re-issued ten times up until 1998 and helped to educate several generations of German nursing students. With the integration of the nursing process into the exam regulations of the nursing act of 1985, it became not just accepted but also required for German nurses to use the nursing process.[313]

In the next pages, I will examine the WHO's role in the transformation of healthcare services in its member states in Europe as well as how the WHO's

---

310 Ashworth et al., *People's Needs for Nursing Care*.
311 Monika Krohwinkel, "Krankenpflegeforschung in Europa. 2. Arbeitstagung europäischer Krankenpflegeforscher in Kopenhagen [Nursing Research in Europe: Second Work Day of European Nursing Researchers in Copenhagen]," *Krankenpflege* 34, no. 1 (1980), 15; Renate Reimann, "Stagnation oder Fortschritt in der Entwicklung der Pflegeberufe? [Stagnation or Progress in the Development of Nursing Occupations?]," *Krankenpflege* 35, no. 1 (1981), 20 & 37; Monika Krohwinkel, "Krankenschwester arbeiten gemeinsam an der Verbesserung der Krankenpflege in Europa. Eine Orientierungshilfe zur Forschungskomponente des mittelfristigen Programms der Weltgesundheitsorganisation für das Krankenpflege- und Hebammenwesen in Europa [Nurses Collaborate to Improve Nursing in Europe]," *Krankenpflege* 34, no. 6 (1980), 195–97; Monika Krohwinkel, "Krankenpflegeforschung in Europa [Nursing Research in Europe]," *Krankenpflege* 33, no. 3 (1979), 83–85; Krohwinkel, "Krankenpflegeforschung in Europa II," 15; Monika Krohwinkel, "Pflegeforschung und ihre Auswirkung in der Praxis im Zusammenhang mit Pflege [Nursing Research and Its Impact on Practice Regarding Nursing]," *Krankenpflege* 38, no. 7–8 (1984), 224–27; Marianne Weber, "Der Krankenpflegeprozeß in der Schweiz: Ergebnisse eines Forschungsprojektes und seine Folgen [The Nursing Process in Switzerland: Results of a Research Project and Its Consequences]," *Krankenpflege* 40, no. 1 (1986), 30–32; Nicole Delmotte, "Der Krankenpflegeprozeß in Belgien. Erfahrungen mit der WHO-Studie [The Nursing Process in Belgum: Experiences with the WHO Study]," *Krankenpflege* 40, no. 1 (1986), 32–35.
312 Verena Fiechter and Martha Meier, *Pflegeplanung. Eine Anleitung für die Praxis [Nursing Care Plan: An Instruction for Practice]* (Basel: RECOM, 1987).
313 KrPflAPrV, "Ausbildungs- und Prüfungsverordnung für die Berufe in der Krankenpflege vom 16. Oktober 1985 [Regulation for Education and Examination in the Occupations of Nursing from October 16th, 1985]," in *Z 5702 A*, ed. Bundesgesetzblatt (1985).

agenda was received in Germany. It should be understood that the nursing process was an instrument to make healthcare professionals, and nurses in particular, manageable and accountable, and to break the professional enclosures, particularly of physicians, by introducing management strategies and the principle of economic activity.

6.3 The WHO's Role in the Implementation of the Nursing Process

The World Health Organization was established in 1946 and succeeded the following international health organizations: The Office International d'Hygiene Publique (OIHP) founded in 1907; the International Health Division (IHD), founded in 1913; and the League of Nations Health Organization (LNHO), founded at the end of the First World War.[314] The rationale upon which the IHD and the LNHO in particular based their work was the belief that wealth could only be established by maintaining or improving health. Hence, they connected citizens' stable health status as a precondition for economic wellbeing on a societal level They argued that diseases would lower the productivity of citizens, increasing poverty and hindering the progress of society.[315] The connection of the health of the individual to societal values and aims was transferred to the WHO when it was established shortly after WWII. The understanding of health as "a state of complete physical, mental and social well-being and not merely the absence of disease or infirmity,"[316] as it was declared in the preamble of its constitution, was postulated during WWII: "For health is more than the absence of illness; the word health implies something positive, namely physical, mental, and moral fitness. This is the goal to be reached."[317] The concept of health, therefore, was broadened by including a social component and by positioning health as the ultimate opposite to sickness. Following this definition, individuals

---

314 Whereas the OIHP can be defined as an observational organization collecting data on border-crossing infection diseases such as cholera and yellow fever, the IHD and the LNHO ascribed themselves more executive functions such as establishing campaigns against diseases and programs to improve health and hygiene in countries and regions. The ideas of such international health organizations were avoiding pandemic infections and improving wealth by improving health. The IHD was an important unit of the Rockefeller Foundation and the LNHO was financially supported by the same foundation in the 1920s and 1930s (Marcos Cueto, Theodore M. Brown, and Elizabeth Fee, *The World Health Organization: A History* (Cambridge: Cambridge University Press, 2019)).
315 Cueto, Brown, and Fee, *The World Health Organization*.
316 WHO, "The First Ten Years of the World Health Organization," (Geneva: World Health Organization, 1958), 459.
317 Gautier, 1943, p. 1, as cited in Cueto, Brown, and Fee, *The World Health Organization*, 33.

could barely reach and maintain this position and always had to strive for it. Health became something that had to be produced continuously. Ascribing such a significance to health and establishing it as political aim relates the WHO's concept of and strategy on health to the biopolitical perspective on governing a society. The body of population should be as healthy as possible in order to build the wealth of a nation. Fostering the health status of the population means governing the individual to constantly attempt to achieve a better health status. From this biopolitical perspective, the individual is made to behave in a more health-conscious fashion by connecting disease to amoral behaviour and hence, by moralizing the individual in regard to living a healthy life (see chapter 5.1).[318]

Furthermore, the Constitution of the WHO not only deems that aiming to stay healthy is a natural need of individuals, it also demands that citizens be responsible for their health: "The health of all peoples is fundamental to the attainment of peace and security and is dependent upon the fullest co-operation of individuals and States."[319] Thus, the political sphere is also integrated into the health of the citizens. In "attain[ing] peace and security," the cooperation of the people to obtain and maintain their health is a key factor. In the aftermath of WWII, this call made it a moral obligation for individuals to act in favour of their health.

A proposal from the US Public Health Service became the foundation of the constitutional document of the WHO. The framework within which the support of the WHO should take place was also adopted from the US instrument of "technical assistance," in that development was understood "primarily [as] a matter of transferring knowledge of science and technology, thus avoiding the need to address the economic interests and social realities that led to underdevelopment."[320] The WHO was not constituted as a funding organization to give financial support to countries to help them establish health promotion programs but instead focused on calls for reorganization and networking among countries to create strategies for the improvement of health among their own citizens.[321]

This instrument of technical assistance was meant to influence the context in which countries made decisions in such a way that the behaviour of them or their decision-makers led to the preferred outcome. From the perspective of governmentality, this meant they were to provide credible information and establish plausible strategies. The WHO was established on the belief that resistance to these strategies or goals would lessen if they were based on scientific knowledge

---

318 Michel Foucault, "The Politics of Health in the Eighteenth Century," in *Power/Knowledge: Selected Interviews and Other Writings 1972–1977*, ed. Colin Gordon (New York: Harvester Press, 1980), 166–82.
319 WHO, "The First Ten Years," 459.
320 Cueto, Brown, and Fee, *The World Health Organization*, 63–64.
321 Cueto, Brown, and Fee, *The World Health Organization*.

as their legitimizing foundation. The power used here is not hard and coercive. In the perspective of the Foucauldian notion of "conduct of conduct," the preferences of complex entities like countries can be shaped in a certain way. Hence, technical assistance based on science and technology provided by the WHO should establish practices for fostering health in different countries. Based on the perceived neutral and apolitical essence of science and technology, countries themselves should establish a national goal for financially and structurally promoting health and for making their citizens responsible for maintaining a good health status. Using technical assistance offered by the WHO should be understood as an early neoliberal attempt to govern governments and their citizens from a supra-national level indirectly and with minimal effort. Therefore, the WHO was not equipped with executive power over its member states, and the idea was that countries themselves should request help from the WHO.[322].

In order to work closely with nations, the constitution of the WHO contained the aspect of regionalization. "The regional offices were responsible for setting regional policies, hiring staff, supervising and carrying out WHO policies in the regions and organizing meetings with representatives of the governments of each member country."[323] Six regions were established, one of which was the region of Europe (acronym EURO) in 1951. In 1957, the WHO bureau of the region Europe was located in Copenhagen. While East Germany's requests for membership were denied, West Germany became a member of the WHO in 1951.[324]

6.3.1 The WHO's Construction of Health as an Economic Product

With the definition declaring that health was more than the absence of disease, the WHO cultivated a discourse of health and prevention in healthcare that focused not only on pathological influences but broadened the issue of health to the whole area of life. According to Lengwiler and Madarász, prevention in the early 20th century was described as a rational, more economic, and more efficient instrument to regulate modern complex societies than repression and sanctions.[325] While in the first half of the century, preventive interventions were focused especially on general conditions of life, after WWII, this focus changed. Individuals were increasingly urged to become responsible for their own health,

---

322 Cueto, Brown, and Fee, *The World Health Organization*.
323 Cueto, Brown, and Fee, *The World Health Organization*, 72.
324 Cueto, Brown, and Fee, *The World Health Organization*.
325 Lengwiler and Madarász, "Präventionsgeschichte," 11–28.

which must be understood as part of the discursive trend of the neoliberal rationale towards individualization and consumerization.[326]

The WHO had an important role in establishing the economy as the preferred mode through which to direct decisions on healthcare by implementing a specific understanding of health. As I will demonstrate, the WHO was a driver of this new perception of health, changing the understanding of how to deal with this perception of health at the level of nation-states and encouraging the logic of the market into national healthcare systems. WHO strategies included supporting and assisting health campaigns, promoting research on people's attitudes to their health status, calling for health education in the curricula of health professionals, and emphasizing the responsibility of the individual. And it demanded a "more effective use of both preventive and curative health services."[327]

Of special interest with regard to the WHO strategies is a report on an organizational study entitled *Methods of Promoting the Development of Basic Health Services*.[328] This study discussed new strategies for implementing health services, effectively transmitting the WHO's agenda into national healthcare systems. The working group of this study proposed to equip these strategies with accounting technologies like mechanisms of control and management to be able to evaluate output after implementation. Moreover, implementing accounting measures should also foster the reorganization of healthcare systems and bring "proper management" of healthcare services.[329] Not only was constituting patients and communities as engaged and responsible partners in maintaining their health a concern of the WHO, but also the integration of efficient management and administration into health services.[330] "[H]ealth services are progressing fast in a direction which would result in the introduction of a health management system which could give confidence that health decisions are being carried out in

---

326 Virginia Berridge, "Medizin, Public Health und die Medien in Großbritannien von 1950 bis 1980 [Medicine, Public Health and the Media in Britain from the 1950s to the 1970s]," in *Das präventive Selbst. Eine Kulturgeschichte moderner Gesundheitspolitik*, ed. Martin Lengwiler and Jeannette Madarász (Bielefeld: transcript Verlag, 2010), 205–28; Lengwiler and Madarász, "Präventionsgeschichte," 11–28; Carsten Timmermann, "Risikofaktoren: Der scheinbar unaufhaltsame Erfolg eines Ansatzes aus der amerikanischen Epidemiologie in der deutschen Nachkriegsmedizin [Risk Factors: The Apparently Unstoppable Success of an Approach from American Epidemiology in the German Postwar Period]," in *Das präventive Selbst. Eine Kulturgeschichte moderner Gesundheitspolitik*, ed. Martin Lengwiler and Jeannette Madarász (Bielefeld: transcript Verlag, 2010), 251–77.
327 WHO, "The Second Ten Years of the World Health Organization 1958–1967," (Geneva: World Health Organization, 1968), 54.
328 WHO, "Organizational Study on "Methods of Promoting Development of Basic Health Services". Report of the Working Group, 16 January 1973," (World Health Organization, 1973).
329 WHO, "Organizational Study," 8.
330 WHO, "Organizational Study."

the most efficient way possible."[331] With the need to evaluate the results of its programs, the WHO established the notion of "output" as the desired result of a program. For example, in a study to promote basic health services, output is defined as "the final return to the individual in health status and in service."[332] This has to be understood as a quantitative and economic rationale related to health and healthcare interventions. The WHO was thus a driving force for economizing healthcare systems by connecting health and healthcare interventions to the logic of the market.

Throughout the late 1960s and the 1970s, a new trend in health programming was adopted by the WHO in order to restructure and improve their health programs. This new method contained a series of collecting data, analysing situations, preparing program proposals and deciding between them, as well as integrating them into the healthcare structure. It was very much structured as a problem-analysis/problem-solving process, required multidisciplinary teams, called for active engagement of the participants and consumers and for evaluating the efficacy of the particular health program.[333]

The WHO recommended using a system analysis approach for the management processes of national health administrations in order to use limited resources in the best possible way. The following characteristics are ascribed to such a system analysis:
- a planning approach that relates input to output;
- an emphasis on quantification;
- rigour in analytical methods;
- orientation towards health problems rather than towards categories of service;
- communication with key government decision-making centres in which comparable methods are used;
- early attention to planning and priority setting;
- improved interdisciplinary collaboration; and
- use of a wide range of analytical models and methods of considerable power.[334]

On the European level, the work of the WHO, as well as its strategies, are recorded in session and annual reports. In the annual report of 1968–1969, and at the same time when concerns of too-costly healthcare emerged (see chapter 2.2), the regional director of Europe stated that the healthcare system was "moving from a 'handicraft' to an 'industrial' approach [...] and that the need for long-term

---

331 WHO, "Organizational Study," 8.
332 WHO, "Organizational Study," 4.
333 WHO, "The Third Ten Years of the World Health Organization 1968–1977," (Geneva: World Health Organization, 2008).
334 WHO, "The Third Ten Years," 43.

planning and better managerial leadership" was becoming obvious.[335] The narrative of a need for healthcare planning was established. "Much attention was now being devoted in Europe to management techniques and questions of communication, and there was an obvious need for planning and evaluation."[336] In consequence, the introduction of a new unit in the Regional Office, which would assist European countries in planning their national health programs, was discussed and confirmed in 1974.[337]

Using the argument that increasing healthcare costs were causing economic tensions, the WHO introduced procedures to manage health on different levels of its work: on the meta-level of the WHO itself, on the medium level with national healthcare systems, and at the micro-level in other smaller healthcare settings. The WHO in the mid-1970s proposed to integrate planning and strategies of management into the curricula of all healthcare personnel.[338] The next section will demonstrate that procedures to reform the structure and organization of health programs of the WHO were very similar to the way the WHO recommended nursing should be restructured. The same problem-solving cycles and evaluation processes can be found both in the new structure of the WHO programs themselves as well as in the reorganization of nursing based on the nursing process.

6.3.2 The Nursing Process as an Instrument to Transform Healthcare Services

The WHO examined nursing for its activity in health programming and described "health" as an important part of nurses' work. From the 1960s on the WHO promoted nursing research "as an essential part of the planning of health services."[339] For example, the WHO called for research in nursing to figure out "the most effective staffing patterns."[340] Auxiliary workers in nursing were predicted to become a more important working group among healthcare workers when national healthcare programs developed further. A European study was conducted in 1961 that discovered that nursing aides in most European countries lacked a systematic education and were poorly integrated into healthcare sys-

---

335 WHO, "Report of the Nineteenth Session of the Regional Committee for Europe 9–13 September," (Budapest: World Health Organization, 1969), 7.
336 WHO, "Regional Committee for Europe. Report on the Twenty-Fourth Session," in *EB55/26* (1974), 8.
337 WHO, "Regional Committee for Europe."
338 WHO, "The Third Ten Years."
339 WHO, "The Second Ten Years," 69.
340 WHO, "The Second Ten Years," 69.

tems.³⁴¹ In the 1970s, the WHO focused on nursing more concretely. They believed that nursing should take an active part in healthcare planning, recommending

> that experiments on nursing care patterns be planned for different population groups, such as the elderly or foreign workers, and be designed in such a way that their adequacy, suitability, efficiency and effectiveness could be evaluated; that health planning as a whole should provide for research and experimentation in new ways of organizing nursing services and nursing education.³⁴²

In the objectives of the planned European programs starting in 1976 and 1977, the WHO stated that it wanted to help health administrations by recommending and supporting both the introduction and strengthening of managerial techniques such as information and evaluation procedures.³⁴³ These were the first steps in developing the medium-term program for nursing and midwifery that ran from 1976 to 1983, which helped to implement the nursing process into nursing in European states. This program was structured to focus on supporting already established activities in the European states concerning the nursing process, nursing education, and the management of nursing services.³⁴⁴

The medium-term program of the WHO was developed during a time when different European countries were raising concerns about rising healthcare costs.³⁴⁵ However, the main official objective was to improve nursing care and the position and status of nursing within healthcare settings by drawing on the argument of the poor status of nursing in Europe. The poor status of nursing, so the argument went, was caused by a dominant focus on treatment with its medically oriented foundation and the vast neglect of care in the healthcare settings. Instead, the WHO program put the emphasis on health education and health information as well as on a stronger focus on parish nursing and on all individuals – whether sick or not.³⁴⁶

The aims of the medium-term program corresponded with the claims that the WHO raised about the reconstruction of healthcare systems: Nurses should look

---

341 WHO, "The Second Ten Years."
342 WHO, "The Third Ten Years," 74.
343 WHO, "Proposed Programme Budget for 1976 and 1977," in *No. 220* (1974); WHO, "Organizational Study."; WHO, "Regional Committee for Europe."
344 Rosemarie Weinrich, "Kurz berichtet aus der Hauptgeschäftsstelle [Brief Report of the Essentials of the Head Office]," *Krankenpflege* 30, no. 2 (1976), 49–50.
345 Weber, "Der Krankenpflegeprozeß in der Schweiz," 30–32.
346 Rosemarie Weinrich, "Wichtiges in Kürze aus der Hauptgeschäftsstelle [Brief Overview of the Essentials of the Head Office]," *Krankenpflege* 30, no. 6 (1976), 183–84; Dorothy C. Hall, "Probleme der Krankenpflegeausbildung in Europa [Problems of Nursing Education in Europa]," *Krankenpflege* 29, no. 10 (1976), 292, 301–03.

for "other patterns in management and organization of nursing service."[347] Nurses should move away from the illness-oriented perspective that was inherent in medicine. Rather, they should shift their focus to promoting health, health education, and to instructing people to live their lives in a healthy way, touching on the concept of lifestyle.[348] The term "lifestyle" was rare in Germany at this time but became more well-known from the end of the 1970s onward. As nursing scholars Thomas Foth and Dave Holmes demonstrate, lifestyle was a key concept of the 1974 Canadian Lalonde report, *A New Perspective on the Health of Canadians*, published under the direction of the Minister of National Health and Welfare, Marc Lalonde. Its central concept of lifestyle spread to European countries. This report outlined a new perspective on health in Canada in order to "stimulate interest and discussion on future health programs for Canada."[349] The report proposed a shift in programming from a structural perspective on healthcare systems to an individual perspective on (potential) patients. The progress in medical knowledge and technology that had been understood as the foundation for the improvement in health of the Canadian people was less important than the change in awareness of health risks or in risky behaviour (e.g. smoking). The notion of lifestyle was thus established as a key concept for managing the health of the Canadian population.[350]

According to Foth and Holmes, the Lalonde report with its focus on the concept of lifestyle functioned to restructure the Canadian healthcare system in a neoliberal way.[351] The lifestyle concept contains within it the perspective that individuals are self-determined and rational subjects. By changing the rationales upon which subjects base their decision-making, their behaviour can be changed. Introducing the concept of lifestyle into policies and programs of healthcare, from the perspective of governmentality, is a neoliberal measure to influence the behaviour of subjects in regard to their health, but it acts less by disciplinary power and more by (self-)regulation. Using the concept of lifestyle as the foundation for new strategies in the healthcare system is an example of the

---

347 "Pflegekräfte und Ärzte müssen bereit sein, nach anderen Mustern im Management und der Organisation von Pflege zu experimentieren" (Hall, "Probleme der Krankenpflegeausbildung," 303; my translation).
348 Hall, "Probleme der Krankenpflegeausbildung," 292, 301–03; Annemarie Ludwig, "3. Delegiertenversammlung des DBfK am 24./25. Sept. 1976 im Bildungszentrum Essen [Third Meeting of DBfK Delegates, September 24th/25th, 1976 in the Training Center Essen]," *Krankenpflege* 30, no. 11 (1976), 327–29.
349 Marc Lalonde, "A New Perspective on the Health of Canadians. A Working Document," (Minister of Supply and Services Canada, 1974/1981), http://www.phac-aspc.gc.ca/ph-sp/pdf/perspect-eng.pdf.
350 Lalonde, "A New Perspective on the Health of Canadians".
351 Thomas Foth and Dave Holmes, "Governing through Lifestyle: Lalonde and the Biopolitical Managemnt of Public Health in Canada," *Nursing Philosophy* 19, no. 4 (2018), 1–11.

neoliberal mode of governing by empowering subjects to make their own decisions and to be responsible for those decisions.[352]

Decreasing the dominant power of medicine and shrinking the powerful enclosures of that profession is closely connected with a "democratization" in the healthcare system.[353] It is here that the nursing vocation seems to have become important to accountants and healthcare managers. To support the empowerment of patients the dominance of the medical profession had to be broken. The Lalonde report, for example, called for shifting certain tasks formerly in the medical scope of practice to less expensive healthcare vocations. The attempts to decrease the medical monopoly in healthcare and increase the self-determination of patients coincided with stronger calls for professionalization in nursing in several Western countries and with the establishment of the medium-term program of the WHO.

With the nursing process, the WHO wanted to introduce administrative mechanisms to make substantial organizational changes in nursing. The content of nursing (what nursing is and does), as well as how nursing is organized, was called into question. The nursing process was an instrument to make nursing service more manageable and calculable by establishing a new language in which it could be expressed. In order to demonstrate the relevance of nursing to society, nurses would need to prove the effectiveness of their work through planning and transparency. The nursing process, seen as the appropriate tool to evaluate the effectiveness of nursing work, was understood as a new process based on rationality and a problem-oriented approach with which nursing care could be estimated, decided on, documented, and planned in its entirety.[354]

Dorothy C. Hall was responsible for the widespread implementation of the WHO's program, promoting it in the 1970s all over Europe. A Canadian nurse who specialized in primary nursing, at that time a new concept of providing holistic nursing care, Hall became a regional officer of the European Bureau of the WHO. In 1976 and 1977, she gave talks and published articles promoting the program as a means to restructure the nursing vocation in Europe. Although she did not focus on the German situation specifically, her talks and publications were translated and published in *Krankenpflege*, the journal of the DBfK, the largest German nurses' association. German nursing scholars took up the discussion and developed it further. Hall argued that nursing had lost the essence that Florence Nightingale had proposed,[355] and that the WHO program's focus was to reactivate what nursing "actually" is. The following presents a detailed

---

352 Foth and Holmes, "Governing through Lifestyle," 1–11.
353 Foth and Holmes, "Governing through Lifestyle," 1–11.
354 Hall, "Probleme der Krankenpflegeausbildung," 292, 301–03.
355 Florence Nightingale, *Notes on Nursing: What It Is and What It Is Not* (New York: Dover Publications, Inc., 1969/1860).

presentation of Hall's arguments because they were constantly repeated by German nursing scholars who used them to legitimize the introduction of the nursing process as well as their calls to restructure nursing care and transform the nursing vocation.

In May 1976, Hall spoke in front of a consortium of nursing teachers in Berlin. Arguing that "the development of the nursing service is 40 to 50 years behind the medical service"[356] she called for an improvement of the nursing situation. (In this talk, she first drew on the situation in Germany but gradually turned her perspective to nursing in general.) The low status of nursing that was too closely tied to a medical perspective and the neglect of its own scope of practice Hall related to an identity crisis. She claimed that nursing would need to become independent of medicine to become an autonomous vocation that was complementary to medical treatment. Hence, as a solution, Hall called for a "Reorientation to our primary task"[357] and reminded her audience that nursing had already been defined more than a century ago with a scope of practice that included health promotion, prevention of illness, and support of the sick and the dying. Against this backdrop, nursing should, according to Hall, establish itself as one of the subsystems of the healthcare system with its own and clearly defined scope of practice. Within this scope of practice, the nursing vocation should focus on nursing *care*, on the promotion of health for individuals and communities, and on the responsibility of the individual for his or her own health. Here, Hall based her argument on the 1948 definition of health, which defined health as not just the absence of illness but as physical, social, and mental wellbeing. Hence, Hall wanted nursing to be directed not just to the sick but also focused on health promotion. Nursing should reorient itself towards the "actual duty of nurses," that is, caring for patients, with a strong emphasis on prevention.

> If the future health services of a society aim to foster and maintain health instead of treating individuals and families after they became sick or wounded; if the role of the individual for his or her own care and healing becomes more and more acknowledged; if the rights and responsibilities of individuals in regard to their health, their families, and the society in which they live become acknowledged and respected; if we are ready not only to control and use our knowledge and technology in an efficient way but also apply it in an ethically correct way; then we need radical changes in our thinking, our education, and our services.[358]

---

356 "Als Folge davon liegt die Entwicklung der pflegerischen Dienste nach vorsichtiger Schätzung 40–50 Jahre hinter der des medizinischen Dienstes zurück" (Hall, "Probleme der Krankenpflegeausbildung," 292, my translation).
357 "Neubesinnung auf unsere primären Aufgaben" (Hall, "Probleme der Krankenpflegeausbildung," 302, my translation).
358 "Wenn die Gesundheitsdienste der Gesellschaft der Zukunft mehr darauf gerichtet sind, Gesundheit zu fördern und zu erhalten, statt einzelne und Familien zu behandeln, nachdem sie krank oder verletzt worden sind, wenn mehr und mehr die Bedeutung der Rolle des

In this quote, Hall proposed a domain of nursing that went well beyond the care of the individual sick person to encompass responsibility for the health of the whole population. Furthermore, she made it a moral obligation for individuals to stay healthy not just for themselves but also for the society that they lived in. This rationale relates to the WHO objectives that called for individuals to cooperate in living a healthy life in order to reach the political aim of stable and peaceful nations. Here as well can be found in the argument of a nurse the critique of the Ordoliberals' and other neoliberals that the current healthcare system made individuals dependent. Hall was proposing a nursing vocation and service that encouraged individuals to become self-reliant and responsible consumers of healthcare services, supporting the neoliberal calls for individuals to be responsible for their health.

Hall's concept of nursing, according to her, existed already in Florence Nightingale's *Notes on Nursing* and only had to be reactivated. She especially emphasized the importance of the caring aspect and of basic nursing care, which she described as the area in which "actual" care and health promotion should start. To re-orient nursing, that is, to be able to find its way back to its already defined body of competencies, Hall promoted the nursing process as an appropriate tool. She described it as one of the newest achievements of nursing, and that it was an instrument for providing holistic care by which healthy and sick people and their families could be assessed, treated, and cared for. With a larger emphasis on health education and prevention as part of this holistic care, patients' whole environments and lifestyles would become relevant to nursing. Furthermore, Hall embedded the nursing process in the call to re-orientate nursing to its primary task, defining it as a foundation for evaluating the effectiveness of nursing actions. The ability to show effectiveness was, according to Hall, a foundation of autonomy in nursing.[359]

Hence, she claimed to integrate the components of the nursing process as well as social nursing care [*Sozialpflege*] and parish nursing into current nursing curricula. In order to strengthen her claim that the nursing process was important for the nursing vocation, Hall connected the argument for holistic, health-oriented, and effective care with the problematization of increasing

---

einzelnen für die eigene Pflege und Heilung gesehen wird und seine Rechte und die Verantwortung, die er im Zusammenhang für seine Gesundheit und die seiner Familie und die der Gesellschaft, in der er lebt, geachtet werden, wenn wir bereit sind, unser Wissen und die Technologie nicht nur in einer wirksamen Weise zu kontrollieren und zu benutzen, sondern auch in ethischer Hinsicht richtig anzuwenden, dann müssen sich radikale Änderungen in unserem Denken, unserer Erziehung und unseren Diensten vollziehen" (Hall, "Probleme der Krankenpflegeausbildung," 301, my translation).

359 Hall, "Probleme der Krankenpflegeausbildung," 292, 301–03; Ludwig, "3. Delegiertenversammlung des DBfK am 24./25. Sept. 1976," 327–29.

hospital costs: "We are aware that hospital costs have reached the highest border in every society. Curiously, we [are] not able to provide services which can estimate the health status of individuals or which help people to maintain an acceptable health status for themselves and for their families."[360] This is, again, an economic argument, which was already inherent in the concept of prevention and which was further emphasized by the goal or output of the WHO's health programs of having the individual back in health and in service. Furthermore, it is an argument to move nursing care and patients out of hospitals and into communities, thus reducing the number of hospital admissions, and hence, costs. Therefore, it is in line with calls from economists and Ordoliberals to reduce costs in the healthcare system.[361]

Hall claimed additionally that nursing service could be reorganized by building on differently qualified nurses and integrating a management perspective into nursing. Arguing from an international perspective, Hall explained that some countries had already rebuilt their nursing service in order to make their healthcare system function more efficiently. Depending on the healthcare system of the country, Hall stated, the number of different types of nurses varied between two and four.[362] Hall thus regarded having only one type of nurse in a nursing system as outdated, arguing that restructuring was needed to provide good and functional healthcare in a modern state.

A few months after Hall's talk, guidelines were published in the journal *Krankenpflege* that nurses were to follow to provide modern healthcare.[363] This article was a shorter and translated version of Hall's *A Position Paper on Nursing* that was first published in 1975 in the WHO/Europe (document Euro/Nurs 75.1) and in 1977 in the *Journal of Advanced Nursing*[364] where she presented her

---

360 "Es ist uns wohl bewußt, daß die Krankenhauskosten in fast jeder Gesellschaft die obere Grenze erreicht haben, doch es ist uns sonderbarerweise nicht gelungen, Dienste zur Verfügung zu stellen, welchen einen Gesundheitszustand abschätzen und den Menschen helfen, sich selbst und ihre Familien auf einem annehmbaren Stand von Gesundheit zu erhalten" (Hall, "Probleme Der Krankenpflegeausbildung," 303; my translation).

361 See for example Siegfried Eichhorn, "Zielkonflikte zwischen Leistungsfähigkeit, Wirtschaftlichkeit und Finanzierung der Krankenversorgung [Conflicts of Objectives between Performance, Efficiency and Financing of Healthcare]," *Das Krankenhaus* 66, no. 5 (1974), 186–96; Walter Hamm, "Programmierte Unfreiheit und Verschwendung: Zur überfälligen Reform der gesetzlichen Krankenversicherung [Programmed Bondage and Dissipation: On the Overdue Reform of the Statutory Health Insurance]," *ORDO Jahrbuch für die Ordnung von Wirtschaft und Gesellschaft* 35 (1984), 42; Walter Hamm, "Verschwendung in Krankenhäusern durch falsche Anreize [Wastefulness in Hospitals Because of False Incentives]," *ORDO Jahrbuch für die Ordnung von Wirtschaft und Gesellschaft* 33 (1982), 363–68.

362 Hall, "Probleme der Krankenpflegeausbildung," 292, 301–03.

363 Dorothy C. Hall, "Überlegungen zum Krankenpflegeberuf [Considerations on the Nursing Vocation]," *Krankenpflege* 31, no. 2 (1977), 40–42.

364 Dorothy C. Hall, "A Position Paper on Nursing," *Journal of Advanced Nursing* 2, no. 3 (1977), 327–28.

thoughts on the nursing profession and analyzed what she believed nursing should look like. She augmented her claims already stated in her 1976 talk by emphasizing the need to introduce research and science into nursing and to change nursing legislation.

Hall defined nursing in this article "as a profession in its own right and a discrete health discipline, [which] is responsible for planning, organizing, implementing and evaluating nursing services as a distinct segment of healthcare, and for educating practitioners to provide these services."[365] Emphasizing that nurses have to play a part in the health education of the population, Hall provided a concrete understanding of professionalization in nursing: Professional nurses grounded their actions in transparency and effectiveness and needed to be accountable for those. This is a very different understanding of and approach to the concept of profession than what the sociology of professions described. This redefinition of what characteristics and role professions should have I will discuss in chapter 8 in more detail.

Basing nursing on scientific research and a rational plan makes the assumption that nurses would gain more influence and respect, making their efforts at health education more successful. This fits with the political aim of the WHO and is an important indication of the role and influence nurses should have in regard to the citizens of a state. Professional nurses can demonstrate that they are relevant and important agents in the national healthcare system by helping to realize the political program of making citizens responsible for their own health. In order to achieve this status, that is, of being perceived as knowledgeable and trustworthy experts, nurses would need to make the effect of their work transparent to those citizens.

In conclusion, the medium-term program for Nurses and Midwifery, which was initiated and operated by the WHO from 1976 to 1983, aimed not only at introducing the nursing process and nursing research into nursing vocations in European states. It was also a program, following the WHO's agenda, to establish management strategies in healthcare systems and to make them more effective and efficient. Moreover, by fostering transparency and accountability in nursing service, the invisible work and tacit knowledge within nursing would be included in a cybernetic process and translated into a calculable language. Arguing from a governmentality perspective, the enclosures of the nursing vocations were opened to a managerial logic, which needs to be understood as a strategy to reorganize healthcare in a neoliberal manner. To encourage acceptance of this program, nurses were promised that nursing would become professionalized.

---

365 In the German translation "profession" is not translated as '*Profession*' but as '*Beruf*' which means occupation or vocation (Hall, "A Position Paper," 327; Hall, "Überlegungen zum Krankenpflegeberuf," 40).

However, contained within this promise was a particular understanding of autonomy and professionalism in nursing, for it needed to be accountable and to prove the effectiveness of its work in order to demonstrate its value in the national healthcare service.

6.4 The German Debate over the Medium-Term Program of the WHO

The WHO's medium-term program reached Germany at a time of several changes in healthcare and nursing. From the second half of the 1960s on, not only did German nursing suffer from the loss of its former religious foundation, but it also increasingly faced the introduction of rationalization strategies.[366] From 1955 to 1966 the German Hospital Institute carried out several job analyses in nursing. In 1967, Eichhorn published the results in a book about hospital business operations. In order to sort the different nursing activities, he used a scheme that had already been developed in the British study, *The Work of Nurses On Hospital Wards*, published by the Nuffield Provincial Hospitals Trust.[367] The Nuffield study was carried out by economists and contained observations and analyses of nurses' work in a stationary hospital setting. According to Peter Miller, such observational studies aim to introduce scientific management into organizations. The field of work is analyzed with seemingly objective observations based on a timely assessment of actions. "The actions of the worker, each and every movement of the worker's body, would be studied so as to optimize the efficiency of each individual action. No matter how minute or apparently trivial the activity, scientific management promised a government of the factory that would be based on the objectivity of expertise."[368] As a result, observers and analysts can claim to be experts in making visible the productive activities and "waste" or non-productive activities of a working field. Hence, economists who are foreign to nursing could create powerful scientific knowledge to constitute an image of nurses' work upon which economic interventions could be implemented, for example, to eliminate "waste." In this way, those studies fostered the economization of nursing service.

---

366 Susanne Kreutzer, "Conflicting Christian and Scientific Nursing Concepts in West Germany, 1945–1970," in *Routledge Handbook on the Global History of Nursing*, ed. Patricia D'Antonio, Julie A. Fairman, and Jean C. Whelan (London, New York: Routledge, 2016), 151–64.
367 Nuffield Provincial Hospitals Trust, *The Work of Nurses in Hospital Wards: Report of a Job-Analysis [Job-Analysis Team Director, H.A. Goddard]* (London: Nuffield Provincial Hospitals Trust, 1953).
368 Peter Miller, "The Margins of Accounting," *The Sociological Review* 46, no. 1_suppl (1998), 174–93: 186.

The Nuffield study was translated and published by the German Hospital Institute in 1954[369] but it seems to have been ignored in the literature afterwards. The study sorted observed and measured nursing activities into the categories of "basic nursing" (e. g., bed making, washing and bathing patients, preparation, distribution and collection of food and drink); "making patients comfortable," (personal attention and conversation with patients, etc.); "technical nursing" (dressings, technical procedures, urine tests, pre- and post-operative care, etc.); and "domestic work" (e. g., housekeeping, cleaning, laundry, etc.).[370]

Although not directly citing the Nuffield study, Eichhorn used the very same categories and part of the literal translation of nursing activities for his overview of activities in nursing.[371] However, there seems to be a difference between basic nursing care elsewhere and its German counterpart, *Grundpflege*. In Germany, the differences between *Grundpflege* [basic nursing care] and *Behandlungspflege* [technical nursing care] had long been integrated into social legislation in regard to how they were paid for. Since *Grundpflege* was declared as less costly than *Behandlungspflege* it had already been considered a lesser form of nursing and thus had been devalued. Even into the present, the different terms are still used in nursing in legislation and by insurance companies.[372]

This increasing dissection of nursing based on the implementation of rationalization strategies and the loss of a religious-based vocational identity from the 1960s on paved the way to a transformation of German nursing into a medical assistance vocation with a very functional differentiated field of tasks. Nurses themselves expressed the following problems: loss of autonomy and identity; the feeling of low societal status of the nursing vocation; increasing nursing shortages; and a weak information flow in the newly established three-shift-system.[373]

---

369 Margarete Steinbrück, *Schwesternarbeit auf der Station: Bericht über eine englische Arbeitsstudie [Nurses' Work on the Ward: Report About an English Working Study]*, ed. Bd. 1. Schriften des Deutschen Krankenhausinstituts e.V. (Karlsruhe/Baden: Braun, 1954).
370 The Nuffield Provincial Hospital Trust, *The Work of Nurses in Hopsital Wards: Report of a Job Analysis* (London: Nuffield Lodge, 1953), 20–28.
371 Nuffield Provincial Hospitals Trust, *The Work of Nurses in Hospital Wards*; Siegfried Eichhorn, *Krankenhausbetriebslehre: Theorie und Praxis des Krankenhausbetriebes Band 1 [Business Operation of Hospitals: Theory and Practice of the Hospital Administration. First Volume]*, 3rd ed., Schriften des Deutschen Krankenhausinstituts E. V. Düsseldorf Band 11 (Köln: Verlag W. Kohlhammer, 1975).
372 Heiner Friesacher, "Wider die Abwertung der eigentlichen Pflege [Against the Devaluation of Actual Care]," *intensiv* 23, no. 4 (2015), 200–14.
373 Susanne Kreutzer, ""Before, We Were Always There – Now, Everything Is Separate": On Nursing Reforms in Western Germany," *Nursing History Review* 16 (2008), 180–200; Susanne Kreutzer, "Krankenbeobachtung. Zur Entwertung einer pflegerischen Schlüsselkompetenz in der Bundesrepublik und Schweden nach 1945 [Patient Observation: On the Devaluation of a Key Competence in Nursing in the Federal Republic of Germany and Sweden after 1945]," in *Gesundheit/Krankheit. Kulturelle Differenzierungsprozesse um Körper, Geschlecht und Macht in Skandinavien*, ed. Lill-Ann Körber and Stefanie von Schnurbein,

The WHO medium-term program promised a solution to the difficulties in German nursing with its aim to improve nursing care and the status of nursing in society.

Strategies to Advertise the Medium-Term Program of the WHO in the German Context

Although articles of the nursing process can be found before the medium-term program of the WHO, this program was an important driver for the reception, publicity, and official implementation of the nursing process in Germany. The program was adapted and further developed for the German context by the German nursing association DBfK in the following years using two different strategies: The first strategy was to promote and support educational events and activities connected to the WHO program. For example, in 1978 the association published a report about a big event as part of the "day of nursing" that provided workshops and presentations related to nursing and politics, healthcare [*Gesundheitspflege*], health education, and public health counselling [*Gesundheitsberatung*]. One of the activities was devoted to "the nursing process as a part of the medium-term WHO program regarding nursing in Europe."[374] Additionally, courses for continuing education dedicated to the nursing process were advertised in the association's publication.[375] These courses were to help integrate the nursing process into the daily work and perception of nurses. The aims of these centralized and decentralized educational courses were to raise awareness among nurses for its necessity in planned and organized nursing care and to make the benefits of it understandable and transferable to their own work. Only when people understood the reasons for this change in practice would behaviour be changed.[376] For example, in one report of such a course, the use of the nursing

---

Berliner Beiträge Zur Skandinavistik, Bd. 16 (Berlin: Nordeuropa-Institut, 2010), 167–88; Susanne Kreutzer, "Sorge für Leib und Seele – Arbeits- und Lebensalltag evangelischer Krankenpflege, 1950er bis 1970er Jahre [Caring for Body and Soul: Daily Work and Life in Protestant Nursing, 1950s to 1970s]," in *Entwicklungen in der Krankenpflege und in anderen Gesundheitsberufen nach 1945. Ein Lehr- und Studienbuch*, ed. Sylvelyn Hähner-Rombach and Pierre Pfütsch (Frankfurt am Main: Mabuse-Verlag, 2018), 91–119.

374 "Der Pflegeprozeß als Teil des mittelfristigen Programms der WHO für die Krankenpflege in Europa" (DBfK, "Großveranstaltung zum Tag der Krankenpflege [Major Event at the Day of Nursing]," *Krankenpflege* 32, no. 3 (1978), 99; my translation).

375 DBfK, "Bayern Fortbildung – Systematische Planung der Pflege [Further Education in Bavaria: Systematic Planning of Nursing Care]," *Krankenpflege* 34, no. 3 (1980), 92; DBfK, "Fortbildungstage [Training Days]," *Krankenpflege* 35, no. 3 (1981), 119.

376 Weinrich, "Ausblick auf die Arbeit des DBfK," 16–18.

process became connected to vocational self-fulfillment [*berufliche Selbstverwirklichung*].³⁷⁷

Prominent nursing scholars, like Monika Krohwinkel and Renate Reimann, emphasized in their articles how the nursing process could be used to improve nursing care if implemented in nursing. Renate Reimann, who was the director of the educational centre of the DBfK in Essen, strongly supported science in nursing and focused on the improvement of nursing care at the bedside. Monika Krohwinkel, an academic scholar who studied nursing science in the UK, strongly promoted research in nursing and was active in European and German nursing research associations. She developed and established the German nursing theory of the activities and existential experiences of life (AEDL). Krohwinkel also published the first large German study on the nursing process using the example of patients who had suffered a stroke.³⁷⁸ This study was based on a multinational study initiated by the WHO and was meant to foster nursing research as well as the "right" utilization of the nursing process in nursing. According to Krohwinkel, her study demonstrated that using the nursing process in the care of patients with strokes helped promote professionalization in nursing, the satisfaction of nurses in regard to their work, and the rehabilitation process of patients. Krohwinkel also concluded that not providing this kind of nursing process-based and rehabilitative nursing care might lead to "costly consequences."³⁷⁹

The second strategy was to report on the progress of the WHO's program. Even before Hall's article was published, reports can be found in DBfK's journal on the program and its aims to redirect nursing care to a focus on health; to strengthen nurses' position in healthcare systems; to achieve autonomy in nursing; and to advise European countries in the planning and executing of nursing education and in developing further education.³⁸⁰ Throughout the years, several reports about the progress of the WHO program in Germany were

---

377 Irmgard Simon, "Ein bayrischer Gruß an alle Fortbildungs-Muffel [A Bavarian Salute to All Continuing Education Grumps]," *Krankenpflege* 33, no. 1 (1979), 15–16.
378 Monika Krohwinkel, *Der Pflegeprozess am Beispiel von Apoplexiekranken: Eine Studie zur Erfassung und Entwicklung ganzheitlich-rehabilitierender Prozeßpflege [The Nursing Process Using the Example of Patients with Strokes: A Study to Capture and Develop Holistic-Rehabilitative Nursing Care in a Process]*, ed. Bundesministerium für Gesundheit, vol. 16, Schriftenreihe des Bundesministeriums für Gesundheit (Baden-Baden: Nomos Verlagsgesellschaft mbH & Co. KG, 1993).
379 "Wenn solche Pflege nicht entwickelt wird, sind kostenträchtige Konsequenzen zu befürchten" (Krohwinkel, *Der Pflegeprozess am Beispiel von Apoplexiekranken*, 276; my translation).
380 Weinrich, "Wichtiges in Kürze," 183–84; Weinrich, "Kurz berichtet aus der Hauptgeschäftsstelle," 49–50.

published.[381] In the first year of the program, Rosemarie Weinrich repeated that the main focus of the WHO program was to bring nursing back to the bedside as well as to redirect it to the care of healthy people. Weinrich was the director of the DBfK from 1973 to 1988 and had nursing experience in Germany as well as in South Africa. She was also a member and vice-chairman of the European Nurses Group (ENG), now the European Federation of Nurses Associations (EFN), and represented this group at the Council of Nurses and the WHO. Furthermore, she was active in the national and international field of vocational politics in nursing and worked on developing a directive for the mutual recognition of nurses throughout the European Economic Community.[382] Her arguments can be understood from a management perspective with which she tried to fight for better working conditions for nurses.

Weinrich argued that these changing perspectives and a focus on health could achieve huge cost savings for the healthcare systems of different countries.[383] She also broached several times in the journal the issue of German participation in this program. However, although the nursing process and the WHO program became well-known in Germany through articles, seminars of further education, and even local research projects, participation in the program was not financially

---

381 Antje Grauhan and fellows, "Mittelfristiges WHO-Programm für Krankenpflege- und Hebammenwesen in Europa [Middle-Term Program of the WHO Concerning Nursing and Midwifery in Europe]," *Krankenpflege* 32, no. 2 (1978), 67–68; Reimann, "Pflegeplanung," 154–57; Lore Kroeker, "Aktuelles aus der Hauptgeschäftsstelle [News from the Headquaters of the DBfK]," *Krankenpflege* 33, no. 1 (1979), 13–14; Krohwinkel, "Krankenpflegeforschung in Europa II," 15; Dr. Mattheis, "Die Rolle der Krankenpflege im Gesundheitswesen [The Role of Nursing in Healthcare]," *Krankenpflege* 34, no. 3 (1980), 80; Rosemarie Weinrich, "Zusammengefasster Arbeitsbericht der Hauptgeschäftsstelle vom 26.4.1980–25.4.1981 [Summarized Working Report of the Head Office from April 26th, 1980 to April 25th, 1981]," *Krankenpflege* 35, no. 6 (1981), 251–54; Rosemarie Weinrich, "Arbeitsbericht der Hauptgeschäftsführerin für das Jahr Oktober 1977 – September 1978, vorgelegt auf der 5. Delegiertenversammlung des DBfK – gekürzt [Working Report of the General Manager for the Year October 1977 – September 1978. Presented on the Fifth Meeting of the DBfK Delegates – Shortened]," *Krankenpflege* 32, no. 11 (1978), 378–80; Lore Kroeker, "Klinische Pflegepraxis. Ermittlung, Entwicklung und Auswertung [Clinical Nursing Practice: Ascertaining, Development, and Evaluation]," *Krankenpflege* 37, no. 2 (1983), 53–54.
382 Birgit Trockel, Irmgard Knäuper and Margret Notthoff, *Who Is Who in der Pflege. Deutschland – Schweiz – Österreich [Who Is Who in Nursing. Germany: Switzerland – Austria]* (Bern, Göttingen, Toronto, Seattle: Verlag Hans Huber, 1999); Weinrich, "Zusammengefasster Arbeitsbericht," 251–54; Council Directive 77/452/EEC, "Council Directive of 27 June 1977 concerning the Mutual Recognition of Diplomas, Certificates and Other Evidence of the Formal Qualifications of Nurses Responsible for General Care, Including Measures to Facilitate the Effective Exercise of the Right of Establishment and Freedom to Provide Services (77/452/Eec)," ed. Council of the European Communities (1977).
383 Weinrich, "Kurz berichtet aus der Hauptgeschäftsstelle," 49–50.

supported by either the Federal Republic or the WHO itself.[384] However, the DBfK remained very committed to integrating the nursing process into German nursing. In its program of action for the 1980s, the nursing process was one of the main components. The DBfK wanted to raise awareness of the nursing process among nurses and integrate it into daily nursing work.[385] In discussions about a new nursing law, which was eventually passed in 1985, the DBfK urged the inclusion of the nursing process in the practical exams for nursing students.[386]

The international aspect of the WHO program was emphasized as well to the readers of the journal – it was an international nursing issue and not just a German program. Weinrich reported on a workshop in Copenhagen organized by the WHO that was attended by members of the Red Cross, the ICN, the International Confederation of Midwives (IDM), the International Catholic Committee of Nurses and Medico-Social Assistants (CICIAMS), the European and Nordic nursing associations, the German union ÖTV, and Public Services International (PSI). There was a European context to the aims of the WHO program: to improve nursing in Europe, to encourage participating states to increase collaboration and information flow among each other, and to encourage institutions in their respective countries to participate in this program.[387]

Resistance

Arguments for the benefits of the nursing process can be found throughout the 1960s, 70s, and 80s in the journal *Krankenpflege*, but those against it were not publicly discussed. Only in articles about the implementation of the nursing process were problems partly reported. Physicians and nurses themselves had some hesitation and doubt about time or organizational constraints. Nurses feared not having enough time to follow the nursing process and physicians feared that such changes in the system would result in them losing the nurse as a helpful assistant.[388]

---

384 Weinrich, "Zusammengefasster Arbeitsbericht," 251–54; Weinrich, "Kurz berichtet aus der Hauptgeschäftsstelle," 49–50.
385 Weinrich, "Ausblick auf die Arbeit des DBfK," 16–18.
386 Rosemarie Weinrich, "Stellungnahme zum Entwurf einer Ausbildungs- und Prüfungsverordnung für die Berufe der Krankenpflege – (KrPflAPrO) [Commentary on the Draft of the Training and Examination Regulations of the Nursing Occupations]," *Krankenpflege* 36, no. 10 (1982), 321–22.
387 Weinrich, "Wichtiges in Kürze," 183–84.
388 Leni Brunner and Sabine Goedeckemeyer, "Modellversuch einer Pflegeplanung auf zwei Stationen – Protokoll (2. Folge) [Pilot Project of a Nursing Care Plan on Two Wards: Protocol (2nd Part)]," *Krankenpflege* 34, no. 3 (1980), 87–90; Leni Brunner and Sabine Goedeckemeyer, "Modellversuch einer Pflegeplanung auf zwei Stationen – Protokoll (3. Folge und Schluß) [Pilot Project of a Nursing Care Plan on Two Wards: Protocol (3rd Part and End)],"

In 1978, a report on a seminar on ongoing education for nurses that focused on the nursing process stated that attendees were concerned that they were already experiencing a shortage of time and that using the nursing process would demand additional resources. Interestingly, the result of the discussion was not that nurses should fight for better working conditions in order to have time for the nursing process but instead they stated that the time available for daily nursing care would not be used optimally.[389]

In 1980, three articles reported on a project to introduce the nursing care plan into daily nursing care.[390] Leni Brunner and Sabine Goedeckemeyer, the two initiators and administrators of this project, described its organization and progress. Here, hints of resistance can be found: Not only did they have to repeatedly explain certain steps of the nursing process and to readjust some, they also discussed problems nurses had in following certain steps. First, they emphasized that assessments of patients in nursing case histories were rarely completed. Nurses appeared unable to observe patients and to ask questions in a goal-oriented way, and were weak in verbalizing nursing problems. Besides the shortage of time, the biggest problem that the authors described, another problem was in following the cybernetic structure of the nursing process. The participants wanted to express nursing interventions before they had articulated problems or goals. The step of setting nursing goals appeared to be especially difficult: The authors described a discussion between them and a nurse who found it more logical and practical to plan nursing interventions based on nursing problems and to set goals after having planned the interventions. "This shows us that the group is not familiar with the possibility of evaluating the nursing process with the nursing goals."[391] Here the authors found the need to repeat how the structure of the cybernetic cycle worked. In their evaluation protocol, the authors reported that the nurses still had problems with setting nursing goals and partly ignored or avoided them in their work.[392]

Finding this type of resistance in the journal is notable because the implementation of the nursing process and the concept of planning nursing care in this regulatory way was never discussed critically between the 1960s and 1980s. In

---

Krankenpflege 34, no. 4 (1980), 122–24; Thompson, "Der Krankenpflegeprozeß," 243–44; Simon, "Ein Bayrischer Gruß," 15–16.

389 Simon, "Ein Bayrischer Gruß," 15–16.
390 Leni Brunner and Sabine Goedeckemeyer, "Modellversuch einer Pflegeplanung auf zwei Stationen – Protokoll (1. Folge) [Pilot Project of a Nursing Care Plan on Two Wards: Protocol (1st Part)]," *Krankenpflege* 34, no. 2 (1980), 46–48; "Modellversuch einer Pflegeplanung II," 87–90; "Modellversuch einer Pflegeplanung III," 122–24.
391 "Das zeigt uns, daß der Pflegeprozeß im Hinblick auf seine Überprüfbarkeit anhand der Pflegeziele der Gruppe noch nicht vertraut ist" (Brunner and Goedeckemeyer, "Modellversuch einer Pflegeplanung II," 88; my translation).
392 Brunner and Goedeckemeyer, "Modellversuch einer Pflegeplanung III," 122–24.

none of the three journals I reviewed did I find an article in which the concept of the nursing process was presented negatively, nor have I found articles in which it was not advertised as something to improve nursing care. However, finding these issues during a project to implement the nursing process into nursing care shows that there was indeed some resistance and bewilderment from bedside nurses.

In the late 1970s and especially in the 1980s the discussions surrounding the implementation of the nursing process highlighted more strongly its relevance for German nursing. The arguments of support for the implementation of the nursing process can be differentiated into two main sections: Progress in nursing (later called professionalization) and the implementation of management strategies into nursing. Many nursing scholars like Rosemarie Weinrich, Monika Krohwinkel, Renate Reimann, Antje Grauhan, Lore Kroeker, Detlef Hohlin, and Christel Bienstein, who published their pleas for the nursing process, played an important role in the politics of the nursing vocation and in the education of nurses. Their articles, therefore, may have had a stronger impact on the readers of the nursing journal *Krankenpflege*, and their arguments are the focus of the next two chapters.

In chapter 7, I will analyze the nursing process and its impact from the perspective of critical accounting and governmentality. The nursing process needs to be understood as a technology to implement a new mode of governing in healthcare and to reconfigure people in healthcare in a neoliberal way. As an accounting tool, the nursing process helped to restructure not only the practices of nursing care in particular but also to constitute a new perception of what nursing practise should look like and, consequently, what the nursing vocation is. Hence, this part of the chapter focuses on the nursing vocation in its role and position in the healthcare system by emphasizing the transformation of nursing practice into calculable nursing actions, that is, the economization of the nursing vocation and of nursing care.

In chapter 8, I focus more on the internal perspective of the nursing vocation. Here, the question of professionalization in nursing is central. I will show how the economization of the nursing vocation redefined what a profession is into an understanding that promoted the neoliberal idea of professions. It will become obvious that this professionalization project in nursing had several contradictions, and these I will discuss based on the perspective of neoliberal governmentality, demonstrating that this process that nurses call professionalization should rather be understood as a de-professionalization.

These next two chapters represent the two opposite positions of the hybrid discourse that developed in German nursing in the second half of the 20th century. This discourse combined discourses from both accounting and nursing in a way that they interpenetrated and strengthened each other. Therefore, separating each of these two sides is – of course – artificial, but I did it this way in order to be able to analyze and discuss these parts in an understandable and structured way. However, several times in the next two chapters the interpenetration of the two sides will become obvious and has to be acknowledged at these specific points in order to understand how this hybrid discourse works.

Chapter 7:
The Benefit of the Nursing Process to the Economization of Healthcare

In this chapter, I will focus especially on the nursing process as an accounting tool to show how nursing became constructed as an important economic service in a market-based hospital organization. The issue of cost explosion in the healthcare system was used as the main argument to reason cost-saving strategies and the need to reorganize healthcare. The cybernetic structure of the nursing process enhanced this transformation. Discussions on the financial problems in the healthcare system can be found throughout the 1970s and 80s in the German journals. Keywords such as "cost explosion" and "cost containment" [*Kostendämpfung*] were used as a foundation to claim changes or to urge for modernization in the healthcare setting.[393] In 1978, Karl Jung, from the Federal Ministry of Work and Social Order, published an article in the nursing journal *Krankenpflege* in which he used the argument of cost explosion to introduce and justify cost containment strategies. He listed the costs of health insurance for the year 1950 (2.3 billion German Mark (DM)), 1970 (58.6 billion DM), 1977 (70.0 billion DM), and for 2000 (estimated 393.0 billion DM), demonstrating a dramatic increase.[394]

From the perspective of governmentality, these numbers have an important role in the neoliberal rationale. Based on the belief that accounting is a neutral and trustworthy form of knowledge that calculates aspects of reality, these numbers appear as a neutral representation of reality and function as economic evidence. They represent the sum of expenses in the respective past years. That means, truth is ascribed to them and they become constituted as hard facts. The

---

[393] These are the same arguments which were raised in the 1960s in the US healthcare system when the nursing process was being developed (Alistar M. Preston, "The Birth of Clinical Accounting: A Study of the Emergence and Transformations of Discourses on Costs and Practices of Accounting in U.S. Hospitals," *Accounting Organizations and Society* 17, no. 1 (1992), 63–100).

[394] Karl Jung, "Führt Kostendämpfung im Gesundheitswesen zu einem Dilemma in der Krankenpflege? [Does Cost Containment in the Healthcare System Lead to a Dilemma in Nursing?]," *Krankenpflege* 32, no. 2 (1978), 49–51: 49.

estimated cost for the year 2000 is also constructed as a hard fact, standing in line with the already calculated representatives of past reality. This, in turn, strengthened Jung's call for countermeasures. He demanded more effective economic behaviour and improved efficiency in healthcare. Although he acknowledged the claim that economic behaviour would likely lead to ignoring the humanism necessary in patient treatment, he delegitimized it in two ways: These claims were being used to secure the interests and privileges of certain healthcare groups or they originated from not knowing that the central problems in the healthcare system were wastefulness and structural weaknesses.[395] Hence, he declared that criticism of cost containment interventions was not valid and even dangerous in the light of the estimated expenses in 2000. He recommended strategies "to reduce avoidable costs, to eliminate wastefulness, and to use strategies of rationalization better."[396]

His strategies were in line with the claim of the WHO to restructure healthcare systems by introducing mechanisms of the market into hospitals especially, and to foster more effective, efficient, and transparent procedures in healthcare.[397] And it is clearly a neoliberal argument to cultivate cost-conscious behaviour and decision-making. This kind of efficient and effective behaviour is valued in Jung's article as a strategy to improve the healthcare system and its performance in regard to patient treatment. At the same time, people critical of these measures become devalued intellectually and even morally by the argument that they are acting either from a knowledge deficit or from the selfishness of certain healthcare groups who value their power and their interests over the interests of others. This puts strong pressure on everyone who questions the narrative of cost explosion. From the perspective of governmentality, this is an example of how an economic rationale was introduced as the basis of good decision-making and behaviour and how it was defended in the healthcare setting.[398]

Even though other dissenting voices doubted that cost explosion was actually taking place, it did not change the discourse of it and cost containment interventions. For example, in 1980, when the notion of "cost explosion" had already

---

395 Jung, "Kostendämpfung im Gesundheitswesen," 49–51.
396 "Es geht darum, die dadurch verursachten vermeidbaren Kosten abzubauen, Verschwendung zu beseitigen, Rationalisierungsreserven auszuschöpfen und damit eine solide Grundlage für die Weiterentwicklung unseres Gesundheitswesens und für die Steigerung seiner Leistungsfähigkeit zu schaffen" (Jung, "Kostendämpfung im Gesundheitswesen," 51, my translation).
397 WHO, "Organizational Study on "Methods of Promoting Development of Basic Health Services": Report of the Working Group, 16 January 1973," (World Health Organization, 1973).
398 See chapter 5.2.1 and for example Nikolas Rose, "Government, Authority and Expertise in Advanced Liberalism," *Economy and Society* 22, no. 3 (1993), 283–99; Michel Foucault, *The Birth of Biopolitics: Lectures at the Collège De France, 1978–79* (Basingstoke, New York: Palgrave Macmillan, 2008).

spread to the healthcare setting, physician Jan Blumenstock wrote in *Krankenpflege:* "The current noticeable cost-containment interventions in hospitals have been prepared with the propaganda of 'cost explosion.' No governmental representative could verify coherently how long this 'cost bomb' was ticking and when it would explode."[399] He argued that only the health insurance system faced increasing costs because hospitals' statutory financial support had decreased after the hospital law of 1972 and health insurance had to cover the rapid increase in daily healthcare costs.[400] From the perspective of professionalism and neoliberal governmentality, this is very interesting because it is an example of competing rationales: Blumenstock, as a physician, criticized the increasing cost-containment interventions that called for restraining medical power and autonomy by introducing managerial language into the medical sphere. Ordoliberals argued for restraining medical dominance in the healthcare setting in order to establish the economy as the dominant mode of governing. Hence, this article of Blumenstock can be read as an attempt to regain control over the mode of governing of the healthcare system.

This attempt, however, was not successful, and the narrative of "cost explosion" in the healthcare system continues today. Nursing scientist Michael Simon argues too, that in retrospect, cost explosion could not be proven for the hospital sector but rather for health insurance. As already described in chapter 2, the health insurance system experienced an increase of costs not because of uneconomic behaviour but because of structural changes within healthcare services with changes in the organization of health personnel and in the financial structure of hospital-based healthcare. The argument of cost explosion was introduced, Simon argues, to implement cost-saving strategies in healthcare in order to shift money away from health insurance to other social insurances such as pension insurance, which had experienced huge financial problems.[401] This is another example of the kinds of strategies used to implement a new mode of governing into the healthcare system. With the problematization of healthcare costs and the establishment of the argument of cost explosion, the im-

---

399 "Die derzeit an den Krankenhäusern spürbaren Kostendämpfungsmaßnahmen sind lange Jahre durch die unter dem Begriff der 'Kostenexplosion' geführte Propaganda vorbereitet worden. Wie lange diese 'Kostenbombe' tickte und wann sie explodierte, konnte von keinem Regierungsvertreter schlüssig belegt werden" (Jan Blumenstock, "Das Märchen von der Kostenexplosion im Gesundheitswesen [The Fairytale About the Cost Explosion in the Healthcare System]," *Krankenpflege* 34, no. 7/8 (1980), 248–49: 248, my translation).
400 Blumenstock, "Das Märchen von der Kostenexplosion," 248–49.
401 See chapter 2; Michael Simon, "Die ökonomischen und strukturellen Veränderungen des Krankenhausbereichs seit den 1970er Jahren [The Economic and Structural Changes of the Hospital Setting since the 1970s]," in *Mutationen des Krankenhauses: Soziologische Diagnosen in organisations- und gesellschaftstheoretischer Perspektive,* ed. Ingo Bode and Werner Vogd (Wiesbaden: Springer Fachmedien Wiesbaden, 2016), 29–45.

plementation of accounting and of cost-containment strategies could be legitimized. With accounting technologies, then, the argument of cost explosion could be proven by using numbers as neutral and trustworthy representations of reality, thereby strengthening the argument for cost-containment strategies and the need for cost-conscious behaviour.

In the articles I found in the journals, it becomes obvious that the argument of cost explosion became a valid rationale in the healthcare setting. The cost containment acts of 1977 and 1981 regulated this rationale by law and provided, in this way, an unquestionable foundation for deep changes in the organization and content of healthcare. This gave rise to the problematization of costs in healthcare, to mechanisms and instruments to measure and calculate the costs of healthcare services, and to legal demands to show a cost-consciousness behaviour. Hence, the introduction of mechanisms of cost containment, then, can be analyzed as disciplinary strategies with the aim to produce cost-conscious healthcare personnel.[402] This is an example of problematization: something, such as healthcare costs, becomes problematized, which leads to the development and implementation of specific strategies, such as cost containment strategies (e. g., accounting technologies, audits, cost-conscious behaviour), to address the established problematization.

Contradictions in daily healthcare occur when the economic principle and cost-saving behaviour is not explicitly subordinated to the patient's interests.[403] However, hospitals were urged to transform into enterprises and nursing practice became integrated into an economic frame and equipped with the language of the market. From the moment that these arguments were accepted as truth, they became taken-for-granted assumptions and hardly anybody could seriously argue against cost explosion in healthcare.

As I will show, nursing leaders carried this argument of cost explosion and cost containment further, quite uncritically, and developed an image of danger around shortcuts and dehumanization in nursing. In order to avoid this danger, different strategies were recommended: reorganize nursing care, make transparent what nurses do to avoid shortcuts, and improve quality and control. Nurses saw a chance to improve nursing care as well as the status of the nursing vocation both in the healthcare system and in society by implementing strategies for cost-saving. They developed concrete plans to restructure healthcare with the help of the nursing process, and participated in economizing their own setting.

---

402 See also Woon Hau Wong, "Caring Holistically within New Managerialism," *Nursing Inquiry* 11, no. 1 (2004), 2–13.
403 Hagen Kühn, "Ethische Probleme der Ökonomisierung von Krankenhausarbeit [Ethical Problems of the Economization of Hospital Work]," in *Dienstleistungsqualität und Qualität des Arbeitslebens im Krankenhaus*, ed. André Büssing and Jürgen Glaser (Göttingen, Bern, Toronto, Seattle: Hogrefe-Verlag, 2003), 77–98.

The focus on health, here, is a central component. Health is constituted as the aim toward which healthcare interventions, e.g. nursing actions, should be directed. Furthermore, health in the understanding of the WHO is an economic good that has to be produced, making the healthcare system a health-producing machine by introducing the logic of the market into healthcare services. This, in turn, reconstitutes what nursing care has to be: transparent and controllable in order to show its effectiveness and even efficiency. In the next section, I will show in more detail how this understanding of nursing became constituted as an unquestionable truth and how it used the nursing process as a key component of "right" and modern nursing.

7.1 Reorganization of Nursing Care in the Hospital

In the late 1950s, effective nursing care was already recognized as being a key part of a hospital: "A hospital cannot defend its right to exist if it cannot provide effective care to its patients."[404] Since nursing is an important part of healthcare in hospitals, it needed to be transformed into a controlled activity when hospitals were reorganized as enterprises. Good nursing care was seen to be planned and rational, using the most appropriate technical standards to maintain continuous improvement.[405] This image of nursing as a controllable activity was established in opposition to its former image, where detailed nursing work was not visible and thus, out of reach of managers, accountants, and economists. In the following decades, nurses themselves argued that a transformation was necessary to prove how essential the nursing vocation was within the context of the dehumanizing environment of the hospital.[406]

The reorganization of nursing service was discussed in regard to strategies of restructuring and calculations based on patients' needs, health as the general aim of nursing service, and the neoliberal rationale in which nursing service should take place.

---

404 "Ein Krankenhaus kann seine Daseinsberechtigung nicht verteidigen, wenn es seinen Patienten nicht eine effektive Pflege zu bieten vermag" (Sirkka Levá, "Eine gute Krankenpflege. Was ist damit gemeint, und wie ist sie zu erreichen? [Good Nursing Care: What Are We Talking About, and How Can It Be Achieved]," *Die Agnes-Karll-Schwester* 11, no. 2 (1957), 54 & 56: 56; my translation).

405 Levá, "Eine gute Krankenpflege," 54 & 56; Friedrich Eichhorn, "Grundgedanken zur Rationalisierung des Pflegedienstes [Basic Ideas on the Rationalization of Nursing Service]," *Die Agnes-Karll-Schwester* 11, no. 3 (1957), 78–82.

406 DBfK, "Bremen, Hamburg und Schleswig-Holstein [Bremen, Hamburg and Schleswig-Holstein]," *Krankenpflege* 33, no. 4 (1979), 132; Friederike Dittrich, "Der Terminal auf der Station [The Computer on the Ward]," *Krankenpflege* 38, no. 9 (1984), 278–79.

7.1.1 Patients' Needs as Foundation for the Reorganization of Healthcare Services

Claims to restructure the hospital and its healthcare responsibilities into an enterprise and economic services can be found as early as the 1960s (see chapter 5.2.1).[407] Moreover, in 1974 a nurse published an article in the hospital journal *Das Krankenhaus* in which she discussed a new organization of healthcare based on the level of care that patients needed. Wards for patients with intensive care needs and wards for minimal care were recommended.[408] These considerations found their way into the nursing journal *Krankenpflege* and were developed further in the 1970s by Detlef Hohlin, who actively discussed a newly structured nursing service and how to calculate the number and kind of nursing personnel needed. Hohlin was a head nurse of a civic hospital in the 1970s who later became a member of the DBfK directory and participated in expert committees of the German Hospital Society (DKG).[409]

Hohlin's articles in this nursing journal coincided with the beginning of the medium-term program of the WHO. The nursing process seems to have provided possibilities to structure nursing service in a new way, as I will show in the following pages.

Organization of Hospital Services

Hohlin drew on the argument of cost explosion and the need to reduce financial costs in his proposal to organize hospitals in such a way that the patient would be continuously transferred to different wards based on his/her intensity of care. He reasoned that creating a newly organized nursing service would acknowledge economic demands. According to him, "the aim of patient-oriented, holistic and individual nursing care which considers psycho-social aspects has to be harmonized exactly with medical necessities/requirements [*Notwendigkeiten*] and economic possibilities."[410] Hohlin called this "progressive nursing care," which was based on the steps of the nursing process and, according to him,

---

407 Siegfried Eichhorn, "Die betriebswirtschaftlichen Aspekte der Leistungssteigerung durch Zusammenarbeit [Economic Aspects to Increase Performance through Collaboration]," *Das Krankenhaus* 58, no. 8 (1966), 315–23.
408 Carola Ramge, "Effizienzverbesserung im Pflegedienst durch Umstrukturierung der pflegerischen Versorgung [Improvment of Efficiency in Nursing Service through Restructuring Nursing Care]," *Das Krankenhaus* 66, no. 5 (1974), 200–04.
409 For information about the DKG see chapter 4.3.
410 "Progressivpflege" (Detlef Hohlin, "Notwendigkeit der Adaption der Krankenhäuser an Strukturänderungen aus pflegerischer Sicht [A Nursing Perspective on the Necessity of Hospitals Adapting to Structural Changes]," *Krankenpflege* 31, no. 9 (1977), 287–90: 290; my translation).

ensured both a good quality of nursing care and a reduction of healthcare costs.[411] In order to achieve that kind of organization of nursing service and progressive nursing care, Hohlin recommended moving away from the medically oriented order of wards to an organization of healthcare services based on patients' needs for nursing care. This, in turn, would mean, however, that the patient could not stay in one place during his/her illness but would need to be moved several times through different healthcare settings depending on the actual medical and nursing needs of the patient; whether the patient needed diagnosis or treatment, whether the patient's condition was serious or not, and whether the patient was more or less dependent on help to satisfy his/her needs.[412] The constant moving of beds was based on the idea that throughout the first steps of the nursing process, a concrete plan would be developed which would transfer with the patient regardless of the nurse who provided this care. The planned nursing care based on the patient's condition could be executed by any nurse. Since the relationship between a patient and a specific nurse – which formerly guaranteed continuous nursing care – was not needed for a smooth transfer of information, the patient could be constantly moved between wards which then could be equipped differently with (expensive) machines and techniques. To optimally address and manage a patient's condition, expensive new technology would not be needed in every ward. Rather, the patient could be moved to the resources and material needed. This kind of organization, hence, should consequently decrease healthcare costs.[413]

This was exactly what a nursing study from Singapore revealed: Following a managerial logic and the nursing manager's demands, nurses at the end of their shifts moved patients between different wards in order to "match" nursing care based on these needs with the ward on which this care could be provided, thus using as few resources as possible. The patient as an individual, however, was hidden by this managerial logic, which directed its focus to medical conditions and aspects of functionality. Moreover, "in daily usage, the term 'bed' [became] so compelling a term that patients and beds [were] often used interchangeably, to the extent that patients [were] not referred to by their names or seen as persons."[414] This daily nursing practice, the movement of beds to achieve the resource-conscious operation of hospitals, called for a cost-conscious nurse rather than a nurse who was knowledgeable about caring for a patient. This reconstitution of nurses as economic entities I will discuss later (see chapter 7.1.3).

---

411 Hohlin, "Notwendigkeit der Adaption der Krankenhäuser," 287–90.
412 Hohlin, "Notwendigkeit der Adaption der Krankenhäuser," 287–90.
413 Hohlin, "Notwendigkeit der Adaption der Krankenhäuser," 287–90; Detlef Hohlin, "Neue Horizonte für die Krankenpflege [New Horizons for Nursing Care]," *Krankenpflege* 30, no. 1 (1976), 13–14.
414 Wong, "Caring Holistically within New Managerialism," 7.

Hohlin wanted nurses to actively participate in the reorganization of healthcare, in the assessment of working conditions and economic demands for the establishment of progressive nursing care. In his considerations of this new organization of healthcare, two aspects stand out: He believed that turning away from the medically based, that is, illness-oriented organization of hospital services to one that was based on a patient's needs would better meet the problems of cost explosion.[415] But this is a critique of the medical profession as an outmoded form of a professional organization, where medical hospital services are seen as less flexible and uneconomic. Hence, when economic thinking became more valuable than the medical orientation in healthcare – as happened with neoliberalism – the nursing vocation perceived the chance to free itself from the medical profession. This could occur only when it could base nursing interventions more on an economic logic than a medical perspective, as I will discuss more in depth later.

According to Hohlin then, nursing autonomy was only realizable within this economic frame.[416] Hohlin's article shows the establishment of the hybridized discourse of nursing and accounting, as the concept of nursing autonomy (which later was transformed into professionalization in nursing) became linked with the need for accountability and cost-consciousness. If nurses wanted to be considered professionals, they had to have self-disciplining mechanisms to execute nursing care in an economic way. This was comparable to the study from Singapore in which it was concluded "that the market-like rationale in health delivery and governance re-codes and re-problematizes the function of the healthcare system, predominantly in terms of a cost-efficient discourse."[417]

Calculating Personnel Demands

Connected to a new organization of hospital services were considerations of healthcare personnel. Nurses were acknowledged as the largest cost factor in healthcare services; they were and still are the largest group working in healthcare. After the 1950s, the nursing vocation changed dramatically. New secularized nurses demanded a higher salary than nurses who had been trained under the motherhouse system (see chapter 3.1). With the nursing shortages in the 1960s and with the modernization of hospitals, the number of hospital nurses rose between 1965 and 1975. In the late 1960s, more nursing aides were employed in the hospital setting and also the number of examined (registered) nurses also

---

415 Hohlin, "Notwendigkeit der Adaption der Krankenhäuser," 287–90.
416 Hohlin, "Notwendigkeit der Adaption der Krankenhäuser," 287–90.
417 Wong, "Caring Holistically within New Managerialism," 12.

increased. The costs of nursing personnel thus increased rapidly within two decades.[418]

Over the course of discussions around the cost containment acts of 1977 and 1981 (see chapter 2.2), pressure mounted to develop another mode of calculating and paying for costs related to hospital operations. The traditional mode of financing the main costs of operating hospitals was payment according to a flat-rate calculation of daily hospital charges for care per patient. This was considered retrospective payment, in that hospitals were paid after treatment had been carried out. In 1986, this changed to a mainly prospective payment,[419] which demanded a calculation of estimated hospital costs based on the calculations from years before. Different from the old method of payment based on the use of hospital beds, in this new mode, profit was possible when the actual costs were lower than the estimated costs. A prominent example was the introduction of Diagnosis Related Groups (DRGs) in the German healthcare system in the 1990s. A patient's diagnosis was connected to the average time a patient with that condition remained in hospital. Time thus became a precious resource: the less time a patient with a certain DRG needed before discharge the more money could be saved. Focusing payment more on patients' diagnoses and needs than on actual care made healthcare personnel eager to discharge the patient as soon as possible.[420] Consequently this method of payment was likely going to lead to decreased time for patient interaction.[421]

By the 1970s, modes of payment were completely different. Nurses themselves were active participants in developing a method on how best to calculate the number of different types of nursing personnel needed in the hospital. Patients' needs and the intensity of care they needed were recommended as a base for these calculations, and these considerations occurred alongside discussions on how to change the calculation for financing hospitals.

With his recommendations for a new organized nursing service, Hohlin shared his thoughts on calculating nursing staff. A nursing assessment, Hohlin stated, would help to find out patients' needs upon which subsequent nursing care could be planned. He also recommended placing similar patients with

---

418 Michael Simon, *Krankenhauspolitik in der Bundesrepublik Deutschland. Historische Entwicklung und Probleme der politischen Steuerung stationärer Krankenversorgung [Hospital Policy in the Federal Republic of Germany: Historical Developments and Problems of the Political Control Stationary Healthcare]*, Studien zur Sozialwissenschaft Band 209 (Wiesbaden: Springer Fachmedien Wiesbaden GmbH, 2000).
419 Simon, "Die ökonomischen und strukturellen Veränderungen des Krankenhausbereichs seit den 1970er Jahren," 29–45.
420 Rolf Rosenbrock and Thomas Gerlinger, *Gesundheitspolitik. Eine systematische Einführung [Health Policy: A Systematic Introduction]*, 3rd. ed. (Bern: Verlag Hans Huber, 2014).
421 Kühn, "Ethische Probleme der Ökonomisierung," 77–98.

similar care needs in the same wards.[422] He based his considerations on the perception that technical nursing care would be provided by nurses whereas basic nursing care could be carried out by nursing aides: "If we assume that on a ward of patients needing normal nursing care, 25 to 30% of those would need basic nursing care then the number of nursing aides should not exceed 25 to 30%."[423] Hohlin drew on the differentiation of nursing care into basic and technical in order to suggest hospital spaces that would meet the different demands on the quantity and level of nursing work. For example, he recommended establishing wards for patients with a diagnosis that demanded a higher level of technical nursing care, for intensive care patients with high demands on both technical and basic nursing care, and for normal patients who had rather less demand on nursing care. Hohlin's purpose for reorganizing hospital wards according to patients' demands on nursing care was twofold. First, he aimed to deploy nurses and nursing aides in an adequate relation to the amount and quality of nursing work needed. This nursing work would be calculated on the needs of specific patients. Second, nursing personnel but also expensive and high quality technical instruments and machines would be disseminated in a cost-conscious way.[424] Both the use of nursing personnel and technical equipment would be set in relation to measured and categorized needs of patients.

Although his thoughts for this new structuring of healthcare in hospitals that was based on patients' needs were never applied in practice, Hohlin continued to work in this area and, together with Lore Kroeker, was active in a working group of the German Hospital Society (DKG) that was preparing a new and future-oriented procedure for the calculation of personnel demands "under the premise of transparency and traceability."[425] The DKG was influential in the development and negotiation of laws for the hospital sector.[426] Kroeker and Hohlin were actively involved in the discussions for restructuring hospital financing, attempting to turn away from the flat-rate calculations of daily hospital charges towards other calculation systems that would reimburse single interventions or

---

422 Hohlin, "Notwendigkeit der Adaption der Krankenhäuser," 287–90.
423 "Geht man davon aus, daß im Normalbereich ca. 25–30% Grundpflege anfällt, so kann der Anteil des in der Krankenpflegehilfe ausgebildeten Pflegepersonals höchstens 25–30% betragen" (Hohlin, "Notwendigkeit der Adaption der Krankenhäuser," 289; my translation).
424 Hohlin, "Notwendigkeit der Adaption der Krankenhäuser," 287–90.
425 "Ermittlung und Berücksichtigung der unterschiedlichen ggf. höheren Pflegeintensität im Pflegezeit- und damit im Personalaufwand unter der Prämisse der Transparenz und Nachvollziehbarkeit" (Detlef Hohlin, "Werden Anhaltszahlen durch neue Berechnungsmethoden abgelöst? Teil I [Will Reference Data Soon Be Replaced by New Methods of Calculation? Part I]," *Krankenpflege* 40, no. 3 (1986), 102–04: 103; my translation).
426 Falk Illig, *Gesundheitspolitik in Deutschland. Eine Chronologie der Gesundheitsreformen der Bundesrepublik [Health Politics in Germany. A Chronology of the Health Reforms of the Federal Republic]* (Wiesbaden: Springer VS, 2017).

intervention groups.[427] The aim was to substitute the payment of hospital care based on daily rates with an analytical calculation based on patients' needs. This new calculation would be based on the requirements of patients for differing amounts of nursing care. A higher intensity need for nursing care would call for more time that would need to be spent with patients and, hence, heavier personnel demands. According to Hohlin, although the working team considered up to seven different nursing categories, it agreed – because of questions about practicability and feasibility – on four.[428]

The categories were concerned with the demand of care a patient needed for his or her daily activities. A fully independent patient was consigned to the first category. Patients with some degree of needing support in order to fulfill their daily needs were sorted into the second or third category. The fourth category would contain fully dependent patients who could not master any of their daily activities. According to the examples provided in the article, the focus was not only put on the physical needs of patients but also on the mental, social, and communicative areas. Furthermore, the importance of the nursing care plan was demonstrated as it was considered a part of each of the four categories, although there was a special emphasis on evaluation steps in categories three and four.[429] According to Hohlin, the nursing care plan would determine nursing interventions leading to individual nursing goals, enabling the "success of each single nursing intervention."[430]

Hohlin recommended that calculating personnel demands in nursing consisted – among other hospital-specific data – of the time needed for nursing care that had been derived from the different nursing categories.[431] Patients' needs are assessed, made visible, controlled and reported with the nursing process. The nursing process is, therefore, an instrument to make patients as well as nursing

---

427 Lore Kroeker, "Referentenentwurf eines Gesetzes zur Neuordnung der Krankenfinanzierung vom 16.7.1984. Anhörung beim Bundesministerium für Arbeit und Sozialordnung am 31.7.1984 – Kurzbericht [Draft of a Law for the Rearrangement of Healthcare Financing, July 16th, 1984. Official Hearing in the Federal Ministry for Work and Social Order, July 31st, 1984]," *Krankenpflege* 38, no. 9 (1984), 289.
428 "Abweichend von zum Teil theoretischen Vorstellungen über bis zu sieben Pflegekategorien einigte sich die Arbeitsgruppe unter anderem auch aus Gründen der praktischen Anwendbarkeit und Durchsetzbarkeit auf vier Pflegekategorien" (Hohlin, "Anhaltszahlen I," 103; my translation).
429 Hohlin, "Anhaltszahlen I," 102–04.
430 "Sie ermöglicht die Kontrolle des Erfolgs der einzelnen pflegerischen Handlung" Detlef Hohlin, "Werden Anhaltszahlen durch neue Berechnungsmethoden abgelöst? Teil II [Will Reference Data Soon Be Replaced by New Methods of Calculation? Part II]," *Krankenpflege* 40, no. 4 (1986), 142–43: 142; my translation).
431 Detlef Hohlin, "Werden Anhaltszahlen durch neue Berechnungsmethoden abgelöst? Teil III [Will Reference Data Soon Be Replaced by New Methods of Calculation? Part III]," *Krankenpflege* 40, no. 5 (1986), 189–90, 207.

care calculable, not only to provide nursing care capable of meeting the determined problems and nursing goals but also to calculate the costs of the care of patients and to estimate the number of differently qualified nursing personnel.

7.1.2 Focusing on Health

The focus on health is already inherent in WHO programs. For example, the WHO built its medium-term program on the importance of healthcare by constructing health as both the actual and traditional focus of nursing care (see also chapter 6). Health in its specific understanding as an individual and political aim is a central aspect of the constitution of the WHO. This understanding became re-affirmed as a social and economic goal in the Declaration of Alma-Ata. More precisely, a certain level of health should be guaranteed or achieved to enable individuals "to lead a socially and economically productive life."[432] Moreover, the individual was not only ascribed the right but also the duty to participate in programs of healthcare.[433] The slogan "Health for All by the Year 2000" originated from the Alma-Ata conference and it became a global strategy.[434] German nurses writing in the nursing journal *Krankenpflege* picked up on the slogan and included it in their aim to further support the application of the nursing process into daily nursing practice.[435]

Moreover, in the second half of the 20th century, international influence on national health discourses grew stronger in general. For example, the International Council of Nurses (ICN), as the overarching professional nursing association, acknowledged in 1986 that because of cost-explosion and subsequent cost-containment strategies in national healthcare systems, nursing's scope of practice in nursing service would change. The focus would be more directed to self-

---

432 WHO, "Global Strategy for Health for All by the Year 2000," 1981), https://iris.wpro.who.in t/bitstream/handle/10665.1/6967/WPR_RC032_GlobalStrategy_1981_en.pdf.
433 WHO, "Declaration of Alma-Ata. International Conference on Primary Health Care, Alma-Ata, Ussr, 6–12 September 1978," 1978), https://www.who.int/publications/almaata_declara tion_en.pdf.
434 WHO, "Global Strategy".
435 Rosemarie Weinrich, "Sitzung des Rates der Ländervertreter – 18. internationaler Krankenpflegekongreß in Tel Aviv [Meeting of the Council of the Representatives of the Countries: 18th International Nursing Congress in Tel Aviv]," *Krankenpflege* 39, no. 9 (1985), 298–301; DBfK Gesamtverband/Redaktion KRANKENPFLEGE, "Die Krankenpflege von heute und morgen – Arbeitspapier des Weltbundes der Krankenschwestern und Krankenpfleger – ICN [Nursing of Today and Tomorrow: Working Paper of the International Council of Nurses – ICN]," *Krankenpflege* 40, no. 9 (1986), 353–56.

care, health, and health education or rehabilitation in nursing based on the nursing process.[436]

Another example is the international influence of the Canadian "Lalonde Report"[437] on national public health considerations. The notion of lifestyle became an especially strong force in the transformation of preventive discourses by emphasizing individual responsibility for remaining healthy.[438]

Health Education

With the strengthening of the neoliberal critique of the welfare state, the former focus on structural modes of prevention such as mass vaccinations or obligatory health promotion programs declined, and the individual's responsibility was increasingly emphasized.[439] Health education as an intervention in this realm promoted self-responsibility and the independence of individuals to make their own decisions. The individual should be informed about how to prevent illness, foster health, and live a healthy lifestyle. However, the individual was also urged to make decisions based upon all available information.[440] Constituting this decision-making as a rational act, the individual was considered responsible for the outcome of decisions.[441]

In the 1960s, health education was discussed in the nursing journal as an important part of nursing service and a specific responsibility of the nursing vocation. According to health experts Wolfgang Fritsche and Christa Topfmeier,

---

436 DBfK Gesamtverband/Redaktion KRANKENPFLEGE, "Die Krankenpflege von heute und morgen," 353–56.
437 Marc Lalonde, "A New Perspective on the Health of Canadians. A Working Document," (Minister of Supply and Services Canada, 1974/1981), http://www.phac-aspc.gc.ca/ph-sp/pdf/perspect-eng.pdf.
438 Virginia Berridge, "Medizin, Public Health und die Medien in Großbritannien von 1950 bis 1980 [Medicine, Public Health and the Media in Britain from 1950s to the 1970s]," in *Das präventive Selbst. Eine Kulturgeschichte moderner Gesundheitspolitik*, ed. Martin Lengwiler and Jeannette Madarász (Bielefeld: transcript Verlag, 2010), 205–28; Martin Lengwiler and Jeannette Madarász, "Präventionsgeschichte als Kulturgeschichte der Gesundheitspolitik [Prevention History as Cultural History]," in *Das präventive Selbst. Eine Kulturgeschichte moderner Gesundheitspolitik*, ed. Martin Lengwiler and Jeannette Madarász (Bielefeld: transcript Verlag, 2010), 11–28; Thomas Foth and Dave Holmes, "Governing through Lifestyle: Lalonde and the Biopolitical Managemnt of Public Health in Canada," *Nursing Philosophy* 19, no. 4 (2018), 1–11.
439 Malte Thießen, "Praktiken der Vorsorge als Ordnung des Sozialen: Zum Verhältnis von Impfungen und Gesellschaftskonzepten im "langen 20. Jahrhundert" [Practices of Prevention as Social Order: About the Relationship of Vaccinations and Societal Concepts in the "Long 20th Century"]," in *Geschichte der Prävention. Akteure, Praktiken, Instrumente*, ed. Sylvelyn Hähner-Rombach (Stuttgart: Franz Steiner Verlag, 2015), 203–27.
440 DBfK Gesamtverband/Redaktion KRANKENPFLEGE, "Die Krankenpflege Von heute und morgen," 353–56.
441 Foth and Holmes, "Governing through Lifestyle," 1–11.

health education occurs "when a) the desired healthy behaviour is the determined goal, b) the applied interventions are adequate to reach the goal, c) and those interventions are utilized purposefully, practically [*zweckmäßig*], and are well-planned."[442] Health education, it was said, has to happen in a rational and goal-oriented process in which the "desired healthy behaviour" should be achieved with appropriate and practical interventions. Nurses were conceptualized as valuable healthcare workers, able to influence the patient's behaviour because they were closer to the patient's life circumstances and enjoyed a more trustworthy relationship to the patient and his or her family. Aiming to influence the patient's behaviour and to provide effective health education [*wirkungsvolle Gesundheitserziehung*] meant that nurses would need to be convincing and use simple and understandable language. By translating scientific knowledge into simple language and into practice, nurses would become key workers in implementing preventive and health-promoting behaviour in patients and family members.[443] Hence, nurses could play an important role in the establishment of a health-conscious and self-responsible individual: The expertise of nurses should indirectly guide and influence the patient in a manner so that being educated, the patient would be able to make his or her own decisions and become self-responsible, thereby following the rationale that the nurses provided through health education. The underlying process to govern the individual in regard to prevention in health contains the same structural pattern as the nursing process. Health education should be structured as a planned process with a concrete goal and with very clear purposeful and practical interventions that are adequate to achieve the goal and should, therefore, be understood in terms of the implementation of the neoliberal rationale.

This is also in line with the mode of health programming of the WHO, which also conceptualized "health" as a goal or output of healthcare (as already defined by the WHO in 1973).[444] Based on the rationality of the cybernetic process, the steps and interventions to achieve this goal can be defined and followed in a simplified and rationalized way. The cybernetic process became a universal pattern in which healthcare, for example, nursing service and health education,

---

442 "Echte Gesundheitserziehung findet statt, wenn a) die gewünschte gesundheitsförderliche Verhaltensweise als Ziel feststeht, b) die angewandten Maßnahmen geeignet sind, das angestrebte Ziel zu erreichen, c) die als geeignet erkannten Maßnahmen gezielt, zweckvoll und planmäßig zum Einsatz gebracht werden" (Wolfgang Fritsche and Christa Topfmeier, "Gedanken zu Inhalt und Methodik der Gesundheitserziehung [Thoughts Upon Content and Method of Health Education]," *Die Agnes-Karll-Schwester* 21, no. 4 (1967), 133–35: 133; my translation).
443 Wolfgang Fritsche and Wolfgang F. Meyer, "Gesundheitserziehung und Gemeindepflege [Health Education and Parish Nursing]," *Die Agnes-Karll-Schwester* 22, no. 1 (1968), 3–6.
444 WHO, "Organizational Study."

could be provided in a clear, rational, and transparent manner that was easy to plan and enabled calculations.

The focus on health was closely connected to the aim of achieving huge cost savings for national healthcare systems. The underlying explanation was that the focus on health would lead to fewer admissions to the hospital, shorter durations of stay for patients, and better care before and after hospitalization. In consequence, the medium-term program of the WHO called for a fundamental rethinking of nursing and fostered the establishment of health education and information as nursing tasks on its agenda.[445]

7.1.3 Economizing Subjects in Hospital Care

In order to transform hospitals into enterprises and nursing care into a commercial service the patient must be conceptualized as a customer or client [*Kunde*]. In a report on an ongoing education seminar, published in the nursing journal *Krankenpflege*, the patient as a person seeking advice, information, and help in the hospital was equated with a person looking for advice, information, and help in a clothing store.[446] In this case, the patient became thought of as a person in need of commercial good "health." By transforming the patient into a customer, nursing care, in consequence, was thought of as a commercial service comparable to the selling of a piece of clothes, with nurses as salespersons. The attendees of this seminar were taught about the nursing process from this economic perspective. According to the report, this economic perspective on nursing was logical for the attendees, and until today, German nursing continues to discuss whether nursing is an economic service and the patient a customer.[447]

---

445 Rosemarie Weinrich, "Kurz berichtet aus der Hauptgeschäftsstelle [Brief Report of the Essentials of the Head Office]," *Krankenpflege* 30, no. 2 (1976), 49–50; Rosemarie Weinrich, "Wichtiges in Kürze aus der Hauptgeschäftsstelle [Brief Overview of the Essentials of the Head Office]," *Krankenpflege* 30, no. 6 (1976), 183–84.
446 Irmgard Simon, "Ein bayrischer Gruß an alle Fortbildungs-Muffel [A Bavarian Salute to All Continuing Education Grumps]," *Krankenpflege* 33, no. 1 (1979), 15–16.
447 E.g. Marita Andrzejak, "Krankenpflege als Dienstleistung [Nursing as Service]," *Krankenpflege* 36, no. 3 (1982), 82–84; Thomas Behr et al., "Positionspapier: Pflege raus aus dem Abseits – Empfehlungen zu einer Refokussierung auf den Kernprozess der Pflege [Position Paper: Nursing Away from the Offset – Recommendations for Re-Focusing on the Core Process of Nursing]," in *Aufbruch Pflege*, ed. Thomas Behr (Wiesbaden: Springer Fachmedien, 2015), 61–81; Heiner Friesacher, *Theorie und Praxis pflegerischen Handelns [Theory and Practice of Nursing Action]* (Göttingen: V&R unipress, 2008); Alexandra Manzei and Rudi Schmiede, "Über die neue Unmittelbarkeit des Marktes im Gesundheitswesen – Wie durch die Digitalisierung der Patientenakte ökonomische Entscheidungskriterien an das Patientenbett gelangen [On the New Immediacy of the Market in the Healthcare System: How Economic Criteria for Decision Making Came to the Bedside Via Digitalization of

However, as nursing scholar Michael Simon argues, an economized administration of the hospital setting can cause flaws and damage, although they are barely recognizable in the economic benchmarks of such an enterprise and therefore, might not be visible in economic analyses of this setting.[448] As an example, nurse-patient relationships could be transformed in such a way with marketization that they could become de-individualized.[449]

As already mentioned, health was considered by the WHO as the output of healthcare services.[450] This narrative was continuously repeated in the nursing journal *Krankenpflege*.[451] The nursing process was seen as an instrument to achieve this output by setting health as the overall aim of nursing action and by reorganizing nursing action in a cybernetic logic that directs all activities in nursing towards this aim. Furthermore, the patient became conceptualized as an empowered individual responsible for his or her own health. The nursing process helped to conceptualize patients as active and empowered individuals who were to be responsible for living their lives in a healthy way.

Nursing documentation – written reports and patient charts – make manifest this newly constructed patient-subject. By making patients visible as economized subjects and defined through patient histories and nursing reports, they become open to strategies of health education and health promotion that could be applied to different areas of their lives. In consequence, the patient could be invaded with the rationale of "lifestyle" in different aspects of his or her life. The integration of this rationale could even be evaluated with the cybernetic cycle of the

---

Patient Records]," in *20 Jahre Wettbewerb im Gesundheitswesen. Theoretische und empirische Analysen zur Ökonomisierung von Medizin und Pflege*, ed. Alexandra Manzei (Wiesbaden: Springer Fachmedien, 2014), 219–39; Arne Manzeschke, "Privatisierung von Krankenhäusern. Ethische Erwägungen zum moralischen Status eines öffentlichen Gutes [Privatization of Hospitals: Ethical Considerations on the Moral Status of a Public Good]," *Pflege und Gesellschaft* 14, no. 1 (2009), 24–38.

448 Simon, "Die ökonomischen und strukturellen Veränderungen des Krankenhausbereichs seit den 1970er Jahren," 41.
449 Friesacher, *Theorie und Praxis pflegerischen Handelns*.
450 WHO, "Organizational Study."
451 Weinrich, "Wichtiges in Kürze," 183–84; Rosemarie Weinrich, "Arbeitsbericht der Hauptgeschäftsführerin für das Jahr Oktober 1977 – September 1978, vorgelegt auf der 5. Delegiertenversammlung des DBfK – gekürzt [Working Report of the General Manager for the Year October 1977 – September 1978. Presented on the Fifth Meeting of the DBfK Delegates – Shortened]," *Krankenpflege* 32, no. 11 (1978), 378–80; Rosemarie Weinrich, "Ausblick auf die Arbeit des DBfK in den 80er Jahren [Outlook to the Work of the DBfK in the 80s]," *Krankenpflege* 35, no. 1 (1981), 16–18; e.g. Monika Krohwinkel, "Pflegepersonal setzt sich für bessere Gesundheit ein [Nurses Campaign for Better Health]," *Krankenpflege* 38, no. 5 (1984), 138–40; Weinrich, "Sitzung des Rates der Ländervertreter," 298–301; Maria Mischo-Kelling, "Gesundheit – Ein pflegerisches Paradigma und Maßstab für Pflegequalität [Health: A Nursing Paradigm and Benchmark for Nursing Quality]," *Krankenpflege* 41, no. 2 (1987), 52–54, 63–64.

nursing process not only by nurses but also by patients themselves, since nursing goals and the nursing care plan should be transparent. Furthermore, the cybernetic structure with its feedback loop could be applied to other situations and areas of life, equipping the individual with self-regulating and self-managing strategies. The introduction of the nursing process enabled the reconstruction of the individual by empowering it to become self-responsible and to work for its healing, and, ultimately, to live a healthy life. An example of a reconstruction of the individual can be found in a 1978 article of the journal *Krankenpflege*. The human being was defined as a "complex man" consisting of "social man" with social needs and "economic man" with economic needs.[452] The needs ascribed to the complex man were defined as basic psychological needs and a need for security, socialization, acknowledgement (*Anerkennung*), and self-fulfilment [*Selbstverwirklichung*]. In order to meet these needs and, hence, provide a good quality of nursing care, the nursing process should be in place with its steps of nursing goals, nursing care plan, patient history, and nursing interventions.[453]

The striving of nurses for professionalization also promoted the establishment of the patient as an economic subject. In the nursing journal *Krankenpflege* professionalization in nursing was connected with a focus on health and prevention and on economic concepts such as effectiveness and efficiency. This argument, however, was not articulated in a conscious and direct way. But it became clear that with the issue of increasing costs the focus on preventive health would be important in order to curtail financial burdens.[454] The nursing vocation in its struggle for recognition and its close relationship with patients established its scope of practice at the intersection of economic issues and patients seeking their help. These two foci strengthened on the acknowledgement that they were an inherent responsibility of nurses themselves and they were included in their agenda of professionalization.[455] Hence, an active and empowered patient who increasingly becomes more responsible for his or her own health is a result of this modern and professional nursing based on the nursing process.

In the 1980s, this kind of economic thinking in nursing developed further. Austrian nurse Friederike Dittrich published an article in the German nursing journal *Krankenpflege* in which she constructed healthcare as a kind of machinery. As the title of the article "Nursing as a Service – Documentation is the

---

452 Regina Dreißiger, "Information im Pflegedienst [Information in Nursing Services]," *Krankenpflege* 32, no. 6 (1978), 200–04: 201.
453 Dreißiger, "Information im Pflegedienst," 200–04.
454 Weinrich, "Arbeitsbericht der Hauptgeschäftsführerin," 378–80.
455 Weinrich, "Arbeitsbericht der Hauptgeschäftsführerin," 378–80; Krohwinkel, "Pflegepersonal setzt sich für bessere Gesundheit ein," 138–40.

Proof"[456] suggests, nursing should be acknowledged as an economic good (a service), but documentation was needed to show that the service was provided. Nursing work, according to Dittrich, is one part of healthcare within the economic system *hospital*. She described the process within the hospital in ergonomic terms: "In a very concretely defined sense of ergonomics the following happens: The patient enters this healing system (hospital), people working inside put an effect upon him (*sic*) with their resources, and he (*sic*) leaves this system in a more positive health situation."[457] Nursing is further conceptualized as a relay point between the offering and establishment of healthcare services.[458] The introduction of input-process-output procedures and managerial vocabulary, as well as increasing standardization and transparency, enables the transformation of nurses' work into a market-oriented part of an enterprise. Using the nursing process enables structuring nursing in this way. Hence, nursing action was not only acknowledged in economic terms but also became constituted as an economic action at the same time.

Both Hohlin and Dittrich presented the work of nurses as an economic component of a health-making machinery. In this perception, it is unquestionable that any work done in the machinery needs to be proven in order to maintain its right to be part of the system. Conceptualizing nursing as an economic good and a service within a market-oriented healthcare system would call for a visible and measurable, hence accountable, nursing activity. Moreover, decision-making in nursing (as part of the nursing process) also becomes subject to business control.[459] Hence, decision-making in nursing, when based on the nursing process, is inherently controlled by market regulations. As soon as professional nursing is conceptualized as nursing care based on the nursing process it can only be valid when acting in an economic way.

---

456 "Pflege als Leistung – Dokumentation ist Beweis" (Friederike Dittrich, "Pflege ist Leistung – Dokumentation ist Beweis [Nursing Is a Service: Documentation Is the Proof]," *Krankenpflege* 38, no. 4 (1984), 142–44: 142; my translation).
457 "Im arbeitswissenschaftlichen, eindeutig definierten Sinn geschieht folgendes: Der Patient tritt in dieses Heilsystem (Krankenhaus) ein, dort wirken arbeitende Menschen mit ihren Hilfsmitteln auf ihn ein, und er verläßt dieses System mit einer positiv veränderten Gesundheit" (Dittrich, "Pflege ist Leistung," 143; my translation).
458 Dittrich, "Pflege ist Leistung," 142–44.
459 This issue is discussed for the physician-patient-relationship by Kühn, "Ethische Probleme der Ökonomisierung," 77–98.

7.2 Making Nursing Service Traceable

The nursing process was introduced as a means to achieve a "goal-oriented, visible, and for the patient, accessible nursing planning and acting based on a specific system."[460] The problem-solving cybernetic cycle is this "specific system" in which nursing action is executed. Instrumental rationality underlies nursing action, in which the acting person balances purpose, resources, and consequences of each action against another. This logic is based on German sociologist and economist Max Weber's understanding of rational action in capitalism, the constant striving of individuals to achieve profit by balancing costs and benefits.[461] Hence, the nursing process brought planned, traceable, and evaluable action into nursing care, action which could be judged on its rationality by people external to this action.

I will now first discuss the call for transparency in German nursing from the 1960s on. It is closely related to the attempts at restructuring healthcare services into economic entities. Implementing the nursing process was meant to make nursing service become understandable to those who did not belong to the nursing vocation. Moreover, the impact of nursing service and hence, its economic value, would then become visible. In the second part, I will show how the nursing process, as a structure that demands instrumental rational action, brought the possibility of a thorough external control into nursing. By comparing the planned nursing goal with the actual output, nursing care becomes controllable. Evaluating nursing care, as well as the quantity and costs of nursing interventions in regard to the achieved nursing output, helps to control the effectiveness and efficiency of nursing care. The more defined and measurable the planned nursing goal and the nursing interventions are, the easier it becomes for people other than the acting nurse to control this nursing care and judge its success.

In articles from the nursing journal *Krankenpflege*, control was presented as an aspect of improved nursing care and increased quality. That means, controllable (or accountable) nursing was seen as a worthy goal and a sign of high

---

460 "In ihrem Vortrag über Pflegeplanung wies Frau Abermeth, Berlin, auf die Bedeutung der Pflegeplanung hin, nämlich: zielorientiertes, sichtbares und für den Patienten einsehbares, pflegerisches Planen und Handeln nach einem bestimmten System" (Ingrid Tietze, "10. Fortbildungskongreß für Krankenschwestern/-pfleger in Berlin [10th Congress for Further Education for Nurses in Berlin]," *Krankenpflege* 33, no. 7/8 (1979), 282: 282; my translation).
461 Max Weber, *Grundriss der Sozialökonomie. III. Abteilung Wirtschaft und Gesellschaft [Layout of Social Economy: Third Division Economy and Society]* (Tübingen: Verlag von J. C. B. Mohr (Paul Siebeck), 1922), 13; Christopher S. Chapman, David J. Cooper, and Peter B. Miller, "Linking Accounting, Organizations, and Institutions," in *Accounting, Organizations, and Institutions: Essays in Honour of Anthony Hopwood*, ed. Christopher S. Chapman, David J. Cooper, and Peter B. Miller (New York: Oxford University Press, 2009), 1–29.

nursing quality. In the third part following, I discuss how the concept of quality in nursing care transformed from a rather humanistic understanding to an economic understanding. Based on the possibility of controlling nursing service, a specific logic of quality in nursing care could be introduced.

7.2.1 Transparency

With the attempts to restructure nursing service into an economic entity, a call for the transparency of nursing actions emerged. These calls could already be found in the 1950s and 1960s, for example, in regard to task analyses in the nursing setting[462] or in regard to effective collaboration between different healthcare workers in order to increase the performance of a hospital.[463] The call for transparency has to be understood as an attempt to open the enclosure of the nursing vocation and of nursing knowledge in order to make accounting mechanisms applicable to it. In an economic entity, transparency is the basis from which to trace the flow of money. In this sense, the nursing process has to be understood as a technology of mistrust. Instead of believing in the statements and decisions of nurses per se, nurses now have to prove that their actions and decisions are effective.[464] Hence, the nursing process shifts the former trust in nurses to the demands that nurses have to be accountable for their actions by making their service and its impact transparent.

The arguments for transparency that I found in the journals were twofold. On the one hand, it was argued that transparency was needed to establish hospitals – and in turn, healthcare in general – as enterprises and to make them work more effectively and efficiently. Since in such an economic entity monetary value is ascribed to visible and effective performances, nursing as a part of the hospital needed to establish structures to show its benefit to the hospital. Furthermore, nursing service also needed to be calculable and predictable in its demands (such as staff requirements) in order for the hospital to work in an economic manner. On the other hand, transparent nursing service was seen as important with the danger of facing shortcuts in a time of political and societal pressure to reduce costs in healthcare. Nurses themselves urged their colleagues to make visible their performance in nursing to justify and fight for their right to exist.

Antje Grauhan, nursing pedagogist and prominent supporter of professionalization in German nursing based on scientific research, advocated for the

---

462 Eichhorn, "Grundgedanken zur Rationalisierung," 78–82.
463 Eichhorn, "Die betriebswirtschaftlichen Aspekte der Leistungssteigerung," 315–23.
464 See chapter 5.2; Rose, "Government, Authority and Expertise," 283–99; Tony P. Gilbert, "Trust and Managerialism: Exploring Discourses of Care," *Journal of Advanced Nursing* 52, no. 4 (2005), 454–63.

nursing process because it could visualize the scope or area of responsibility of nurses' work. She complained that nurses were not keen to present their work to the public in an understandable way. As she admitted: "Nurses preferred to perform nursing care rather than writing and talking about it."[465]

The issue of documenting nursing service has to be discussed critically. Documentation practice, especially in the structure of the nursing process that provides specific formulas for assessment, nursing care planning, recording interventions and reactions of the patient, is disentangled from the actual nursing situation. It should not be understood as a direct representation of what nurses (and the patient) did but more as a reality on its own which carries its own truth and logic. With documenting procedures, nursing actions become transparent and are transformed into an accounting activity. Nursing action then becomes constituted as an output-oriented and problem-solving service aiming at producing health. Hence, nursing documentation needs to be understood as an accounting procedure in which nursing action becomes accountable. This newly constituted reality of nursing service, consequently, becomes applicable to the neoliberal rationality, that is, it enables the governing of nurses (and the patient) in their actions and decisions on the mode of economy. Therefore, the written formulas that form nursing documentation are less of an image of the work of nurses and more a tool that constitutes the scope of practice and responsibilities of nurses.[466]

In the course of her cost-containment discussions, Grauhan constructed a dangerous picture of a nursing vocation in the future that does not record exactly and elaborately its actions and decisions. In this image, this nursing vocation could only provide poor nursing care since it would suffer from huge material and personnel shortcuts. "The discussion about benchmarking and the success of nursing services is urgent not only in Germany but in all European countries. The so-called cost-explosion forces us to think about potential savings in healthcare everywhere."[467] The nursing process, then, is presented as *the* instrument making

---

465 "Krankenschwestern haben es vorgezogen, Pflegedienst zu leisten anstatt darüber zu schreiben und zu reden" (Antje Grauhan and fellows, "Mittelfristiges WHO-Programm für Krankenpflege- und Hebammenwesen in Europa [Middle-Term Program of the Who Concerning Nursing and Midwifery in Europe]," *Krankenpflege* 32, no. 2 (1978), 67–68: 67; my translation).

466 See for the role of medical records: Marc Berg, "Practices of Reading and Writing: The Constitutive Role of the Patient Record in Medical Work," *Sociology of Health & Illness* 18, no. 4 (1996), 499–524; see for the crucial role of records in psychiatric care: Thomas Foth, *Caring and Killing. Nursing and Psychiatric Practice in Germany, 1931–1943* (Göttingen: V&R unipress, 2013).

467 "Die Diskussion über Maßstäbe zur Bewertung des Erfolgs pflegerischer Dienstleistungen ist heutzutage nicht nur in der Bundesrepublik, sondern in allen Ländern Europas dringlich. Überall zwingt die sogenannte Kostenexplosion im Gesundheitswesen zu Gedanken über

nursing work and its impact on the patient transparent. The possibility to evaluate nursing work based on clear and measurable defined nursing goals promised to create "hard" and understandable facts of the necessity and the benefit of good nursing service. Presenting a positive impact of nursing care to the public was especially important to make clear that the nursing vocation was valuable for society. In order to achieve this, it was necessary to implement the nursing process and focus on careful nursing documentation; to use epidemiological data; to produce transparent and verifiable data; to establish a special nursing vocabulary; and – most importantly – to make changes in nursing visible to the public.[468] Arguing in this way, it becomes clear that nursing, per se, is not accepted as an integral and important part of healthcare anymore unless it can make its importance understandable to lay people outside nursing. Hence, Grauhan urged nurses to develop and establish a language that transcribed nurses' work in simplified and measurable terms.

This shift in the public consciousness that now required nursing to become transparent was also characterized by Rosemary Donley, an American nursing scientist and pedagogist who wrote on human needs and the nursing process:

> During the 1970s, evaluation became a keyword in discussions about education and the health professions. In former times it was accepted that education, nursing, and medicine were good in themselves and worthy of support. These values are in transition and the work of these professions, and often of the professional himself (sic), is challenged and examined. In the health field, the loss of faith in professionals and institutions has had noticeable effects. Questions on the efficacy and effectiveness of treatments, once reserved for clinical trials of new drugs, are being raised about the length of stay in hospitals and use of certain surgical treatments.[469]

This need for evaluation has not only forced nurses into having their work evaluated, but it has also forced them to open their corpus of knowledge in order to have their work accepted and to demonstrate its value. Opening up this knowledge in nursing service worked in favour of the "de-mystification" of the nursing vocation as was demanded by German economist Siegfried Eichhorn.[470] But nurses themselves (see Grauhan's arguments above) were also eager to open up their knowledge to the public. The issues of de-mystification and increasing

---

Sparmöglichkeiten" (Grauhan and fellows, "Mittelfristiges Who-Programm," 67; my translation).
468 Grauhan and fellows, "Mittelfristiges Who-Programm," 67–68.
469 Rosemary Donley, "The Need for Rationality, Conceptualization, and Problem Solving," in *Human Needs 3 and the Nursing Process*, ed. Helen Yura and Mary B. Walsh (Norwalk, Conn.: Appleton-Century-Crofts, 1983), 85–116: 101.
470 Siegfried Eichhorn, "Zielkonflikte zwischen Leistungsfähigkeit, Wirtschaftlichkeit und Finanzierung der Krankenversorgung [Conflicts of Objectives between Performance, Efficiency and Financing of Healthcare]," *Das Krankenhaus* 66, no. 5 (1974), 186–96: 192.

transparency and standardization will be discussed in the following chapter under the perspective of professionalization.

Although calls were raised constantly to make nursing action transparent, it seems that nurses still struggled with their attempts to make their work visible and they experienced disadvantages in the hospital setting. In 1984, Weinrich blamed economic considerations in healthcare for the perception of nursing as a sacrificing vocation. Nurses faced increased demands in the hospital setting to take over more and more tasks without receiving more resources. She claimed that nursing should be recognized the same as any other group of hospital workers with the right to the same working conditions and performance-based salary. She repeated Grauhan's claims of the necessity to convince the public of the importance of nursing by showing them what nursing does:

> To this end, it is necessary to make nursing visible and present it in measurable terms as a human service which can only be seen as a whole. The extent of the services and the corresponding qualifications of nursing personnel [should be] determined based only on the care dependency of the human being. They have to be reflected in a goal-oriented and planned nursing care as it is already described in the nursing process.[471]

Weinrich hoped that this would come along with the development of a new self-awareness of nurses' own work and a badly needed raise of self-esteem in nurses themselves.[472]

Ingo Schomburg, nurse pedagogist, used this same argument when reporting on his own experiences in applying the nursing process in daily nursing care. Although he believed that there were several structural problems, he praised the fact that the steps of the nursing care plan and subsequent documentation enabled nurses to make visible and measurable their work. "Nursing documentation is a milestone which cannot be overstated when proving the work of nursing personnel to committees which are responsible to make decisions regarding nursing service."[473] He put hope in the instrument of the nursing process

---

471 "Dazu ist es notwendig, daß Krankenpflege sichtbar gemacht und messbar dargestellt wird als eine Dienstleistung am Menschen, die nur als Ganzes gesehen werden kann. Das Ausmaß der Leistungen und die dazu notwendigen Qualifikationen des Pflegepersonals werden allein durch die Pflegebedürftigkeit des Menschen bestimmt und müssen in gezielter und geplanter Pflege ihren Niederschlag finden, wie es bereits im Krankenpflegeprozeß beschrieben wird" (Rosemarie Weinrich, "Bedeutung und Stellenwert der Krankenpflege in unserer Gesellschaft [Role and Importance of Nursing Care in Our Society]," *Krankenpflege* 38, no. 1 (1984), 2–3: 3; my translation).
472 Weinrich, "Bedeutung und Stellenwert der Krankenpflege," 2–3.
473 "Die Pflegedokumentation ist der Meilenstein in der Argumentation, wenn es darum geht, die Arbeit des Krankenpflegepersonals anderen Gremien, die über uns entscheiden, nachdrücklich zu belegen" (Ingo Schomburg, "Pflegeplanung und ganzheitliche Pflege im Stationsalltag – Pflegemodellstation und Arbeiten mit dem Krankenpflegeprozeß [Nursing Care Plan and Holistic Care in the Daily Routine of the Ward: Training Ward and Working

to be the first step towards analyzing work which should, then, prove the intensity of nurses' work and could be used for new calculations for personnel demands.[474]

Nurse Sabine Thiel published an article in 1986 on the nursing care plan and nursing documentation, arguing that nurses themselves would be the fiercest opponents of nursing documentation because they believed they would not have enough time. The author listed all the advantages of using the nursing process that had been presented in the nursing journal for years: the guarantee of individualized nursing care, holistic nursing care, and improved flow of information. However, her strongest argument was that more and more patients would sue healthcare personnel and that it would be more often nurses and physicians themselves who had to prove that they provided good care, as opposed to earlier when it was the patient who had to show incorrect nursing and medical care.[475]

Hence, working in a transparent manner became conceptualized as the right mode through which to provide nursing care. It was constituted as good nursing care because it guaranteed a focus on individuality, and was considered a good healthcare service in the enterprise of "hospital" because it could articulate its personnel demands and its impact on the healing process of the patient in measurable and understandable terms. Moreover and very importantly, it was argued that nursing documentation was a legal instrument in order to prevent nurses, and hence, hospitals, from being sued. The argument can be understood in regard to the call for empowered patients. It can be seen both as a precondition of constituting an empowered patient – by making nursing service open to legal actions of the patient – and as a counter reaction– because healthcare services need to secure themselves against empowered patients. Here, the stability and "trust" in the relationship between patients and nurses is not established by nursing action based on proximity, experience, and empathy, but by the possibility of legal complaints. This removes the patient from a subordinate position to nurses and makes him/her able to evaluate and judge the healthcare received.

The argument of patients suing nurses legitimized even more the call for more visibility in nursing action, in which the nursing process played a specific role. On the one hand, the nursing process was appreciated as a possible way to reorganize nursing care and redirect its focus to healthy citizens in order to save money in a time of a so-called cost explosion in the healthcare system. On the other hand, the necessity of the nursing process was also explained with the need to make nurses' work visible and to save the nursing vocation from shortcuts in material and staff.

---

with the Nursing Process]," *Krankenpflege* 38, no. 7–8 (1984), 231, 236–38: 238; my translation).
474 Schomburg, "Pflegeplanung und ganzheitliche Pflege," 231, 236–38.
475 Sabine Thiel, "Pflegeplanung und Pflegedokumentation [Nursing Care Plan and Nursing Documentation]," *Krankenpflege* 40, no. 1 (1986), 9–12.

While the nursing process was valued as an instrument for saving costs, it was also appreciated as a measure to save the nursing vocation from the consequences of cost savings.

The Danger of Invisibility

Alongside the issue of more visibility, the scope of nursing practice, in general, was much discussed in the 1980s. More concretely, several articles were published on how to make the "right" nursing performances visible. Warnings forecasted that failing to hold onto certain activities in their scope of practice would make those activities disappear from nursing's field of responsibility. Consequently, as nursing scientist Sabine Bartholomeyczik asserted, there would be neither time nor resources for those activities anymore.[476] In those warnings, nurses and nursing were conceptualized as victims of health policy and the trend of financial constraints.

The reason why nursing activities would be in danger of disappearing were found (1) in the low self-perception of nurses which would perpetuate nurses' inability to successfully present their work; (2) in the problem that a lot of nursing activity could be ascribed to other workers in healthcare, to accountants, or patients' family members; (3) in the problem that nursing activity was not recognized as an integral part of nursing care by patients and other healthcare personnel or even from nurses themselves; (4) in the very nature of nursing work. Demands in nursing underwent a continuous flow and thus nurses themselves would have to constantly judge, decide, execute, evaluate, and adapt – hence, change – their activity. As soon as the patient's needs were satisfied, the work that had led to the satisfaction would lose its meaning – and would disappear.[477]

A solution to this danger of disappearing was seen in using the nursing process and in the expression of nurses' actions in well-defined activities covering everything in their work. The nursing process (applied to every patient) was conceptualized as the key element needed to sum up all single activities in order to make nurses' work visible. With the use of the nursing process the foundation of nursing care could be made explicit. Furthermore, writing down nursing actions would enable an understanding of their work and the ability to reconstruct nursing procedures afterwards. The steps of nursing documentation and the

---

[476] Sabine Bartholomeyczik, "Arbeitsplatz Krankenbett [Bedside Workplace]," *Krankenpflege* 41, no. 5 (1987), 158–61.

[477] Dittrich, "Pflege ist Leistung," 142–44; Weinrich, "Bedeutung und Stellenwert der Krankenpflege," 2–3; Bartholomeyczik, "Arbeitsplatz Krankenbett," 158–61; Antje Grauhan, "Berufsethische Normen in der Krankenpflege [Ethical Norms in Nursing]," *Krankenpflege* 39, no. 7–8 (1985), 231–33.

goal-oriented structure of the nursing process would enable nurses to demonstrate their performance.[478]

Activities in danger of disappearing from nurses' scope of practice were, for example, attention and listening to the patient, patient consultation, recognizing and answering needs and fears, and good body care.[479] Under the time pressures in daily nursing, those activities could lose their importance against the more visible tasks in nursing like correctly performed secretarial work [*Schreibtischarbeit*] and medical assistance. As one solution, Weinrich recommended that good quality patient-oriented care be a vocational norm in nursing rather than the number of visible performances of nurses, as well as thorough documentation [*ausführliche Dokumentation*] especially in times of stress and crisis.[480]

Attempts to establish a standardized terminology in nursing was also endangering those aspects of nursing and nursing work that were not "rational" or were non-verbalizable. A standardized terminology needs to be understandable and non-repetitive, able to recognize and cover familiar issues or issues of implicitness. In order to develop such a nursing language, Dittrich recommended using existing forms and documents in the hospital: "There is already a number of forms and models for nursing documentation which become increasingly easier, more exact, and more standardized."[481] She referred to examples of surgery protocols and accounting forms of health insurance companies. The author recommended adapting those documents to nursing. That means, accounting documents should not just be introduced into the nursing field but become a foundation for the establishment of a specific nursing language. Besides making nursing accountable, the application of such documents and development of a nursing language – not as a unique terminology but based on an already existing terminology of the hospital – could open possibilities of making connections between the management of a hospital and concrete nursing activities in order to calculate manpower requirements based on the calculated care needs of patients and corresponding nursing activities.[482] Such a standardized terminology and documentation system would certainly benefit nursing by integrating nursing

---

478 Dittrich, "Pflege ist Leistung," 142–44; Bartholomeyczik, "Arbeitsplatz Krankenbett," 158–61.
479 Rosemarie Weinrich, "Rechtsnormen und ethische Normen in der Krankenpflege [Legal Norms and Ethical Norms in Nursing]," *Krankenpflege* 39, no. 7–8 (1985), 234–36; Bartholomeyczik, "Arbeitsplatz Krankenbett," 158–61.
480 Weinrich, "Rechtsnormen und ethische Normen," 234–36.
481 "Es gibt bereits eine Reihe von Vordrucken und Mustern für die Pflegedokumentation, die immer einfacher, genauer und einheitlicher werden" (Dittrich, "Pflege ist Leistung," 144; my translation).
482 Dittrich, "Pflege ist Leistung," 142–44.

service into the economic structure of a hospital and avoiding the danger of completely disappearing.

But Dittrich not only discussed needing the nursing process to avoid the danger of disappearing but she also emphasized that its use had a beneficial aspect to the development of the nursing vocation itself. Being able to retrace nursing procedures would increase knowledge and competence of nurses and nursing leaders, and improve education, research, and science. According to the author, it would also improve the self-esteem of nurses as well as awareness of their performance, and increase their work satisfaction.[483] Hence, Dittrich saw another danger in the way that the nursing vocation might not develop further and might receive unmotivated members when nurses themselves did not acknowledge their work by making it visible.

However, a nursing documentation that is based on administrative forms of the enterprise hospital has to be written in objective and positivistic terms. Transcribing nursing experience into objective terms negates the recognition of implicit knowledge and non-verbalizable structures, which can hardly be considered in this kind of standardized documentation.[484] For example, some emotional aspects of nursing care are often not recognized anymore as parts of professional nursing.[485]

In summary, nurses viewed the issue of visibility critically, and drew especially on the dangers of leaving nursing activities invisible. Although some authors expressed some reservations regarding the call for visibility,[486] the trend itself was not dismissed. Rather, it was noted that tasks such as office work or medical assistance were made visible but activities such as caring for the patient empathetically, and listening and responding to him or her, were being ignored. "Not

---

483 Dittrich, "Pflege ist Leistung," 142–44.
484 Marie Heartfield, "Nursing Documentation and Nursing Practice: A Discourse Analysis," *Journal of Advanced Nursing* 24, no. August (1996), 98–103; Patricia Benner and Christine Tanner, "Clinical Judgement: How Expert Nurses Use Intuition," *American Journal of Nursing* 87, no. 1 (1987), 23–31; Susanne Kreutzer, "Krankenbeobachtung. Zur Entwertung einer pflegerischen Schlüsselkompetenz in der Bundesrepublik und Schweden nach 1945 [Patient Observation: About the Devaluation of a Key Competence in Nursing in the Federal Republic of Germany and Sweden after 1945]," in *Gesundheit/Krankheit. Kulturelle Differenzierungsprozesse um Körper, Geschlecht und Macht in Skandinavien*, ed. Lill-Ann Körber and Stefanie von Schnurbein, Berliner Beiträge zur Skandinavistik, Bd. 16 (Berlin: Nordeuropa-Institut, 2010), 167–88.
485 André Büssing and Jürgen Glaser, "Arbeitsbelastungen, Burnout und Interaktionsstress im Zuge der Reorganisation des Pflegesystems [Workload, Burnout, and Interaction Stress in the Course of the Reorganization of Nursing Systems]," in *Dienstleistungsqualität und Qualität des Arbeitslebens im Krankenhaus*, ed. André Büssing und Jürgen Glaser (Göttingen, Bern, Toronto, Seattle: Hogrefe-Verlag, 2003), 101–29.
486 Grauhan, "Berufsethische Normen," 231–33; Dittrich, "Der Terminal auf der Station," 278–79.

the *quantity* of visible performances but the *quality* of good patient-centred nursing care should be the vocational norm," Antje Grauhan argued.[487] Rather than advocating against the trend towards visibility, these nurses argued for making the "real" tasks of nursing visible, such as giving attention to the patient by washing and talking with him or her.

7.2.2 Control

The issue of control was often presented as one of the reasons why the nursing process would be needed to improve nursing care. The nursing process promised to enable control both from an external perspective in the sense of visibility, transparency, and ultimately accountability, and from an internal perspective of the nurses themselves. Hence, it can be seen as a disciplinary tool to make nurses act in the "right" way. In 1977, an article explicitly discussing the concept of control compared two different concepts of it. The concept "trust is good, control is better"[488] was dismissed because of the strong focus on hierarchical observation. The second concept was based on cybernetics and was favoured by the authors. They defined control as a "principle of organization and regulation in terms of a value-free gathering of [results] to be able to interfere in a goal-oriented way."[489] Although in this article the nursing process as such was not named at all, the authors recommended understanding control as a principle of nurses' work and applying the cybernetic structure to all working areas in nursing: to the material aspects of ward work such as the functionality and appropriateness of drugs and other working material; to the organizational aspects such as information flow, nursing or shift plans, rational forms and effective work processes [*Arbeitsabläufe*]; to the personnel aspects such as responsibilities of the individual nurse, nursing skills, nursing education on the ward; and to the nursing care of the patient such as evaluating nursing goals on the basis of nursing reports.

Hence, cybernetic logic and its inherent concept of control were presented as applicable to highly different types of nurses' work. As benefits of this kind of

---

487 "Nicht die *Quantität* der sichtbaren Leistungen, sondern die *Qualität* einer guten patientenzentrierten Pflege sollte die berufliche Norm sein" (Grauhan, "Berufsethische Normen," 234; italics in original; my translation).
488 "Vertrauen ist gut, Kontrolle ist besser" (Rada Mrda and Josef Göbbels, "Kontrolle – Zur Diskussion gestellt [Control: An Issue for Discussion]," *Krankenpflege* 31, no. 4 (1977), 136–37: 136; my translation).
489 "Kontrolle ist so gesehen Ordnungs- und Steuerungsprinzip im Sinne von wertfreiem Erfassen von Entwicklungsergebnissen bzw. Zwischenergebnissen, um erforderlichenfalls zielorientiert einwirken zu können" (Mrda and Göbbels, "Kontrolle," 136; my translation).

control, the authors predicted a lower number of mistakes and therefore, an increase of quality in nursing. But they also saw a kind of "democratic" control, meaning that it was not directed from a specific person or position, such as a leader who stands outside of this control, but at everybody in the organization, including the leadership.[490] This understanding of control as a cybernetic regulation is separated from the individual. It has its origin in the cybernetic structure, and not in a leader, which makes it an impersonal structure, apparently value-free, and, consequently, hard to criticize. Moreover, the nurses themselves implement and use this controlling structure as part of self-responsibilization and self-governing. They are not subordinated to a leader who tells them what to do, when work has to be done, in what manner and to what outcome. But nurses themselves organize their work and, based on the cybernetic structure, control their activity. From the perspective of neoliberal governmentality, this kind of control constitutes nurses as self-responsible actors who receive the space and structure to identify themselves with the objectives of the healthcare organization they work in. Within flat hierarchies, nurses become empowered and activated to decide and act "freely" within this cybernetic control. That means, this kind of control fosters creative nurses whose individual objectives are in line with the goals of the hospital. The freedom of those nurses, however, should not be understood as a total freedom but rather as a defined space based on the economic logic in which they are encouraged to pursue their adapted aims and to develop new projects.

Moreover, the control of other healthcare vocations or professions is also possible. Cybernetic logic enables a close collaboration with other workers. It is not only nurses' work that becomes transparent to physicians, therapists, etc., but the strategic language based on input, process, output, and the cybernetic logic can be found in other working areas as well. An example is the therapeutic process that is used for clinical reasoning in other vocations like the physical therapists. It too follows the cybernetic logic and, hence, is very similar to the nursing process.[491] Hence, this cybernetic framework allows a more precise and concrete interaction between different healthcare professionals.[492] Creating strategic plans with other healthcare workers is structurally supported in order to

---

490 Mrda and Göbbels, "Kontrolle," 136–37.
491 E.g. WCPT, "Position Statement of the World Confederation for Physical Therapy," 2007, https://www.wcpt.org/sites/wcpt.org/files/files/WCPT_Description_of_Physical_Therapy-Sep07-Rev_2.pdf.
492 See also an example in which "Cybernetic Communication" in nursing homes is recommended to ensure effective and timely communication between physicians and nurses although despite time constraints: Taghrid Chaaban et al. "Cybernetic Communications: Focusing Interactions on Goal-Centered Care," *Nursing Science Quarterly* 34, no. 1 (2021), 30–32.

produce healthy patients. This collaboration, now called multi-professionalism, was already foreseen by Dorothy Hall in the 1970s.[493]

Control of nurses' work happens especially through documentation and evaluation of nursing care. For example, every entry on a chart has to be signed. This signature becomes an important foundation of control for several reasons: every nurse signing the interventions to be completed feels more responsible for what he/she has done, the signing nurse is accountable for any problems or questions that emerge in regard to the planned or documented care, and it shows the work to be done and could be a starting point to measure the actual and the anticipated workload.[494] This sense of control is even stronger when nurses work in group care, in which one nurse is responsible for planning and executing all of the care for a specific group of patients. In this concept, the nurse-patient relationship becomes more intense. In consequence, as nursing teacher Erika Lingenberg stated, nurses tend to put more control on themselves and "may work more accurately."[495] They will more likely follow the established nursing care plan. The organization of nursing care in patient groups on the ward was and still is presented as the ideal in nursing.

A strong emphasis is laid on the step of evaluation when it comes to the aspect of control. However, the careful development and documentation of the nursing care plan and nursing goals are an important foundation for the evaluation of nursing care. Hence, in order to control and evaluate nursing action, it is important to document the "kind and extent of interventions with the reasoning for the choice of interventions [in order to evaluate] the success."[496]

The nursing process is conceptualized as an improvement for nursing in three ways: it would make nursing accountable and integrable into the enterprise hospital; it would develop nursing further in a professional sense, and it would foster the satisfaction of nurses with their work. Since it appeared to be a solution to all of the three problematizations that occurred in nursing at that time, the nursing process could hardly be ignored or even rejected by nurses. The interesting perception here is that accountability in nursing and, as such, a loss of

---

493 Dorothy C. Hall, "Überlegungen zum Krankenpflegeberuf [Considerations About the Nursing Vocation]," *Krankenpflege* 31, no. 2 (1977), 40–42.
494 Cornelia Send, "Mittel für die Durchführung der individuellen Pflege (III) [Instruments for Providing Individual Nursing Care III]," *Krankenpflege* 29, no. 9 (1975), 368.
495 "Kontroll*möglichkeit* schließt natürlich auch die des Personals ein. Diese Tatsache mag einige veranlassen, sorgfältiger zu arbeiten" (Erika Lingenberg, "Gruppenpflege – Ergebnis eines Arbeitsgesprächs [Nursing Care in Groups: Results of a Working Meeting]," *Krankenpflege* 34, no. 4 (1980), 118–22: 120; italics in original; my translation).
496 "Gute Beispiele haben wir in Krankengeschichten, Operationsprotokollen, Abrechnungsformularen für Krankenkassen – in der Art gleich, im Inhalt der Pflege angepaßt, muß die Dokumentation Art und Umfang der Maßnahmen mit Begründung und Erfolgsauswertung angeben" (Dittrich, "Pflege ist Leistung," 144; my translation).

autonomy within the vocation to an external control, was connected with an increase of professional competence and higher self-esteem of the members of the profession. It was promised that both would go hand in hand.

7.2.3 Quality

During the course of increasing discussions surrounding cost-containment interventions in the 1970s, a concern over humanism in hospitals emerged. Special training programs were advertised for further education under topics such as "Methods for Humanization of the Hospital: Individual Nursing Care"[497] or "Humanity in the Hospital," which contained sessions on "the individual nursing care plan" [*individuelle Pflegeplanung*], and "Humanity and nursing aspects under an economical saving perspective in the hospital" [*"Humanität und pflegerische Aspekte unter wirtschaftlich sparsamen Gesichtspunkten im Krankenhaus"*].[498] Although a specific definition of humanism was not provided in the nursing articles, it was always conceptualized as being contrary to economization, rationalization, and the mechanization of healthcare. As theologist Werner Wehrenpfenning had stated in 1966 in the hospital journal *Das Krankenhaus*: "[T]he danger of dehumanization of the hospital caused by rationalization and mechanization of the hospital operation ... [is] ... that the hospital unnoticeably deforms itself to a 'health factory' through technology which resists any form of inspiration or animation."[499]

The nursing process and its elements were conceptualized as factors of relief to the policies of increasing economization in the hospital setting. In the hectic daily work of hospital routines, the nursing process would still enable the provision of individualized nursing care through its tracking system. This systematic procedure would guarantee quality nursing care even in a three-shift system with fluctuation of nursing staff, shorter working hours, and a relatively high number

---

497 "Methoden zur Humanisierung des Krankenhauses: Individuelle Pflege I [Methods to Humanize the Hospital: Individual Nursing Care, Part I]," *Krankenpflege* 27, no. 6 (1974), 252: 252.
498 "Humanität im Krankenhaus" (DBfK, "Bremen, Hamburg und Schleswig-Holstein," 132; my translation).
499 "[D]ie Gefahr der Dehumanisierung des Krankenhauses, hervorgerufen durch Rationalisierung und Technisierung des Krankenhausbetriebes [...] ist, daß das Krankenhaus sich unmerklich durch die jeder Art Beseeltheit widerstehenden Technik zur 'Gesundheitsfabrik' verformt" (Werner Wehrenpfennig, "Krankenhäuser an zwei Fronten engagiert. Gedanken zum Hauptthema des vierten deutschen Krankenhaustages "Leistungssteigerung im Krankenhaus durch Zusammenarbeit" [Hospitals Engaged on Two Frontiers: Thoughts on the Topic of the Fourth German Hospital Day "Increasing Performance in the Hospital through Collaboration"]," *Das Krankenhaus* 58, no. 5 (1966), 168–70: 169; my translation).

of part-time nurses.[500] Hence, if humanism was enabled in healthcare at the same time as dehumanizing structures and procedures were being implemented, there was no need to stop this economization. Almost two decades later, Claudia Bischoff emphasized in her dissertation that patient-oriented care might be misused as a "human alibi towards the critics from outside in order to maintain all conditions and structures which make nursing care inhuman."[501]

In order to achieve a satisfactory level of nursing care, nurses were called on to provide high-quality information, meaning properly written reports in which nurses expressed themselves clearly and limited themselves to the essentials in regard to nursing goals.[502] A high-quality report from one shift to the next was deemed necessary to let everybody know about the planned care and its goals, to evaluate the success or effects of interventions, to avoid nursing errors, to optimize nursing care, and to decrease the duration of hospitalization.[503]

Quality in nursing, therefore, until the 1970s, was strongly connected to the idea of humanism as described above. Hence, quality in care was conceptualized as a countermeasure to ease the economic pressures that had an impact on this care. However, by the 1980s and on, the idea of quality became increasingly understood in economic terms. The emergence of this new understanding of quality coincided with its use more often in the nursing journals. Quality became a component of a commercial service, containing within it the criterion of efficiency, meaning that it shifted from a component to ease the consequences of economization to a component of economization. The concept of quality assurance was tied to cost reductions in healthcare. Quality assurance was developed in the US because the healthcare system there called for a higher financial contribution from patients. Hence, American patients were thought to be more

---

[500] Cornelia Send, "Mittel für die Durchführung der individuellen Pflege (I) [Instruments for Providing Individual Nursing Care I]," *Krankenpflege* 29, no. 7 (1975), 274; Margit Schellenberg, "Die Bedeutung einer patientenorientierten Pflegeplanung [The Importance of a Patient-Oriented Nursing Care Plan]," *Krankenpflege* 31, no. 9 (1977), 291–93; Hohlin, "Notwendigkeit der Adaption der Krankenhäuser," 287–90; Hohlin, "Neue Horizonte," 13–14.

[501] "Unter den gegebenen Bedingungen ist zu vermuten, daß hinter der "unzeitgemäßen" Forderung nach Patientenorientierter Pflege auch noch andere als humane, patientenbezogene Interessen stehen: daß nämlich Krankenhaus und Medizin die Patientenorientierte Pflege als humanes Alibi gegenüber Kritik von außen (miß-)brauchen, um alle diejenigen Bedingungen und Strukturen aufrechtzuerhalten, die die Krankenversorgung erst inhuman machen" (Claudia Bischoff, *Frauen in der Krankenpflege: Zur Entwicklung von Frauenrolle und Frauenberufstätigkeit im 19. und 20. Jahrhundert [Women in Nursing: About the Development of the Female Role and Female Employment in the 19th and 20th Century]*, vol. 3rd (Frankfurt am Main; New York: Campus-Verlag, 1997), 11; my translation.

[502] Schellenberg, "Die Bedeutung einer patientenorientierten Pflegeplanung," 291–93.

[503] Renate Reimann, "Information im Dienst des Kranken [Information at Patient Service]," *Krankenpflege* 33, no. 7/8 (1979), 249–53.

critical about quality in healthcare. However, "even in European countries now increasing financial costs in the healthcare system have led [us] to consider and initiate quality assurance of medical and nursing performances."[504]

Quality assurance was a concept that also enabled hospitals to compete with each other. In order to be competitive, the healthcare institution needed to increase quality or at least guarantee a stable quality of its work. Factors said to increase or guarantee the quality were an increase in efficiency and a more stringent cost reduction. The development of programs of quality assurance in healthcare called for standardized procedures, such as nursing care based on the nursing process with its sophisticated and practicable documentation system, the development of practicable evaluation criteria that were easy to use, and distinct criteria and standards for medical and nursing performances.[505] The nursing process is thus deeply embedded in the aims of quality assurance and, hence, was a precondition of establishing a competitive hospital that provided a more efficient and more economical healthcare. Here, efficiency and economical healthcare became equated with quality in healthcare. Hence, quality in the 1980s became a new role in the hospital setting. It was not conceptualized anymore as opposite or complementary to efficiency and cost-saving, nor was it presented as something to possibly ease the dire consequences of cost-savings such as poor nursing care. Rather, it became something through which to develop an efficient and inexpensive nursing care. Effective, cost-conscious, and efficient nursing care came to be understood as high quality nursing.

7.3 Digitalization

From the middle of the 1980s on, computing in nursing became more prevalent and discussions occurred on whether and how to connect daily nursing care with a hospital-wide electronic communication system. All the articles discussing computing in nursing and its application through the nursing process aimed to encourage nurses to participate in the development and in the introduction of electronic programs into the nursing area. "We are not able to stop this devel-

---

504 "Auch in den europäischen Ländern haben in heutiger Zeit die steigenden Kosten im Gesundheitswesen dazu geführt, verstärkt über Qualitätssicherung medizinischer und pflegerischer Leistungen im Gesundheitsdienst nachzudenken und initiativ zu werden" (Karin Heuwer and Helga Laurinat, "Qualitätssicherung medizinischer und pflegerischer Leistungen im Gesundheitsdienst [Quality Assurance of Medical and Nursing Performances in the Healthcare Service]," *Krankenpflege* 39, no. 7–8 (1985), 238 & 42: 239; my translation).
505 Heuwer and Laurinat, "Qualitätssicherung," 238 & 42.

opment, but it is our responsibility to make those very expensive systems useful to nursing. We do not have a lot of time left."[506]

Two different arguments can be found: One was the hope to ease the workload for nurses because computing programs would run administrative tasks. It was connected to the promise to have more time for the patient (Merkel, 1984). The other argument, very central in the articles, was rather a warning: if nurses did not participate in the development of such programs it would cause negative consequences. The predicted consequences were either that nursing would not benefit from the positive effects of computerization;[507] would not have its interests considered;[508] that nursing activities that were not integrated into the electronic system would disappear from the official scope of nursing practice;[509] or that administrative activities already done by nurses would make nurses the main people operating the computing system on the ward.[510]

Here, the need for being visible became even more pertinent. The issue that nursing still lacked a concrete definition of what it was and a distinct corpus of nursing activities predicted an even greater danger as the hospital setting became computerized. Having only the visible part of a scope of practice become digitalized would likely result in a situation in which only digitalized activities could be counted as the scope of practice. The digitalization of information leads to a new reality and defines what belongs to this reality and what does not belong to it. Digitalized material such as that digitalized from a system of nursing documentation might become even more powerful than paper-written job-descriptions. Non-digitalized activities that fall out of a scope of practice might become non-existent in this new reality. This becomes even more possible if the computer system combines nursing documentation with calculations of personnel costs, as was recommended in the hospital journal *Das Krankenhaus* in 1990.[511]

---

506 "Wir werden die Entwicklung nicht aufhalten können, aber daß diese dann vorhandenen, sehr teuren Systeme auch für die Krankenpflege von Nutzen sind, liegt an uns. Sehr viel Zeit haben wir nicht mehr" (Rupert Ringelhann, "Eindrücke von der Interhospital '85 in Düsseldorf [Impressions from the Interhospital '85 in Dusseldorf]," *Krankenpflege* 39, no. 7–9 (1985), 236–38: 238; my translation).
507 Ringelhann, "Eindrücke von der Interhospital '85 in Düsseldorf," 236–38.
508 Christa Merkel, "Können Arbeitserleichterungen im Pflegebereich durch verbesserte Informationsweitergabe (EDV) erwartet werden? [Can an Ease of Work Be Expected in Nursing Thanks to a Better Information Flow (Computing)?]," *Krankenpflege* 38, no. 9 (1984), 282–84.
509 Dittrich, "Der Terminal auf der Station," 278–79.
510 Dittrich, "Der Terminal auf der Station," 278–79.
511 Jörg Lanig and Günther Hanke, "PIK – Ein Bund-Länder EDV-Verfahren für den Pflegedienst im Krankenhaus [PIK – A Federal-'Länder' Computing Procedure for Nursing Service in the Hospital]," *Das Krankenhaus* 82, no. 3 (1990), 131–34.

The benefits of digitalization in nursing were seen in the possibility of making nursing performance visible, to have data available at the moment of decision, to categorize patients according to their nursing demands and dependency, to link this information with time values derived from observations, and to calculate and assign personnel.[512] Hence, much data would be available both for the daily work on the ward that was based on patient demand and for the general planning of the roster. According to Dittrich, about 80 percent would be foreseeable and only 20 percent of new data would need to be regularly retrieved.[513]

Therefore, with the increasing pressure of digitalization, nurses were more and more forced to define their scope of practice and to identify all the activities it contained. Moreover, those activities needed to be articulated very concretely and in a unified form to make them digitizable.[514] However, here as well the nursing process with its cybernetic and problem-solving structure fit into a computing system. In an introductory article about computing in nursing care, computer programming was compared to the problem-solving process. This process, according to the author, could be compared with any problem-solving process found anywhere in daily life: "As the problem of 'how do I prepare a Rhenish Sauerbraten?' can be solved with the help of a recipe, and the problem of 'how do I knit a winter sweater' with a knitting guideline, also the computer has to receive a series of instructions which will lead to the desired outcome."[515]

Dittrich was sure that the introduction of the logic of computing into nursing as such would not be a huge problem:

> All the people working in the hospital are managers and work according to this principle, that means determining the actual situation, setting realistic goals for the target state, planning, executing, evaluating. The nursing procedure follows the very same

---

512 Dittrich, "Der Terminal auf der Station," 278–79; Participants of a continuing education course, "EDV in der Krankenpflege – Chance oder Bedrohung [Computing in Nursing: Chance or Threat?]," *Krankenpflege* 38, no. 9 (1984), 304–06; J. G. Veldhorst-Groenewegen and G. van der Reep, "EVA – Ein patientenorientiertes Instrumtent für Pflegeadministration [EVA: A Patient-Oriented Tool for Nursing Administration]," *Krankenpflege* 38, no. 9 (1984), 301–04; Merkel, "Können Arbeitserleichterungen im Pflegebereich durch verbesserte Informationsweitergabe (EDV) erwartet werden?," 282–84.
513 Dittrich, "Der Terminal auf der Station," 278–79.
514 Participants of a continuing education course, "EDV in der Krankenpflege," 304–06.
515 "Wie man z. B. das Problem "Wie bereite ich einen rheinischen Sauerbraten zu?" mit Hilfe eines Rezeptes lösen kann und wie man das Problem "Wie stricke ich mir einen Winterpulli?" mit Hilfe einer Strickanleitung bewältigen kann, so muß auch der Computer eine Folge von Anweisungen erhalten, die dann zum gewünschten Ergebnis führen" (Roland Trill, "Grundlagen der EDV – Eine Einführung für Krankenpflegekräfte [Basics of Computing: An Introduction for Nurses]," *Krankenpflege* 38, no. 9 (1984), 279–81: 280; my translation.

pattern and starts with the assessment of nursing demands: setting the goal – planning; executing – evaluating, all in cooperation with the patient.[516]

Hence, the cybernetic, goal-oriented structure, according to Dittrich, underlay all procedures in the hospital, and the nursing process, as the regulatory cycle for nursing care, would ease the way for nursing care to become digitalized.

Moreover, the nursing process was said to guarantee the individualized presentation of each patient within the standardized terminology of a computing system. It was argued that patients with their individual healthcare problems could be translated into single nursing processes. These processes already contained the standardized steps and cybernetic logic and could be easily inscribed into the standardized structure of the computing program. Hence, the computing program, then, consists of many single cybernetic working projects which can be organized based on their inputs (patients caring needs) and their outputs (becoming healthy after such and such nursing task).[517] This understanding of digitalized individual nursing care has its roots in the argument that the nursing process enables the provision of patient-oriented and individual nursing care. As a consequence, it was logical to believe "that the individual situation of the patient [could] be clearly demonstrated in these frames."[518]

However, the potential for individually oriented nursing care from computerized planning of nursing care can be questioned. In a qualitative study published in 1990, American nurses argued that they were forced to pick already preformulated phrases from a list to create a nursing care plan rather than write their own thoughts based on the individual situation of the patient. It was too time-consuming to deal with all the error messages that resulted, something that did not happen when they used the pre-programmed digitalized phrases. Using only the pre-digitalized phrases, however, makes the nursing care plan more a sum of entries that fit the best available rather than a plan that fits the patient.[519]

In conclusion, while the digitalization of nursing care makes manifest the cybernetic organization in which it is now understood that nursing has to take

---

516 "Sie alle im Krankenhaus Tätigen sind Manager und arbeiten daher nach dem Management-Prinzip, d.h. Feststellung des Ist-Zustanden, realistische Zielsetzung des Soll-Zustandes, Planung, Durchführung, Auswertung. Der Pflegevorgang folgt genau diesem Muster und beginnt mit der Erhebung des Pflegebedarfes: Zielsetzung – Planung; Durchführung – Auswertung, alles in Zusammenarbeit mit dem Patienten selbst" (Dittrich, "Der Terminal auf der Station," 279; my translation).
517 Veldhorst-Groenewegen and van der Reep, "EVA," 301–04.
518 "Wir glauben, daß die individuelle Situation des Patienten voll in diesen Formen deutlich gemacht werden kann" (Veldhorst-Groenewegen and van der Reep, "EVA," 303; my translation).
519 L. Barbara Harris, "Becoming Deprofessionalized: One Aspect of the Staff Nurse's Perspective on Computer-Mediated Nursing Care Plans," *Advances in Nursing Science* 13, no. 2 (1990), 63–74.

place, it also reinforces the fact that certain components of nursing cannot be made visible, thus calling into question the idea of transparency. Computing systems need a clearly distinctive and rationalized language through which they can be programmed. Hence, making nursing care visible in a computer system and constituting it as a real image of nursing care (upon which nursing care can be judged, measured, and calculated) leads to strong pressure for nurses and patients to adapt to this computerized image.[520] German nursing scientist Manfred Hülsken-Giesler calls this the "mechanization of nursing care."[521]

7.4 Accountable Nursing – A Summary

The nursing process enabled dissecting nursing actions into distinct tasks and structuring them into a manageable and transparent cycle. Hence, it led to a fragmentation of nursing service and made this service measurable. Former non-visible activities in nursing were made transparent and enabled the establishment of hospitals and other health enterprises by integrating accounting terminology and an economic logic into nursing. Understanding nursing service in the language of accounting led to the constitution of nursing as an activity of accounting. In consequence, nursing could become transformed into a commercial service which is (and wants to be) accountable, controllable, and cost-conscious. Nurses appreciated this change as a chance to eventually show the public, physicians, managers, and themselves the content, impact, and value of nursing care. By doing that, nurses followed the neoliberal call to disclose their knowledge and to implement mechanisms of distrust such as the nursing process.

The nursing process was constituted as a core tool to provide efficient healthcare services – and not just for nurses. It was argued to be a concept valid for all working people in the hospitals such as a physicians, who should partly base their diagnosis and treatment plans on nursing information.[522] With the constitution of the nursing process as the core or essence of modern nursing service, nursing became construed differently: It was no longer a diffuse assemblage of different tasks that could not be analyzed but rather a well-defined

---

520 See for the US context Harris, "Becoming Deprofessionalized," 63–74 or Carol Romano, Kathleen A. McCormick, and Linda McNeely, "Nursing Documentation: A Model for a Computerized Data Base," *Advances in Nursing Science*, no. 1 (1982), 43–56.
521 "Maschinisierung der Pflege" (Manfred Hülsken-Giesler, *Der Zugang zum Anderen. Zur theoretischen Rekonstruktion von Professionalisierungsstrategien pflegerischen Handelns im Spannungsfeld von Mimesis und Maschinenlogik [Access to and Approach of the Other: For a Theoretical Reconstruction of Professionalization Strategies of Nursing Care in the Tension between Mimesis and Machine Logic]*, ed. Hartmut Remmers, vol. 3, Pflegewissenschaft und Pflegebildung (Göttingen: V&R unipress, 2008), 283; my translation).
522 Veldhorst-Groenewegen and van der Reep, "EVA," 301–04.

combination of identifiable and distinct components that could be analyzed and separated from each other – and at the end could be related to monetary values. The nursing process as an accounting tool could restructure nursing service in such a way that it became applicable to the administrative organization and made nurses in their work accountable.

However, nurses also recognized the problems in trying to verbalize all nursing activity in objective, rational, and even digitizable terms. One of the aims of defining a distinct modern scope of practice and of strengthening nurses' autonomy was to develop a discrete nursing terminology which would need, however, to follow the rational and cybernetic logic of the nursing process. The nursing process, more and more, became synonymous with nursing care and was proposed to frame nurses' scope of practice. As a recent quantitative study on the professional perception of German nurses in hospitals reveals, aspects such as social and emotional compassion become less and less acknowledged as part of this scope of practice.[523]

The negative consequences of the reduction of complexity, of the dominance of rationality, and the introduction of external controls were rarely discussed in the nursing journal *Krankenpflege*. Rather, it was argued that an accountable nursing vocation was a better vocation than it had been before. In the next chapter, I will analyze the impact of the nursing process on the development of the nursing vocation, on its agenda of professionalization, and on its self-perception as a nursing profession.

---

523 Bernard Braun, "Auswirkung der DRGs auf die Versorgungsqualität und Arbeitsbedingungen im Krankenhaus [Impact of DRGs on the Quality of Care and Working Conditions in the Hospital]," in *20 Jahre Wettbewerb im Gesundheitswesen. Theoretische und empirische Analysen zur Ökonomisierung von Medizin und Pflege*, ed. Alexandra Manzei and Rudi Schmiede (Wiesbaden: Springer Fachmedien, 2014), 91–113.

Chapter 8:
The Impact of the Nursing Process on the Concept of Professionalism in Nursing

Nurses in the nursing journal *Krankenpflege* ascribed great hopes to the nursing process, ranging from the improvement of nursing care for the patient to the achievement of autonomy and professionalism in nursing. It is important to note that the subordination of the nursing vocation under economic constraints and the striving for professionalization in nursing developed interdependently and belong to the same hybrid nursing discourse. I will show in this chapter that the understanding of what a profession is became redefined with the implementation of the nursing process. Nurses themselves, starting with Dorothy C. Hall, promoted this redefined understanding of professionalism. However, they did not realize that the perception of profession they were promoting was totally different from the traditional concept of the classic professions, that it was, even more, the exact opposite of what physicians' understanding was of professionalism. It is this new understanding of professions on which the professionalization project of German nurses is built. And still today, German nurses promote this understanding when they call for the professionalization of nursing.

The Narrative of a Weak Nursing Vocation

The question is, why were nurses so willing to implement an accounting tool such as the nursing process with the hope of professionalizing? Why did they even start the project of professionalization? It is interesting to ask this because the medical profession, with its traditional understanding of professionalization, fought against accounting mechanisms and tried to resist neoliberal attempts to open the enclosure of medical knowledge.

I argue that the appreciation of nurses for this new development is based on a specific perception that nurses have regarding their own vocation. As nursing scientists Sioban Nelson and Suzanne Gordon show, nurses constantly deny their past accomplishments. Nurses in former times, as the authors state, thought critically, had a lot of responsibility, and found solutions in critical times in order to care for patients, helping them to heal and to survive. However, regardless of these contributions to nursing and their positive impact throughout time, Nelson and Gordon argue that nurses have tended to ignore their past or label it as "bad" nursing. This has provided nurses with a reason to argue that today they should move away from their past in order to improve or professionalize nursing. In consequence, so Nelson and Gordon contend, nursing seems to reinvent itself constantly and does not build on its past accomplishments.[524]

I found something similar happening in the articles of the nursing journal *Krankenpflege*. Between the 1960s and the 1980s, they created an image that nurses had been under medical power for several decades. The Christian character of nursing as the traditional foundation in German nursing was constructed as the opposite of professional nursing. As it was argued, the Christian call for obedience and submissiveness had led to a weak nursing vocation, which was predestinated to be subordinate to the medical profession.[525]

However, it was not clear for how long nurses had lost their "actual" focus or if a specific event had occurred after which the nursing vocation had become subordinated. What specific information was provided was connected to the "actual" scope of practice, referencing Florence Nightingale.[526] It seems that a historical narrative was created in the nursing journal that romanticized the time in which Florence Nightingale was an active nurse. Her definition of nursing was used as the "actual" content of nursing. The call for redirecting or refocusing nursing in the 1970s and 1980s became connected to the claim to modernize nursing. The necessity of modernizing nursing was argued on the basis of new scientific knowledge and technical and medical innovations, which required an expanded scope of practice in nursing and the introduction and use of sciences.[527] This, ultimately, led to the process that is now called "professionalization" in German nursing.

The image of a subordinated Christian nursing has been strongly criticized, since Christian nurses saw themselves with a distinct scope of autonomous practice and as complementary partners with physicians in healthcare. With the

---

524 Sioban Nelson and Suzanne Gordon, "The Rhetoric of Rupture: Nursing as a Practice with a History?," *Nursing Outlook* 52, no. 5 (2004), 255–61.
525 Rosemarie Weinrich, "Bedeutung und Stellenwert der Krankenpflege in unserer Gesellschaft [Role and Importance of Nursing Care in Our Society]," *Krankenpflege* 38, no. 1 (1984), 2–3; Sabine Bartholomeyczik, "Gesundheit als Voraussetzung patientenorientierter Krankenpflege [Health as a Precondition for Patient-Oriented Nursing Care]," *Krankenpflege* 40, no. 5 (1986), 178–80.
526 E.g. Weinrich, "Bedeutung und Stellenwert der Krankenpflege," 2–3.
527 Rosemarie Weinrich, "Der Wandel im bisher üblichen Verständnis von Krankenpflege [The Change in the Common Perception of Nursing]," *Krankenpflege* 35, no. 4 (1981), 156–58; Claudia Bischoff and Bernd Wanner, "Krankenpflege an der Hochschule? [Nursing at University?]," *Krankenpflege* 38, no. 2 (1984), 64–66.

disappearance of the Christian foundation in nursing care, this distinct scope of practice vanished, leaving nurses without any image other than as a physician's assistant.[528] The narrative that established nursing as a traditionally weak vocation, however, ignored the contributions and status of Christian nursing, but rather criticized it and instead praised the introduction of science and rationality into nursing via the nursing process as a precondition for modernization and professionalization. I argue that it was this self-perception that made nurses more receptive than physicians to the introduction of accounting strategies and tools, such as the nursing process. The desire to move away from the "bad" past to a better future may have encouraged the take up of those processes even more, which consequently led to an economization of nursing.

The Diffuse Understanding of the Profession of Nurses

Although the aim to professionalize was not questioned at all in the nursing journals there was never a critical discussion about the status and organization of existing professions and how such a professional level could be achieved. It was never exactly defined either what the respective authors understood as professionalism in nursing. Rather, nurses in their arguments for professionalization demonstrated quite different and sometimes even contradictory perceptions. When the topic of professionalization was mentioned in the articles of the nursing journal and the hospital journal it was often – especially at the beginning – described as improving the nursing vocation and its status, or as modernizing nursing. Over the course of the 1980s, the term "professionalization" could be found more often. But it was used more as a keyword or a key argument to validate the importance or "rightness" of the strategies and concepts that should be applied to the nursing vocation. However, "autonomy or independence," "scientific knowledge and university education," and "acknowledgement in society" can be found repeatedly as elements in the understanding of professional

---

528 E. g. Susanne Kreutzer, "Krankenbeobachtung. Zur Entwertung einer pflegerischen Schlüsselkompetenz in der Bundesrepublik und Schweden nach 1945 [Patient Observation: About the Devaluation of a Key Competence in Nursing in the Federal Republic of Germany and Sweden after 1945]," in *Gesundheit/Krankheit. Kulturelle Differenzierungsprozesse um Körper, Geschlecht und Macht in Skandinavien*, ed. Lill-Ann Körber and Stefanie von Schnurbein, Berliner Beiträge zur Skandinavistik, Bd. 16 (Berlin: Nordeuropa-Institut, 2010), 167–88; Susanne Kreutzer, *Arbeits- und Lebensalltag evangelischer Krankenpflege. Organisation, soziale Praxis und biographische Erfahrungen, 1945–1980 [Daily Work and Life of Protestant Nursing: Organization, Social Practice, and Biographical Experiences, 1945–1980]* (Göttingen: V&R unipress, 2014); Karen Nolte, "Pflege von Sterbenden im 19. Jahrhundert. Eine ethikgeschichtliche Annäherung [Caring for the Dying in the 19th Century: An Ethical-Historical Approach]," in *Transformationen Pflegerischen Handelns. Institutionelle Kontexte und soziale Praxis Vom 19. bis 21. Jahrhundert*, ed. Susanne Kreutzer (Göttingen: V&R unipress, 2010), 87–107.

status. These elements are in line with those in the theoretical approaches of the sociological theories of professions.

This chapter draws on the same issues that were discussed before under an accounting perspective, only now they are related to the question of professionalization or de-professionalization in nursing. I will critically analyze the discursive formation in which the nursing process is acknowledged to be an instrument of professionalization. Furthermore, I will show why I question the argument of professionalization in nursing through applying the nursing process in nursing care. To begin with, I analyze the desire and attempts of nurses to gain autonomy by establishing a distinct scope of practice. The nursing process is constituted as the central tool with which the establishment of this scope of practice can be realized: to turn away from the medical orientation; to direct power to the patient; to implement rationality and accountability into nursing; to foster nursing research. As a conclusion of this chapter, I will critically discuss developments in the perspective on professionalization and de-professionalization.

8.1 Autonomy Via a Distinct Scope of Practice

Right from the start of the medium-term program of the WHO, Dorothy C. Hall defined autonomous nursing on the basis of the steps of the nursing process. Improving nursing care and its status in society and in healthcare was the aim of this European program. The call for autonomy for nurses is especially directed at the decisions that are taken in nursing and by nurses.

In Germany, this perception of nursing was carried further and its dissemination to the public became part of the DBfK agenda for the decade of the 1980s.[529] This was to be achieved with the following steps: "create a description of the vocation; undertake preparations to establish a college of nurses; make the nursing process better known and help to introduce it."[530]

The nursing process was legally introduced in German nursing in 1985 when it was integrated into the training and exam regulations of the nursing act.[531] With

---

529 Rosemarie Weinrich, "Ausblick auf die Arbeit des DBfK in den 80er Jahren [Outlook to the Work of the DBfK in the 80s]," *Krankenpflege* 35, no. 1 (1981), 16–18.
530 "Als erste Schritte wurden vorgeschlagen: ein Berufsbild zu erstellen, Vorarbeiten zu leisten für die Einrichtung einer Pflegekammer, den Pflegeprozeß bekannt zu machen und zu dessen Einübung zu verhelfen" (Helga Laurinat, "Bericht über die 7. Delegiertenversammlung [Report of the 7th Delegates Meeting]," *Krankenpflege* 34, no. 6 (1980), 207: 207; my translation).
531 Rosemarie Weinrich, "Stellungnahme zum Entwurf einer Ausbildungs- und Prüfungsverordnung für die Berufe der Krankenpflege – (KrPflAPrO) [Commentary on the Draft of the Training and Examination Regulations of the Nursing Occupations]," *Krankenpflege* 36,

this new nursing act, the nursing process by law became an important part of German nursing care. However, a new autonomous scope of practice for the German nursing vocation was just defined recently in a new nursing act.[532]

8.1.1 Stepping Away from the Medical Profession: The Focus on Health and Basic Nursing Care

The Medical Orientation of Nursing as an Obstacle for Professionalization

The medical orientation of nursing was defined as one of the reasons why the nursing vocation struggled in its professionalization process. It was, hence, one of the issues that had to be resolved in order to be able to professionalize. In 1982, Weinrich tried to suggest that it had already happened by comparing two vocational profiles of nursing that the DBfK released. The first one was from the year 1974, the second from 1981. In the first, nursing was presented as a mediator between the physician and the patient and as being responsible for an optimal course of treatment. Evaluating the second vocational profile, Weinrich praised the shift to autonomy in nursing. "[I]n the 70s the unexpected happened [...]: The nursing vocation started off for independence."[533] This autonomous vocation was now "a separate part of the healthcare service [...and] responsible for the planning, executing, and evaluating of nursing care as well as for its own education."[534] Here, the steps of the nursing process were used to define autonomous nursing. It seems that with the latter DBfK vocational profile, the concept of autonomous nursing was slowly becoming synonymous with the nursing process.

But nurses themselves were also accused of leaning on a medical orientation in nursing:"[P]rofessional competence in nursing was almost completely measured on the correctness of the physical care of the patient which was delegated by

---

no. 10 (1982), 321–22; KrPflAPrV, "Ausbildungs- und Prüfungsverordnung für die Berufe in der Krankenpflege vom 16. Oktober 1985 [Regulation for Education and Examination in the Occupations of Nursing from October 16th, 1985]," in *Z 5702 A*, ed. Bundesgesetzblatt (1985).

532 PflBRefG, "Gesetz zur Reform der Pflegeberufe (Pflegeberufereformgesetz) vom 17. Juli 2017 [Law for the Reformation of the Occupations in Nursing from July 17th, 2017]," in *Teil I Nr. 49*,, ed. Bundesgesetzblatt (ausgegeben zu Bonn am 24. Juli 2017).

533 "In den 70er Jahren geschah dann das Unerwartete [...]: Der Pflegeberuf begab sich auf den Weg in die Unabhängigkeit" (Rosemarie Weinrich, "Gedanken zum Berufsbild Krankenpflege [Thoughts About the Vocation of Nursing]," *Krankenpflege* 36, no. 1 (1982), 2–3: 2; my translation).

534 "Als eigenständiger Beruf und selbständiger Teil des Gesundheitsdienstes ist sie für die Planung, Ausführung und Bewertung der Krankenpflege [...] verantwortlich" (Weinrich, "Gedanken zum Berufsbild," 2; my translation).

physicians."[535] Contrary to this medical perception of nursing, all the concepts underlying the nursing process were said to be, as Krohwinkel emphasized, humanistic and carrying the perception of nursing being "a holistic problem-solving and relation process with the key elements of problem-solving and communication."[536] Hence, using and applying the nursing process should make nurses become conscious of their working field of responsibility and should free themselves from their assisting role to physicians.

Redirection on Health

The direction of the nursing vocation towards health as the central aim of nursing service is in line with the WHO construction of the concept "health" as the output and goal of healthcare services. As I showed in chapter 6.3.1, a purely economic logic and the neoliberal rationale underlie this WHO call for health, containing within it the understanding of self-responsible patients who are eager to maintain their own health and of healthcare systems that are efficient and effective. This concept of health was brought into the nursing vocation with the introduction of the nursing process. Nurses received this redirection enthusiastically and saw it as a chance to eventually free themselves from the medical profession and to set it as a foundation for an autonomous nursing vocation.[537] Redirection involved a focus on prevention and rehabilitation as well.[538] Establishing health and rehabilitation as nurses' own area of responsibility within the healthcare system spoke against the medical perspective, strengthening attempts to reposition nursing as opposite to medicine.

The aim of the WHO was moved forward with the program "health for all by the year 2000" that began in the early 1980s. The WHO's call to direct healthcare services towards health also made German nursing feel international pressure to

---

535 "Das hat mancherorts dazu geführt, daß professionelle Kompetenz in der Krankenpflege fast ausschließlich an der Exaktheit der von Ärzten delegierten physischen Versorgung von Patienten gemessen wurde" (Monika Krohwinkel, "Pflegepersonal setzt sich für bessere Gesundheit ein [Nurses Campaign for Better Health]," *Krankenpflege* 38, no. 5 (1984), 138–40: 138; my translation).
536 "… als ganzheitlichen Problemlösungs- und Beziehungsprozeß. Schlüsselelemente solcher Pflege sind also Problemlösung und Kommunikation" (Krohwinkel, "Pflegepersonal setzt sich für bessere Gesundheit ein," 138; my translation).
537 Dorothy C. Hall, "Probleme der Krankenpflegeausbildung in Europa [Problems of Nursing Education in Europe]," *Krankenpflege* 29, no. 10 (1976), 292, 301–03.
538 Weinrich, "Der Wandel im bisher üblichen Verständnis," 156–58; DBfK, "Berufsbild Krankenpflege [Job Description: Nursing]," *Krankenpflege* 34, no. 2 (1981), 64–66; Bischoff and Wanner, "Krankenpflege an der Hochschule?" 64–66; Rosemarie Weinrich, "Sitzung des Rates der Ländervertreter – 18. internationaler Krankenpflegekongreß in Tel Aviv [Meeting of the Council of the Representatives of the Countries:18th International Nursing Congress in Tel Aviv]," *Krankenpflege* 39, no. 9 (1985), 298–301.

reposition itself. In a report on the 18th ICN international nursing congress in Tel Aviv, Weinrich described the recent and upcoming changes in nursing, drawing on the changing role of nurses and the redirection to health. Weinrich predicted that this turn away from traditional nursing, with its focus on illness, towards health education would need a long time in traditionally based Germany. But she pointed out that ignoring this unstoppable progress would more than ever attribute the concepts of "underdevelopment" [*Unterentwickeltheit*] and "backwardness" [*Rückständigkeit*] to the German healthcare system.[539] According to Weinrich, some third-world countries were already a step ahead of Germany in regard to their healthcare system,[540] using shame to put potential pressure on the members of the German healthcare system. Here, the motive for the transformation of nursing was not presented as an intrinsic endeavour to improve but rather was influenced by changes in other countries, which were understood as progress towards modern nursing. In comparison, German nursing was viewed as outdated. Hence, the nursing process was meant to prevent nurses not only from a medical orientation but also from moving backwards. Health education and health information should become part of nurses' scope of practice,[541] meaning that the professionalization project of German nursing was grounded in the WHO concept of health.

In German-speaking countries, the redirection of nursing to health caused a discussion about the designation of nurses. Translated, nursing meant caring for the sick (*Krankenpflege*) and the designation of a "nurse" was translated as "sister of sick people" or "carer of sick people" [*Krankenschwester/Krankenpfleger*]. Both imply caring for the sick, explicitly excluding healthy people from the area of a nurse's responsibility. This focus on health also raised discussions around renaming the German nursing vocation. (Although these discussions were welcomed with curiosity and enthusiasm, it took another three decades before the nursing act of 2002 established a new designation of German nursing that is now translated as "caring for healthy and sick people"[542]).

By following the aim of the WHO, the nursing vocation followed its aim to professionalize at the same time. By working on its aim to professionalize the German nursing vocation, it inherently followed the neoliberal directive to

---

539 Weinrich, "Sitzung des Rates der Ländervertreter," 300.
540 Weinrich, "Sitzung des Rates der Ländervertreter," 298–301.
541 DBfK, "Großveranstaltung zum Tag der Krankenpflege [Major Event at the Day of Nursing]," *Krankenpflege* 32, no. 3 (1978), 99; Friederike Dittrich, "Pflege ist Leistung – Dokumentation ist Beweis [Nursing Is a Service: Documentation Is the Proof]," *Krankenpflege* 38, no. 4 (1984), 142–44.
542 KrPflG, "Krankenpflegegesetz vom 16. Juli 2003 (BGBl. I S. 1442), das zuletzt durch Artikel 1a des Gesetzes vom 17. Juli 2017 (BGBl. I S. 2581) geändert worden ist [Nursing Act 2003]," (2003).

transform healthcare services. As one example, the focus of nursing care was based on the nursing process to motivate the patient and enable him or her to live a healthy lifestyle.[543]

Valuation of Basic Nursing Care and Patient-Orientation

The nursing process was a central component of the calls for the reorientation of nursing. As nursing historian Marianne Schmidbaur states, the concept of patient-oriented nursing care became a matter of discussion in German nursing during the medium-term program of the WHO. This concept could satisfy various interests in the nursing vocation and became established as the central aspect of a vocational identity in nursing.[544] In the different articles, different terms were used in order to explain the concept of patient-oriented nursing care, such as "individual care," "patient-centred care," or "planned nursing care."

Hedi Siebers, director of a school of nursing and an active member of the DBfK, clearly presented planned nursing care as an alternative and in opposition to the medical-scientific foundation of nursing care. The nursing process was seen as a tool to establish this type of nursing care, which considered the needs of the patient and his or her family.[545] This perception of nursing was even stipulated in a job description developed by the DBfK. Nursing was defined as an autonomous and independent profession that was responsible for the planning, executing, documenting, and evaluating of individual nursing care,[546] and it was through these actions that nurses would find independence and autonomy. Therefore, politically active nurses criticized the tendency of some nurses to seek out more medical tasks.[547] They believed that fully educated nurses especially

---

543 Annemarie Ludwig, "3. Delegiertenversammlung des DBfK am 24./25. Sept. 1976 im Bildungszentrum Essen [Third Meeting of Dbfk Delegates, September 24th/25th, 1976 in the Training Center Essen]," *Krankenpflege* 30, no. 11 (1976), 327–29; Weinrich, "Ausblick auf die Arbeit des DBfK," 16–18; Maria Mischo-Kelling, "Gesundheit und Lebensqualität – Ein Anliegen der Pflege für die Zukunft [Health and Quality of Life: A Concern of Nursing for the Future]," *Krankenpflege* 40, no. 5 (1986), 180–84; Thomas Foth and Dave Holmes, "Governing through Lifestyle: Lalonde and the Biopolitical Managemnt of Public Health in Canada," *Nursing Philosophy* 19, no. 4 (2018), 1–11.
544 Marianne Schmidbaur, *Vom "Lazaruskreuz" zu "Pflege Aktuell": Professionalisierungsdiskurse in der deutschen Krankenpflege 1903–2000 [From "Lazaruskreuz" to "Pflege Aktuell": Discourses on Professionalization in German Nursing Care 1903–2000]* (Königstein: Helmer, 2002).
545 Hedi Siebers, "Krankenpflegeausbildung der achtziger Jahre. Auszüge eines Vortrags [Nursing Education in the 1980s: Extracts of a Presentation]," *Krankenpflege* 34, no. 2 (1980), 65–66.
546 DBfK, "Berufsbild Krankenpflege," 64–66.
547 Renate Reimann, "Stagnation oder Fortschritt in der Entwicklung der Pflegeberufe? [Stagnation or Progress in the Development of Nursing Occupations?]," *Krankenpflege* 35, no. 1 (1981), 20 & 37; Weinrich, "Gedanken zum Berufsbild," 2–3.

were wanting to move away from basic nursing care and to attain a "higher" position through providing more technical (more medical) nursing care [*Behandlungspflege*]. In this understanding, basic nursing care should be executed more by nursing aides and 1st year nursing students.[548] "Their own work was measured against the work of the physician – the more physicians' tasks were taken over, the faster they achieved a higher status."[549] This fascination with the medical scientific perspective, it was argued, would not only lead to a decreasing quality of basic nursing care but would also leave nurses as assistants to physicians.[550]

Hence, the solution to this problem was to shift the focus away from the medical perspective and direct it to basic nursing care to have it become the "actual" responsibility of nursing. This was promoted by nurses such as Renate Reimann and Rosemarie Weinrich.[551]. According to Weinrich, nursing should reorient itself to this its primary task – practical nursing care. "Only the return to practical nursing care as the core of actual professional activity can bring real vocation-related satisfaction."[552] The nursing process should help to carry out this shift: "Basic nursing got a suitable upgrading because of the model of the nursing process. 'Patient consultation' has become a continuous part of seminars,"[553] which was especially perceived as an inherent task of professional nursing since communication and the recognition of psycho-social issues were considered to be supportive of healing and could not be carried out better than from a vocation that established the closest relationship with a patient.[554] Furthermore, more and more courses were offered with pure nursing topics. According to Weinrich, this was a sign of an increasing demand for nursing-related information instead of more medically oriented courses.[555]

---

548 Reimann, "Stagnation oder Fortschritt," 20 & 37.
549 "Die eigene Arbeit wurde an der des Arztes gemessen – je mehr von seinen Aufgaben übernommen wurden, desto eher 'war man wer'" (Weinrich, "Bedeutung und Stellenwert der Krankenpflege," 2; my translation).
550 Renate Reimann, "Krankenpflege zwischen Tradition und Forderung [Nursing between Tradition and Demand]," *Krankenpflege* 36, no. 1 (1982), 5–7.
551 Weinrich, "Ausblick auf die Arbeit des DBfK," 16–18; Reimann, "Stagnation oder Fortschritt," 20 & 37.
552 "Die Rückbesinnung auf die praktische Krankenpflege als Kernstück der eigentlichen Berufstätigkeit kann allein echte Zufriedenheit im Beruf bringen" (Weinrich, "Ausblick auf die Arbeit des DBfK," 17; my translation).
553 "Die 'Grundpflege' (allgemeine Pflege) erhielt durch das Modell des Krankenpflegeprozesses eine ihr angemessene Aufwertung. Das 'Patientengespräch' wurde zu einem festen Bestandteil von Seminarangeboten, die Spezialisierungseuphorie ist versachlicht, die praktische Schüleranleitung bekommt in der Ausbildung ein stärkeres Gewicht" Reimann, "Stagnation oder Fortschritt," 37; my translation).
554 Sabine Bartholomeyczik, "Arbeitsplatz Krankenbett [Bedside Workplace]," *Krankenpflege* 41, no. 5 (1987), 158–61.
555 Weinrich, "Der Wandel im bisher üblichen Verständnis," 156–58.

This emphasis on basic nursing care seems to be a specific German discourse, with its origins in the Christian tradition and understanding of nursing care. It is interesting that this re-focus on these very basic responsibilities for patients that were perceived as "actual" nursing care emerged at the same time that the Christian image of nursing was blamed for having weakened the nursing vocation and making it into a medical assistance vocation. The reason can be found in the new constitution of basic nursing care that was established with the nursing process. While before, basic nursing care had been grounded in a holistic caring with a focus on the soul, the new basic nursing care was a cybernetically structured process with distinct, defined, and possibly standardized nursing tasks that could be related to specific nursing goals. In other words, while the traditional focus on basic nursing care was based on the logic of the Christian religion, the new concept of basic nursing care was based on the logic of standardization, transparency, effectiveness, and efficiency. It has to be understood as a neo-liberally transformed basic nursing care for an empowered patient-subject.

Countries belonging to the European Community encouraged the German nursing vocation to introduce the nursing process into nursing care to establish a comparable standard in nursing education. In the 1970s, the European Community released the directive for recognizing nurses of member states. With this directive, nurses were allowed to work in different European countries. However, the required skills and competencies defined in the directive had to be achieved in the nursing education programs of the respective countries.[556] In 1987, the European Nursing Group (ENG) wanted to change the required skills and competencies of this directive and published a memorandum on basic vocational education in nursing. In the memorandum, the ENG made clear that the role of nurses in the future would include being responsible for planning, organizing, and executing nursing care. Furthermore, they predicted that nursing would be increasingly important in prevention, health improvement, and health education. In order to achieve this, nursing education should be based on the nursing process.[557] Hence, the question of whether or not the nursing process should be established in the German education of future nursing students in Germany was not a question just for Germany but at the European level.

---

556 EC, "Council Directive of 27 June 1977 Concerning the Coordination of Provision Laid Down by Law, Regulation or Administrative Action in Respect of the Activities of Nurses Responsible for General Care (77/453/Eec)," (Official Journal of the European Communities1977).

557 Europäische Krankenpflegevereinigung, "Memorandum zur Grundausbildung in der Krankenpflege [Memorandum on Basic Vocational Training in Nursing]," *Krankenpflege* 41, no. 7/8 (1987), 278–80: 278.

8.1.2 Influencing the Patient: The Focus on Cybernetic Holism

In this chapter, I will describe the impact nurses have on the patient through the concept of the nursing process. The nursing process, here, is understood as a tool with which nurses gain detailed insights into the life of patients, where a new patient image is constructed, and where patients can be influenced to behave and change their life in a way that they become self-responsible for their decisions in regard to their health. It was thought, therefore, that the concept of health education should become part of nurses' scope of practice. Patients should learn how to deal with their own illness in order to become a useful part of society again.[558] The constitution of an empowered subject in a neoliberal society calls for mistrusting traditional professions such as the medical profession. An enclosed medical profession seeks a compliant and less knowledgeable patient rather than an empowered one. An empowered patient is seen as a threat to the classic enclosures of medicine because this patient questions the decisions and practices of physicians and asks for transparency in treatment procedures. As I described in chapter 5.2.2, the empowerment of patients has to be understood as a cause of de-professionalization.[559] However, as I will show on the following pages, understanding how to make a patient live a healthy life comes across in the nursing journals as making patients compliant rather than empowering them.

Making the Patient Live a Healthy Life

Using the nursing process calls for collecting patient information. The nursing history should refer to different areas of the patient's life as part of the concept of patient-oriented instead of illness-oriented nursing care.[560] The concept of holism dominated discussions in understanding patient-oriented care based on the nursing process. While the nursing process calls for a continuous collection of information relevant to patients – especially with the need to document nursing

---

558 Sirkka Levá, "Eine gute Krankenpflege. Was ist damit gemeint, und wie ist sie zu erreichen? [Good Nursing Care: What Are We Talking About, and How Can It Be Achieved]," *Die Agnes-Karll-Schwester* 11, no. 2 (1957), 54 & 56; Barbara Schattat, "Bericht über meine ersten Monate in USA im Rahmen des Schwestern-Austauschprogramms [Report on My First Months During a Nurse Exchange in the USA]," *Die Agnes-Karll-Schwester* 15, no. 8 (1961), 263–64.
559 Paul A. C. Parkin, "Nursing the Future: A Re-Examination of the Professionalization Thesis in the Light of Some Recent Developments," *Journal of Advanced Nursing* 21, no. 3 (1995), 561–67; Janet L. Storch and Shirley M. Stinson, "Concepts of Deprofessionalization with Application to Nursing," in *Political Issues in Nursing: Past, Present, and Future*, ed. Rosemary White (Chichester: John Wiley & Sons Ltd, 1988), 33–44.
560 Liselotte Hölzel-Seipp, "Der praktische Krankenpflegeprozeß [The Practical Nursing Process]," *Die Agnes-Karll-Schwester, der Krankenpfleger* 23, no. 5 (1969), 201–03.

care and write reports – the assessment and history of the patient were defined as the basis of the nursing process.[561] Although throughout the 1970s there is no official recommendation about which information should be gathered, several articles recommended considering the psycho-social condition, biography, and hygienic habits of patients, alongside their physical condition.[562]

For example, in 1975 in a detailed guideline on how to use the nursing process, it was recommended that nurses should collect data on the personal, familial, and vocational background, and about habits surrounding sleep or stimulants or attitudes towards illness. Based on the collected information, nurses should develop a patient chart that was considered an objective image or mirror of the patient. Every healthcare worker could help to complete it – almost like a puzzle. Moreover, a consequence of this documentation was that all healthcare personnel like nurses, physicians, pastors, and social workers could access the patient's detailed information.[563]

Leni Brunner and Sabine Goedeckemeyer, who initiated and administered a project to implement the nursing process in certain wards of a hospital, emphasized that specific questions would be important concerning the physical, psychic, and social situation of the patient as well as the way he or she dealt with the illness and what impact the admission had on the personal environment of the patient.[564] They even recommended using the personal crisis of the patient to gain more insights. Because at admission the patient "is anxious, he (*sic*) is worried about the situation, and he (*sic*) is very willing to tell us important things about himself."[565] In this intense situation, the nurse would start the nursing process to assess the patient based on his or her information.[566] Additionally, during hospitalization, nurses should observe the patient and the patient's behaviour, giving advice on every single component of the patient's daily life.[567]

---

561 Luise Wittmann, "Die Pflegeplanung in der Intensivpflege [The Nursing Care Plan in Intensive Care]," *Krankenpflege* 31, no. 5 (1977), 178–80.

562 Wittmann, "Die Pflegeplanung," 178–80; Cornelia Send, "Mittel für die Durchführung der individuellen Pflege (I) [Instruments for Providing Individual Nursing Care I]," *Krankenpflege* 29, no. 7 (1975), 274; Renate Geschwilm, "Pflegeplanung [Nursing Care Plan]," *Krankenpflege* 31, no. 9 (1977), 293–94; Detlef Hohlin, "Neue Horizonte für die Krankenpflege [New Horizons for Nursing Care]," *Krankenpflege* 30, no. 1 (1976), 13–14.

563 Send, "Mittel für die Durchführung der individuellen Pflege (I)," 274.

564 Leni Brunner and Sabine Goedeckemeyer, "Teil der Pflegeplanung – Das Erstgespräch (1. Teil) [Part of the Nursing Care Plan: The Initial Meeting (1st Part)]," *Krankenpflege* 35, no. 4 (1981), 152–54.

565 "Er hat Angst, er macht sich Sorgen, und er ist sehr bereit, uns wichtige Dinge zu seiner Person zu sagen" (Brunner and Goedeckemeyer, "Teil der Pflegeplanung," 152; my translation).

566 Brunner and Goedeckemeyer, "Teil der Pflegeplanung," 152–54.

567 Hölzel-Seipp, "Der praktische Krankenpflegeprozeß," 201–03.

With this kind of intimate knowledge of the patient, nurses should plan and execute activities in order to make the patient willing to adopt a healthy lifestyle.

Nurses can gather very private information to use it in the rational and cybernetic planning of healthcare. The nursing process can also be understood as a structure to help the nurse to influence patients in potentially each area of their lives. With the combination of the knowledge derived from patient information and their knowledge of medicine, epidemiology, nursing management, and health education, nurses can exercise a powerful influence on patients and direct them toward the desired behaviour. The nursing process and the striving for holistic and individual care enable nurses to gain increasingly broader insights into patients' minds and ways of living. The power of nurses over their patients (even healthy people) lies in the apparently rational and scientific structure of the nursing process and the redirection of nursing to health. With the promotion of health and a healthy lifestyle as a newly acknowledged part of their scope of practice, nurses became responsible for influencing both patients and those who were not sick. For example, Weinrich endorsed integrating health education in schools and companies into nurses' field of responsibility.[568]

In the light of the emerging call for empowerment of the patient, this seems to be contradictory. Nurses usually asserted their influence on patients in situations where they were less able to be self-determined. This is a nursing phenomenon that can also be found in the 19th century, where a trust in God and God-fearing behaviour seems to have been of utmost importance for deaconesses. They used the suffering of the patient – and even refused the relief of nursing and medical interventions – in order to (re-)establish trust in God of the dying patient.[569] Hence, with their religious foundation and their position as "mothers" in a family-like structured hospital, nurses were powerful in relation to the patient. As the foundation of nursing turned towards the sciences, the foundation of nursing power turned to scientific knowledge.[570] The agenda of nurses also shifted from guiding the patient towards living a pious life to guiding the patient to live a healthy life in order to maintain or rebuild the patient's functionality for society.

---

568 Weinrich, "Der Wandel im bisher üblichen Verständnis," 156–58.
569 Nolte, "Pflege von Sterbenden im 19. Jahrhundert," 87–107; Walter Klein, "'Sie sehen mir alle mit freundlichen Gesichtern entgegen': Die Beziehung zwischen Patienten und Krankenschwestern im Saarbrücker Bürgerhospital in der Mitte des 19. Jahrhunderts ['They All Look at Me with Friendly Faces': The Relationship between Patients and Nurses in the Public Hospital of Saarbrücken in the Middle of the 19th Century," *Medizin, Gesellschaft, und Geschichte: Jahrbuch des Instituts für Geschichte der Medizin der Robert Bosch Stiftung* 21 (2002), 63–90.
570 See Susanne Kreutzer, "'Before, We Were Always There – Now, Everything Is Separate': On Nursing Reforms in Western Germany," *Nursing History Review* 16 (2008), 180–200.

Fragmented Holism

Besides the attempt to gain deep insight into a patient's whole life situation, however, there was also another tendency that seemed to be contrary. Recommendations can be found in the nursing journal *Krankenpflege* for deliberate data collection. Only relevant information should be written in the nursing documentation. In order to review and evaluate the nursing goals, the nursing report should contain "clear expressions and restrict itself to relevant aspects."[571] This call was repeated in an article about using the digitalized variant of the nursing process. Nurses should avoid over-completing nursing documentation because too much data would cause a lack of clarity, it was argued. The more information collected, the more it would become difficult to determine relevance. Then errors and misunderstandings would occur and as well it would entail a loss of time and energy.[572] Gathering information from the patient should not be undertaken in an unstructured way, but should rather be done from the structured and goal-oriented perspective of the nursing process – for example, by keeping in mind the prepared nursing goals or the areas of life which seemed to be important for nursing interventions. Information with a relevance for the nursing process should be collected in depth, whereas other information irrelevant to the nursing process should be left aside for the sake of clarity.

Here, a distinct understanding of holism is to be found. Holism in nursing is not constructed on its own but is a sum of a specific number of different components. These components can best be described by the nursing theories of Juchli (her theory of the 12 activities of daily life was published in the 1980s), Krohwinkel (her theory of the 13 activities and existential experiences of life was published in the 1990s) and also go back to Maslow's pyramid of needs. Hence, it was perceived that nursing care could be separated into highly distinct and single nursing tasks. Nursing historian Susanne Kreutzer calls this "modernization as fragmentation."[573] The nursing process, while calling for this dissection of nursing, brings these demarcated nursing tasks together afterwards and structures them into a cybernetic cycle. This leads to a different form of holism, which is defined by the sum of the definitions and demarcations of its declared components.

---

571 "Klare Ausdrucksweise und auf das Wesentliche beschränkte Einträge helfen uns, die Pflege im Blick auf das Ziel zu überprüfen und auszuwerten" (Margit Schellenberg, "Die Bedeutung einer patientenorientierten Pflegeplanung [The Importance of a Patient-Oriented Nursing Care Plan]," *Krankenpflege* 31, no. 9 (1977), 291–93: 292; my translation).
572 J. G. Veldhorst-Groenewegen and G. van der Reep, "EVA – Ein patientenorientiertes Instrumten für Pflegeadministration [EVA: A Patient-Oriented Tool for Nursing Administration]," *Krankenpflege* 38, no. 9 (1984), 301–04.
573 "*Modernisierung als Fragmentierung* "(Kreutzer, *Arbeits- und Lebensalltag evangelischer Krankenpflege*, 182; my translation).

Creating such components is a rational act of thinking and decision-making. Areas that cannot be captured rationally are likely to vanish in this creational act. Hence, those aspects might not be included in this holism. This new holism used in the nursing process is already a shaped and definite understanding of holism. This newly constituted concept of holism is shaped by the WHO's concept of health as the "return [...] in health status and in service."[574] But in comparison to a call for empowered patients, it seems rather that patients should be disciplined or forced to be self-determined.

8.1.3 Becoming Autonomous: The Focus on Rationality and Accountability

According to the articles of the nursing journal *Krankenpflege*, nurses appreciated being able to possess an instrument like the nursing process that gave them a voice.[575] They valued the idea that they could make themselves and their work understandable to others outside the nursing vocation. They also considered that the evaluation of nursing care and the self-reflection and self-control that went with it helped to improve their knowledge and competencies.[576]

It seems that the rationality inherent in the cybernetic cycle of the nursing process made the nursing process a helpful tool to claim and establish autonomy in the vocation. In 1969, Liselotte Hölzel-Seipp, a German-trained nurse and later Assistant Professor for nursing at Wayne State University, Michigan, presented the nursing process as an important concept of modern nursing. As Hölzel-Seipp described it, nursing would no longer be based on intuition but more and more on knowledge derived from natural and social sciences. Societal and economic changes – higher life expectancy, a steadily shorter duration of hospitalization, higher costs of hospitalization, and higher demands for rehabilitation – would call for progress and improvement of nursing techniques, such as the introduction of the nursing process.[577] So several years before the WHO medium-term program started, single voices could be heard in the nursing journal suggesting an image of good and up-to-date nursing care based on scientific

---

574 WHO, "Organizational Study on "Methods of Promoting Development of Basic Health Services". Report of the Working Group, 16 January 1973," (World Health Organization, 1973), 4.
575 Wilma Jansen, "Überblick über die wesentlichen Referate [Overview of the Essential Presentations]," *Krankenpflege* 32, no. 6 (1978), 197–200.
576 Tony Gilbert, "Reflective Practice and Clinical Supervision: Meticulous Rituals of the Confessional," *Journal of Advanced Nursing* 36, no. 2 (2001), 199–205; Renate Reimann, "Information im Dienst des Kranken [Information at Patients' Service]," *Krankenpflege* 33, no. 7/8 (1979), 249–53.
577 Hölzel-Seipp, "Der praktische Krankenpflegeprozeß," 201–03.

knowledge and the nursing process that had the ability to meet economic demands.

After the start of the WHO medium-term program, a rational and conscious nursing care became more clearly connected with autonomy and professionalization. As Renate Reimann emphasized in 1979, "a planned, problem-oriented nursing care is the foundation for the recognition of nursing as an autonomous and independent vocation."[578] A scientific foundation and thus, a rationalized language, would become the foundation of a modernized nursing vocation. By showing its effectiveness, so went the argument, nurses could rightfully claim to be allowed to work autonomously.[579] This desire to express oneself in rational and understandable terms came along with the increasing devaluation of non-rational knowledge or tacit knowledge such as intuition.[580] As nursing historian Susanne Kreutzer argues, with the focus on more theoretical knowledge and the introduction of new measurements such as x-rays, sonography, and laboratory tests, "hard facts" became increasingly dominant. They could be articulated in a rational and so-called objective language and were standardizable. Those hard facts were more successful in being acknowledged as truth than subjective reports of patient observation based on soft and blurred descriptions. Here, the foundation changed upon which nurses could claim an independent body of knowledge.[581] Moreover, by shifting to such a rationalized, objectivized and even standardized language, nurses might not even have realized that they constrained themselves by following uncritically and bluntly this formalized knowledge. They more likely perceived this shift as being and acting professionally.[582]

Non-transparent and non-rational knowledge and information can hardly be used by nurses who want to be acknowledged as members of such a nursing profession. However, being unable to use this knowledge can be seen as a loss of autonomy, which is actually contrary to nursing arguments for professionalization. As Kreutzer demonstrated, the devaluation of implicit knowledge

---

578 "[...] eine geplante, problemorientierte Pflegeausüburng (sic) ist das Fundament für die Anerkennung der Krankenpflege als eigenständigem Beruf" (Renate Reimann, "Pflegeplanung – Was bedeutet geplante Pflege in der Berufspraxis [Nursing Care Plan: The Meaning of Planned Nursing Care in the Daily Professional Practice]," *Krankenpflege* 33, no. 5 (1979), 154–57: 157; my translation).
579 Hölzel-Seipp, "Der praktische Krankenpflegeprozeß," 201–03; Reimann, "Information im Dienst des Kranken," 249–53; Antje Grauhan and fellows, "Mittelfristiges WHO-Programm für Krankenpflege- und Hebammenwesen in Europa [Middle-Term Program of the WHO Concerning Nursing and Midwifery in Europe]," *Krankenpflege* 32, no. 2 (1978), 67–68.
580 Kreutzer, "Krankenbeobachtung," 167–88.
581 Kreutzer, "Krankenbeobachtung," 167–88.
582 See Annemarie Kesselring, "Psychosoziale Pflegediagnostik: Eine interpretativ-phänomenologische Perspective [Psycho-Social Nursing Diagnosis: An Interpretative-Phenomenological Perspective]," *Pflege* 12, no. 4 (1999), 223–28.

and the attempt to be accountable based on rationalized knowledge led to the disappearance of a former key competence in nursing: patient observation. This key competency was based on the sum of different kinds of knowledge and experiences, not all of which could be expressed rationally. However, at one time, this competence, as well as the intuitive knowledge of nurses, was acknowledged to constitute a distinct autonomous scope of practice for nurses. It was perceived as a kind of "mystical" knowledge which could neither be explained nor be acquired by everybody.[583]

The enclosed form of professional knowledge, that is, the exclusivity of expertise, is an important characteristic of the traditional understanding of professions. This exclusive knowledge can be defined as expert knowledge that enables members to achieve and defend a powerful position against other professions and vocations.[584] This enclosed and mystic knowledge of healthcare workers like physicians and nurses was criticized by economist Siegfried Eichhorn in 1966 and also by neoliberal scholars as obstacles to the implementation of economic behaviour in these healthcare workers.[585] Transferring this to the history of the German nursing vocation forces us to acknowledge that up until the 1950s, nurses possessed a distinct autonomous field of practice and enclosed

---

[583] Kreutzer, "Krankenbeobachtung," 167–88; Jette Lange, Susanne Kreutzer, and Thomas Foth, "Pflege berechenbar machen – Der Pflegeprozess als Accounting Technology in historischer Perspektive [Making Nursing Accountable: The Nursing Process as Accounting Technology in a Historical Perspective]," in *Neue Technologien in der Pflege – Grundlegende Reflexionen und pragmatische Befunde*, ed. Manfred Hülsken-Giesler, et al. (Göttingen: V&R unipress, 2022), 231–253.

[584] E. g. Alexander M. Carr-Saunders and Paul A. Wilson, *The Profession* (London: Frank Cass & Co. Ltd., 1964); Eliot Freidson, *Professionalism: The Third Logic* (Chicago: University of Chicago Press, 2001); Andrew Delano Abbott, *The System of Professions: An Essay on the Division of Expert Labor* (Chicago: University of Chicago Press, 1988). An interesting angle, here, is provided by the Australian nursing study in which nursing documentation was analyzed discursively. The author argues that the disappearance of nurses from nursing documentation by writing in a specific objective and rational manner can be understood as nurses' resistance to power relations with other healthcare workers. Rather it seems that nurses still rely very much on their oral traditions when meeting with the nurses of the next shift. "A pay-off of invisibility may be that it allows nurses a space separate from that of other disciplines in which to exist and flourish" (Marie Heartfield, "Nursing Documentation and Nursing Practice: A Discourse Analysis," *Journal of Advanced Nursing* 24, no. August (1996), 98–103: 24).

[585] Siegfried Eichhorn, "Die betriebswirtschaftlichen Aspekte der Leistungssteigerung durch Zusammenarbeit [Economic Aspects to Increase Performance through Collaboration]," *Das Krankenhaus* 58, no. 8 (1966), 315–23; Walter Hamm, "Programmierte Unfreiheit und Verschwendung: Zur überfälligen Reform der gesetzlichen Krankenversicherung [Programmed Bondage and Dissipation: On the Overdue Reform of the Statutory Health Insurance]," *ORDO Jahrbuch für die Ordnung von Wirtschaft und Gesellschaft* 35 (1984), 42; Nikolas Rose, "Government, Authority and Expertise in Advanced Liberalism," *Economy and Society* 22, no. 3 (1993), 283–99.

field of expert knowledge. Based on their Christian image of caring for the soul, their work organization based on devoting their lifetime to the ward, and their powerful motherhouse institution, nurses at that time – more than today – could claim an autonomous space of work and decision-making.[586] It also forces us to acknowledge that it was nurses themselves who called for a "de-mystification" of nursing knowledge by striving for transparency and rationality. This has led to the increasing disappearance of nurses' exclusive knowledge and to the diminishing of non-rational parts of nursing knowledge in the nursing vocation. Hence, it has heavily weakened the foundation on which nurses could claim autonomy.

Another example of nurses themselves restricting their area of autonomy can be found in job descriptions for nurses, nursing mentors, and nursing leaders, which were published in 1986 by teachers of the nursing school Agnes Karll [*Krankenpflegehochschule Agnes Karll*]for ongoing education with the aim of creating a business organization [*Betriebsgestaltung*]. Their considerations were based on the professional image of nursing released by the DBfK. The steps of the nursing process have been described as patient-related nursing activities. These steps (especially the step of planning for nursing interventions) were to be executed depending on the healthcare organization and its operational guidelines.[587] This means that the steps of the nursing process should not focus on the patient exclusively nor should they grant complete autonomy to nursing action. Rather, as the authors recommended, the steps of the nursing process should be a compromise between the patient's needs, the autonomy of nurses, and the organizational requirements.

Individuality in a Standardized Pattern

This contradiction of praising rationality touches closely on another interesting contradiction I found emerging in the 1970s and especially in the1980s in both the nursing journal *Krankenpflege*, as well as in the hospital journal *Das Krankenhaus*. The concept of standardization increasingly became an important part of improvement in healthcare. Rationality, objectivity, transparency, and a scientific character were ascribed to standardization. Interestingly, the aspect of individuality was also included in this discursive theme. One very visual example was the development of standardized dishes to individualize food distribution in hospitals. Standardization would enable combining standardized dishes, which,

---

586 Kreutzer, *Arbeits- und Lebensalltag evangelischer Krankenpflege*.
587 Marita Andrzejak et al., "Konzeptionen zur Betriebsgestaltung auf der Grundlage des Berufsbildes Krankenpflege des DBfK [Conception for Business Organization Based on the Professional Image of Nursing Released by the DBfK]," *Krankenpflege* 40, no. 3 (1986), 125.

in turn, would increase the choices a hospital could offer patients with regard to their food preferences.[588] In the case of the nursing process, standardization is constituted as the foundation to provide individualized nursing care, as I will show now.

Renate Reimann, in her article on planned nursing care in 1979, focused particularly on the autonomy of the nursing vocation and rather dismissed the independence and the individual competence of the single nurse or the individuality of a nursing care situation: "Colleagues who could not attend the creation of the plan have to be informed about the plan. Hence, it will not be permitted that everybody uses his/her individual experiences in the treatment of the patient."[589] Furthermore, she had already emphasized elsewhere that only documented activities could be understood as valuable and acceptable information. The situatedness of nursing care, that means, being immersed in the concrete situation of nursing care, she did not consider as reliable or necessary to retrieve information upon which individual nursing care could be executed.[590]

This is a very static perception of how a nursing care plan should be created and how nurses should work with it. This perception needs to be understood as the tendency to exclude the individual nurse from the nurse-patient relationship, to neutralize the individuality of single nurses, and standardize nursing care. It can also be perceived as an attempt to provide continuous and individual nursing care in times of high nurse fluctuation and shorter nursing shifts. In consequence, the German Hospital Society (DKG) published a recommendation to implement a documentation and information system in the hospital with which the nursing process of the patients could be recorded. It seems to have been important to the DKG to disseminate it to hospital managers as well as nurses because this recommendation was published in both the hospital journal *Das Krankenhaus* and in the nursing journal *Krankenpflege*.[591]

---

588 Siegfried Zacharias, "Dekor-Design auf Porzellangeschirr ist nicht Selbstzweck [Decor Design on Procelain Dishes Is Not an End in Itself]," *Das Krankenhaus* 72, no. 7 (1980), 215–16.
589 "Auch Kollegen, die zur Zeit der Absprache abwesend waren, müssen über die Planung informiert werden. Es wird also nicht zugelassen, daß jeder bei dem Patienten seine individuellen Erfahrungen in der Behandlung anwendet" (Reimann, "Pflegeplanung," 154; my translation).
590 Renate Reimann, "Teil II: Das Bildungsangebot für zukunftsorientierte Krankenpflege [Part II: The Educational Program for a Future-Oriented Nursing Care]," *Krankenpflege* 31, no. 5 (1977), 160–61.
591 DKG, "DKG-Vorstand verabschiedet Muster einer Pflegedokumentation und Anpassung des Zeitaufwandes für Apothekenpersonal [Board of the German Hospital Society Passes the Draft of a Nursing Documentation and Adaption of the Expenditure of Time for Pharmacy Staff]," *Das Krankenhaus* 77, no. 6 (1985), 236–37; DKG, "Struktur und Organisation des pflegerischen Dienstes im Krankenhaus [Structure and Organization of the Nursing Service in the Hospital]," *Krankenpflege* 38, no. 9 (1984), 306–07.

A recent Australian study using discourse analysis aimed to reveal the function of nursing documentation as part of nursing practice. According to this study, nurses regularly disappear in the records and "write about observations and responses in a manner that is passive. Such intentions leave the record devoid of meaning as anything more than a record of information that assists the other healthcare providers."[592] In this perspective, this individual nursing care, then, can only claim individuality in regard to the patient and dismisses the relational aspect of the nursing process. As nursing scientists Buus and Traynor argued, both of the different and partly contrary logics of the nursing process – the nursing process as a relational process (as described by Orlando[593]) and the nursing process as a cybernetic and scientific process (as developed by Yura and Walsh[594]) – can be found in nursing care. The contradictions between both usually stand side by side without solving them; a phenomenon they call "doublethinking."[595] In the perception of Reimann and the DKG, the nurse is understood as being exchangeable in the nursing process. The nursing process as a cybernetic organization of nursing care, hence, is clearly emphasized. The importance of making the single nurse disappear lies in the perception that only objective and rational action is scientific and standardizable.

And it seems that the idea of standardization is also transferred to the patient, primarily by reconstituting the patient and the patient's care as components of a standardized process but also by using already established phrases to write the nursing care plan. For example, one of the first articles with a detailed description of the nursing process predicted that the development of nursing care plans would become routine. Certain special schemes for the nursing care plan would come into being which then could be applied and adapted to the individual situation of the patient.[596] In order to handle the effort that has to be put in an individual nursing care plan, other nurses also recommended using checklists or standardized phrases.[597]

---

592 Heartfield, "Nursing Documentation," 102.
593 Ida Jean Orlando, *The Dynamic Nurse-Patient Relationship: Function, Process, and Principles* (New York: Putnam, 1961).
594 Helen Yura and Mary B. Walsh, *The Nursing Process: Assessing, Planning, Implementing, and Evaluating; the Proceedings of the Continuing Education Series Conducted at the Catholic University of America, March 2 through April 27, 1967* (Washington: Catholic University of America Press, 1968).
595 Niels Buus and Michael Traynor, "The Nursing Process: Nursing Discourse and Managerial Technologies," in *The Nursing Process: A Global Concept*, ed. Monika Habermann, Leana R. Uys, and Barbara Parfitt (Edinburgh; New York: Elsevier/Churchill Livingstone, 2006), 31–46.
596 Cornelia Send, "Mittel für die Durchführung der individuellen Pflege (III) [Instruments for Providing Individual Nursing Care III]," *Krankenpflege* 29, no. 9 (1975), 368.
597 Reimann, "Pflegeplanung," 154–57; Ingo Schomburg, "Pflegeplanung und ganzheitliche Pflege im Stationsalltag – Pflegemodellstation und Arbeiten mit dem Krankenpflegeprozeß

The contradiction between standardization and providing individual care in regard to the nursing process was never articulated and, hence, not solved. Applying nursing care to the standardized cybernetic process restructures this nursing care in a standardized series of well-defined steps. However, nurses valued the nursing process in its structure as *the* tool to provide individualized nursing care.[598] This contradiction inherent in the nursing process was not discussed publicly. The silent solution for this contradiction seems to have been the subordination of the individual under the standardized structure. A glance in the scientific literature reveals that this tendency can be found in other circumstances as well, like, for example, in the term "Individualized Standardization"[599] as a combination of the different logics in the healthcare system. Or it underlies the practice to integrate free text entries into electronic programs, calling it "individualization through standardization."[600]. In all these circumstances, an already shaped understanding of individuality is established that fits into standardized tools and concepts in healthcare and enables a working process that is perceived modern and professional.

8.1.4 Establishing Nursing Research: The Focus on Cost-Containment

The call for establishing research in nursing was already made in the medium-term program of the WHO. It was another strategy besides the nursing process to work on the aim of improving nursing in Europe. The German nurses Renate Reimann and Monika Krohwinkel were very active in advertising and supporting research in German nursing. Renate Reimann established a foundation for nursing research and Monika Krohwinkel published several articles about nursing research especially at the beginning and middle of the 1980s. The

---

[Nursing Care Plan and Holistic Care in the Daily Routine of the Ward: Training Ward and Working with the Nursing Process]," *Krankenpflege* 38, no. 7–8 (1984), 231, 236–38; Sabine Thiel, "Pflegeplanung und Pflegedokumentation [Nursing Care Plan and Nursing Documentation]," *Krankenpflege* 40, no. 1 (1986), 9–12.

598 E. g. Send, "Mittel für die Durchführung der individuellen Pflege (III)," 368; Geschwilm, "Pflegeplanung," 293–94; Reimann, "Das Bildungsangebot für zukunftsorientierte Krankenpflege," 160–61.

599 Lena Ansmann and Holger Pfaff, "Providers and Patients Caught between Standardization and Individualization: Individualized Standardization as a Solution Comment on "(Re) Making the Procrustean Bed? Standardization and Customization as Competing Logics in Healthcare"," *International journal of health policy and management* 7, no. 4 (2017), 349–52: 349.

600 Mary Kennihan et al., "Individualization through Standardization: Electronic Orders for Subcutaneous Insulin in the Hospital," *Endocrine practice: official journal of the American College of Endocrinology and the American Association of Clinical Endocrinologists* 18, no. 6 (2012), 976–87: 976.

European-wide, WHO-initiated research project on the nursing process was particularly discussed. This European-wide study was meant to analyze the nursing process in concrete nursing care situations and, additionally, aimed to reform nursing education and the general introduction of nursing research into nursing.[601] Although Germany did not participate in this study, Krohwinkel established and managed a German study of the nursing process, which focused on the application of the nursing process in the case of patients with stroke. It was published in 1993.[602]

Krohwinkel also promoted the introduction of nursing research in nursing education and published recommendations for nursing teachers. Providing a flow chart with the steps of a research project, she explained the process of doing research according to the steps of the nursing process. The first step of the research process was, according to Krohwinkel, the assessment of the current situation and the preparation of the next steps. The second step contained, among others, decisions about the research localities and the development of a research plan. In the third step, the research would be carried out and findings gathered. The final step contained the analysis, interpretation, and application of the results.[603] These four steps are very similar to the four steps of the nursing process as they were recommended by the WHO. Only the feedback-loop is missing. Hence, it is not surprising that Krohwinkel recommended using the steps of the nursing process to help nursing students to understand how to undertake nursing research.[604]

The argument to establish nursing research was twofold: On the one hand, it was argued that nursing research would prevent the nursing vocation from cost-

---

601 Monika Krohwinkel, "Krankenpflegeforschung in Europa. 2. Arbeitstagung europäischer Krankenpflegeforscher in Kopenhagen [Nursing Research in Europe: Second Work Day of European Nursing Researchers in Copenhagen]," *Krankenpflege* 34, no. 1 (1980), 15; Monika Krohwinkel, "Krankenschwester arbeiten gemeinsam an der Verbesserung der Krankenpflege in Europa. Eine Orientierungshilfe zur Forschungskomponente des mittelfristigen Programms der Weltgesundheitsorganisation für das Krankenpflege- und Hebammenwesen in Europa [Nurses Collaborate to Improve Nursing in Europe]," *Krankenpflege* 34, no. 6 (1980), 195–97.
602 Monika Krohwinkel, *Der Pflegeprozess am Beispiel von Apoplexiekranken: Eine Studie zur Erfassung und Entwicklung ganzheitlich-rehabilitierender Prozeßpflege [The Nursing Process Using the Example of Patients with Strokes: A Study to Capture and Develop Holistic-Rehabilitative Nursing Care in a Process]*, ed. Bundesministerium für Gesundheit, vol. 16, Schriftenreihe Des Bundesministeriums für Gesundheit (Baden-Baden: Nomos Verlagsgesellschaft mbH & Co. KG, 1993).
603 Krohwinkel, "Krankenschwester arbeiten gemeinsam an der Verbesserung der Krankenpflege in Europa," 195–97.
604 Monika Krohwinkel, "Wie kann Krankenpflegeforschung uns helfen, besser zu pflegen? [How Can Nursing Research Help Us to Provide Better Nursing Care?]," *Krankenpflege* 34, no. 1 (1980), 14–15.

containment strategies. On the other hand, the need for nursing research was argued to support strategies of saving costs in healthcare.

The Need for Nursing Research to Prevent Cost-Containment Strategies

The argument for research to prevent the nursing vocation from cost-cutting procedures is closely related to the argument for transparency in and the effectiveness of nursing service.[605] For example, Renate Reimann stated that the introduction of science and the conduct of scientific studies should "scientifically prove that a shorter hospital admission period could be caused by a specific nursing activity."[606] It is not surprising, therefore, that from the 1980s on, the focus of research in nursing was predominantly directed to management in nursing. Rosemarie Weinrich in particular called for more and better management knowledge and structure in nursing. The DBfK action program in the 1980s clearly determined the attempt to initiate more research projects. "The DBfK will campaign to foster, support, and put into practice research projects [in nursing] which increase knowledge in nursing and which help to improve nursing care and nursing management especially regarding the care service based on the perspective of the nursing process."[607]

Krohwinkel carried this perception of professional nursing further. Using exact analyses in regard to the situations and requirements at the bedside would make the actual and possible impact of nursing visible, including the conditions for such nursing care.[608] Hence, nursing research was promoted as a tool to avoid cuts in nursing staff. As Krohwinkel explained, nurses in the past were unable to

---

605 Krohwinkel, "Krankenschwester arbeiten gemeinsam an der Verbesserung der Krankenpflege in Europa," 195–97; Renate Reimann, "Probleme der Bestimmung und Messung von Pflegequalität [The Problems of the Determination and Measurement of Quality in Nursing]," *Krankenpflege* 32, no. 5 (1978), 166, 179–80; Reimann, "Pflegeplanung," 154–57; Krohwinkel, "Pflegepersonal setzt sich für bessere Gesundheit ein," 138–40.
606 "So wäre es z. B. sehr wichtig, wenn wissenschaftlich nachgewiesen werden könnte, daß eine Verkürzung der Verweildauer auf spezielle pflegerische Leistungen zurückgeführt werden kann" (Reimann, "Probleme der Bestimmung und Messung von Pflegequalität," 166; my translation).
607 "Der DBfK wird sich einsetzen für die Förderung, Unterstützung und Durchführung solcher Forschungsprojekte, die das Wissen in der Krankenpflege erweitern und zur Verbesserung von Krankenpflegepraxis und Krankenpflegemanagement beitragen, insbesondere im Hinblick auf die Betreuungsleistungen nach den Vorstellungen des Pflegeprozesses" (Weinrich, "Ausblick auf die Arbeit des DBfK," 18; my translation).
608 Krohwinkel, "Pflegepersonal setzt sich für bessere Gesundheit ein," 138–40.

fight against personnel cuts, but nursing research could help nurses to argue and to plan.[609]

The Need for Nursing Research to Support Cost-Containment Strategies

Interestingly, nursing research was not only perceived as being potentially able to secure nursing care from painful cost-containment strategies. It was constituted also as a foundation upon which costs in healthcare could be saved by the effective employment of nursing aides. The knowledge derived from the research projects would enable giving those nursing aides a concrete frame from which they could satisfyingly carry out their practice on the healthcare team, as Weinrich declared in 1981.[610] She repeated this thought in 1985. Due to economic changes, the scope of nursing practice would expand and the demand for nursing service increase, but the number of qualified nursing staff would decrease. Therefore, she recommended reducing activities that did not belong to nursing and to use the nursing process as a help to differentiate between those activities:

> It is undisputed that qualified work can only be executed by appropriately qualified personnel. However, the question still has to be answered whether all work that is executed by examined nurses actually has to be done by them. Or maybe, with a more detailed look, it can be done by unqualified personnel because no qualification is needed for it. A good nursing plan and documentation could be of great help. It should be based on the already recommended nursing process.[611]

However, Weinrich did not provide concrete information about which work would call for qualified nurses and which for nursing aides. But she predicted that this differentiation would ease the nursing shortage (for considerations for the reorganization of nursing service see chapter 7.1). Moreover, the difference between qualified and unqualified nurses, already established by the 1960s, was now applied to the nursing process (and the differentiation between basic and technical nursing care) instead of between those tasks at the bedside and those that could be carried out more remotely. With the creation of an assistant vo-

---

609 Monika Krohwinkel, "Pflegeforschung und ihre Auswirkung in der Praxis im Zusammenhang mit Pflege [Nursing Research and Its Impact on Practice Regarding Nursing]," *Krankenpflege* 38, no. 7–8 (1984), 224–27.
610 Weinrich, "Ausblick auf die Arbeit des DBfK," 16–18.
611 "Es ist unumstritten, daß qualifizierte Arbeiten nur von dafür qualifiziertem Personal vorgenommen werden können. Die Frage bleibt jedoch zu beantworten, ob alle Arbeiten, die von examinierten Pflegekräften ausgeführt werden, auch von diesen übernommen werden müssen oder ob bei genauem Hinsehen vieles nicht auch von unausgebildetem Personal erledigt werden kann, weil es dazu keiner besonderen Qualifikation bedarf. Eine gute Pflegeplanung und Pflegedokumentation könnten in diesem Bereich eine große Hilfe sein. Sie sollten auf dem schon früher vorgeschlagenen Pflegeprozeß basieren" (Weinrich, "Sitzung des Rates der Ländervertreter," 301; my translation).

cation to cover work unnecessary for a qualified nurse to undertake, the nursing vocation created a hierarchical space in the area of nursing. This accompanied a devaluation of those tasks that were taken over by these nursing aides and it was here that the devaluation of basic nursing care occurred. This was probably not intended and contrary to hopes for a reorientation of nursing to its so-called "primary task."[612] However, it was already in the mindset of nurses such as Hohlin, for he declared in his considerations on restructuring hospital nursing care that on a ward with only 30 percent of basic nursing care needed, 30 percent of the staff employed should be nursing aides (see chapter 7.1.1).[613] Hence, the upgrading of the nursing vocation by the establishment of nursing aides accompanied the changing perceptions and content of qualified nurses' scope of practice.

Both arguments for nursing research carry within them the neoliberal argument to establish nursing care as an economic service, which has to prove its effectiveness and which has to show scientifically the necessary conditions to provide efficient nursing care. Interestingly, no concrete scheme was provided in the articles about how to use the results of nursing research to argue against shortcuts. Krohwinkel even emphasized that examples of this research already existed. However, those cuts in nursing personnel, as she stated, would not be based on logical considerations or research but rather on questionable economic thinking.[614] This contradiction is not solved in the articles. Rather, a diffuse understanding was conveyed about what nursing research could do against economic attempts like cost-containment interventions. Nevertheless, nursing research, especially in the 1980s, was continuously praised as an improvement in daily nursing and was conceptualized as part of good and modern nursing.[615]

---

612 Hall, "Probleme der Krankenpflegeausbildung," 302.
613 Detlef Hohlin, "Notwendigkeit der Adaption der Krankenhäuser an Strukturänderungen aus pflegerischer Sicht [A Nursing Perspective on the Necessity of Hospitals Adapting to Structural Changes]," *Krankenpflege* 31, no. 9 (1977), 287–90.
614 Krohwinkel, "Krankenschwester arbeiten gemeinsam an der Verbesserung der Krankenpflege in Europa," 195–97; Krohwinkel, "Pflegeforschung und ihre Auswirkung," 224–27.
615 Jennifer Hunt, "Pflegeforschung – Bringt sie etwas? [Nursing Research: Is It Helpful?]," *Krankenpflege* 38, no. 7–8 (1984), 227–31; Reimann, "Pflegeplanung," 154–57; Krohwinkel, "Krankenschwester arbeiten gemeinsam an der Verbesserung der Krankenpflege in Europa," 195–97; Krohwinkel, "Pflegeforschung und ihre Auswirkung," 224–27; Weinrich, "Ausblick auf die Arbeit des DBfK," 16–18; Marianne Weber, "Der Krankenpflegeprozeß in der Schweiz: Ergebnisse eines Forschungsprojektes und seine Folgen [The Nursing Process in Switzerland: Results of a Research Project and Its Consequences]," *Krankenpflege* 40, no. 1 (1986), 30–32; Roland Trill, "Anforderungen an ein EDV-gestütztes Kommunikationssystem für den Pflegebereich [Requirements for a Computing-Based Communication System in Nursing]," *Krankenpflege* 40, no. 9 (1986), 342–44.

8.2 Professionalization or De-professionalization – A Summary

As already mentioned above, the professionalization project in nursing was established by nurses at the very same time as neoliberal changes became more dominant in Germany. Neoliberalism, however, draws on the principle of the free market and fosters competition in society. Enclosed professions were seen as obstacles to this principle of competition. The introduction of accounting strategies and management processes into professions attempted to open their enclosures.[616] From the 1960s on, in Anglophone countries discussions were raised about the concepts of profession and professionalization, beginning with Wilensky's question "The Professionalization of Everyone?" in 1964 and Marie Haug's counterquestion "The Deprofessionalization of Everyone?" in 1975.[617] These two articles frame the discussion around professionalization and de-professionalization. One position is that with continuous development and progress in different vocations, every vocation seems to have professionalized, for example, by establishing academic education and developing scientific knowledge. This progress in a vocation, however, cannot be understood as professionalization but rather as adapting to societal developments and keeping up with the progress of other vocations in the same field.[618] The attempts to academize nursing education in Germany can be understood in this manner because Germany has experienced this same kind of academic drift in the last decades.

The second position within this frame of professionalization or de-professionalization is, however, more interesting from the perspective of this study. Publications focusing on de-professionalization mainly use the medical profession as an example. The indicators for a de-professionalization are various but mostly connected to each other.

The following pages contain a critical reflection on the question of whether the developments in the 1970s and 1980s in German nursing can be identified as professionalization or de-professionalization. For that reason, I compare the arguments for de-professionalization I found in the literature with the arguments I could find in my empirical material. As I will show, this comparison reveals that the indicators pointing towards the de-professionalization of a classical pro-

---

616 Rose, "Government, Authority and Expertise," 283–99; Peter Miller and Nikolas Rose, "Political Power Beyond the State: Problematics of Government," in *Governing the Present: Administering Economic, Social and Personal Life*, ed. Peter Miller and Nikolas Rose (Cambridge, Malden: Polity Press, 2008), 53–83.
617 Harold L. Wilensky, "The Professionalization of Everyone?," *American Journal of Sociology* 70, no. 2 (1964), 137–58; Marie R. Haug, "The Deprofessionalization of Everyone?," *Sociological Focus* 8, no. 3 (1975), 197–213.
618 Wilensky, "Professionalization of Everyone?," 137–58; William J. Goode, "Encroachment, Charlatanism, and the Emerging Profession: Psychology, Sociology, and Medicine," *American Sociological Review* 25, no. 6 (1960), 902–65.

fession such as medicine were understood by German nurses as strategies for a professionalization of the nursing vocation. Despite that, I do not agree, however, with the belief that professionalization in nursing would cause a de-professionalization in medicine.[619] Rather, I argue that the development of the nursing vocation speaks to a trend that is contrary to professionalization, although German nurses still view their attempts to be in line with a professionalization of nursing.

8.2.1 Implementation of Mechanisms of Mistrust

The mechanization of the physicians' workplace was described as an indicator of de-professionalization because it led to a decline in the value and trust of physicians' own diagnostic competence and professional expertise. It accompanied a higher trust in "hard" and objective data which can be calculated and measured,[620] along with the implementation of antitrust interventions such as DRGs, audit systems, and the increase of bureaucracy.[621] Moreover, whereas in the past the physician owned his/her own (simple) apparatuses, now he or she cannot afford expensive technologies and is dependent on capitalistic and bureaucratic systems in which he or she is employed. In consequence, a formerly exclusive medical decision about the purchase of medical equipment becomes now an agreement or compromise between the physician and administration. "Rather than controlling simple technologies as was true in the past, physicians are finding themselves in positions whereby they are more likely to be controlled (and their autonomy reduced) by advanced technologies and the technicians who design them, control them, and interpret their results."[622]

Understanding the nursing process as an accounting tool (as I showed in chapter 7), means to acknowledge that the nursing process was installed as a technology of mistrust. The call for transparency originated from attempts to make nursing care calculable and understandable for people outside the vocation

---

619 E. g. Ellen Annandale, "Proletarianization or Restratification of the Medical Profession? The Case of Obstetrics," *International Journal of Health Services* 19, no. 4 (1989), 611–34; Julian Wolf and Werner Vogd, "Professionalisierung der Pflege, Deprofessionalisierung der Ärzte oder vice versa? [Professionalization of Nursing, Deprofessionalization of Physicians, or Vice Versa?]," in *Professsionskulturen – Charakteristika unterschiedlicher professioneller Praxen*, ed. Silke Müller-Hermann, et al. (Wiesbaden: Springer Fachmedien, 2018), 151–73.
620 Heinrich Bollinger and Joachim Hohl, "Auf dem Weg von der Profession zum Beruf: Zur Deprofessionalisierung des Ärzte-Standes [On the Way from a Profession to a Vocation: About the Deprofessionalization of the Physicians]," *Soziale Welt* 32, no. 4 (1981), 440–64.
621 George Ritzer and David Walczak, "Rationalization and the Deprofessionalization of Physicians," *Social Forces* 67, no. 1 (1988), 1–22.
622 Ritzer and Walczak, "Rationalization and the Deprofessionalization of Physicians," 12.

and to prove its effectiveness to them. Even more, the nursing process enables comparisons between and among resources used and the costs with the outcome (or benefits) of nursing service, and it relates specific nursing actions to individual nurses. With the nursing process, nursing action and nursing outcome could be judged after being disentangled from its situatedness and its unique relationship between the nurse and the patient. It is not the nurse and the patient who should judge the individual nursing situation in which they were engaged with each other, based on unclear and non-transparent criteria, but it is the cybernetic dynamic that should evaluate and regulate nursing service based on the criteria of input and output.[623] This accompanied the introduction of cybernetic control in nursing. However, this control should not be understood as merely repressive. It appears as a democratic control that is directed to everybody and is non-hierarchical. The incorporation of this kind of control (which happened concurrently with the implementation of the nursing process) constructs a self-responsible subject that governs itself according to this cybernetic control. This control produces a space in which the subject is free to act and decide, not perceiving itself as controlled but empowered and autonomous. This is likley why nurses called for transparency that was inherent in the nursing process as they perceived it as an improvement in their vocation. It made the nursing vocation and the individual nurse accountable, understood by nurses as a characteristic of professionalism in nursing.

Computerization in nursing, however, as the digitalization of this technology of mistrust, was partly perceived as a dangerous process that would likely overrun the nursing vocation. Hence, it was seen as more of a threat to the autonomy of the "emerging nursing profession," and as a force nurses had to subordinate themselves to in order to keep up with and shape in a helpful way for them.

8.2.2 The Decline of Monopolized Knowledge

Another indicator is the decline of autonomy and power in society in general, and in this case, over the patient in particular.[624] This indicator can actually be understood as the consequence of factors already described above. The disappearance or devaluation of monopolized knowledge and the process of the "demystification of knowledge,"[625] is caused by the drive for rationality, trans-

---

623 Now this is possible in a very standardized and calculative manner through the Nursing Outcomes Classifications (NOC) (Sue Moorhead, *Nursing Outcomes Classification (NOC)*, 4th ed. (St. Louis, Mo: Mosby Elsevier, 2008)).
624 Ritzer and Walczak, "Rationalization and the Deprofessionalization of Physicians," 1–22.
625 "Entmystifizierung des Wissens" (Maren Siepmann and David A. Groneberg, "Der Arztberuf als Profession – Deprofessionalisierung [The Medical Vocation as Profession: De-

parency, and accountability, as well as by the increasing availability of (scientific) knowledge.[626]

As mentioned, German nurses were active participants in opening up their knowledge base. Intuition based on tacit knowledge was no longer the foundation for nursing decisions, it was argued, but transparent, objective, and possibly standardized knowledge. The fear of cuts in financial and material resources led to the perception that nurses needed to prove the effectiveness of their service to the public, which can be understood as indicating declining trust and hence, declining power of the nursing vocation.[627] This becomes obvious as well in the warnings that patients could sue nurses or hospitals when they were not satisfied with the nursing care provided.[628] However, this should not neglect the fact that nurses were still powerful in the patient-nurse relationship. Being in a vulnerable situation the patient was and still is subject to a nurse's influence. Now however, nurses became agents of the neoliberal agenda in reconstructing the patient into a neoliberal subject, for example, through health education. Although the nursing vocation experienced a decline in its former autonomy as established under the Christian rationale,[629] within the frame of the neoliberal discourse, nursing service became reconstituted by the nursing process in a way that provided nurses a space in which they could act freely and powerfully towards their patients.

Furthermore, with the reconstitution of the nursing vocation into an economic entity based on the neoliberal rationale, nurses also put pressure on the enclosures of the medical profession. In the articles of the 1970s and 1980s, this aspect was briefly mentioned. However, a recent study of the relationship between physicians and nurses in German hospital care revealed that the integration of management strategies into nursing service and their acting in favour of managerial thinking apparently makes nurses "better" than physicians when thinking of them as parts of the hospital enterprise. Nursing managers especially perceive themselves and the nursing vocation as more valuable members of the hospital than physicians because of nurses' organizational competence and their willingness to value the general organization of

---

professionalization]," *Zentralblatt für Arbeitsmedizin, Arbeitsschutz und Ergonomie* 62 (2012), 288–92: 289; my translation).

626 Haug, "Deprofessionalization," 197–213; Siepmann and Groneberg, "Der Arztberuf als Profession," 288–92; Storch and Stinson, "Concepts of Deprofessionalization," 33–44.

627 See Rosemary Donley, "The Need for Rationality, Conceptualization, and Problem Solving," in *Human Needs 3 and the Nursing Process*, ed. Helen Yura and Mary B. Walsh (Norwalk, Conn.: Appleton-Century-Crofts, 1983), 85–116.

628 Reimann, "Information im Dienst des Kranken," 249–53; Thiel, "Pflegeplanung und Pflegedokumentation," 9–12.

629 See chapter 8.1.3; Kreutzer, "Krankenbeobachtung," 167–88; Nolte, "Pflege von Sterbenden im 19. Jahrhundert," 87–107.

the hospital. Those nursing managers equated themselves with the administration of the hospital and believed they were in the opposite position to physicians who would rather follow their own particular interests.[630] This should not be understood as a professionalization of the nursing vocation that was leading to a de-professionalization of the medical profession. Rather, in their attempts to free themselves from the dominance of physicians, nurses took on managerial logic and were subordinated under economic logic. In turn, this neoliberal force of nurses puts even more pressure on the medical profession and makes it harder for physicians to defend their enclosures.[631]

8.2.3 Subordination Under Economic Premises

The subordination of nursing's own work under economic premises, that is, the "emphasis on quantifiable costs,"[632] as well as the establishment of standards and control mechanisms, has been identified as a main indicator for de-professionalization. It is defined as de-professionalization because it leads to a higher regulation of the professional individual and of the profession in general. The professional is no longer free to make decisions based on his or her professional knowledge but always has to take into account external forces such as aspects of the economy or organizational requirements. Connected to this are increasing calls to act upon the criteria of performance and to re-define professional success as the efficiency of medical interventions in relation to the health of the public. Hence, the medical profession loses its autonomy to define what good medical care is – at least partly – to the economic sphere.[633]

In the articles I analyzed, nurses welcomed the transformation initiated by the WHO. While the rationale of the WHO has to be understood as an attempt to economize healthcare systems, nurses saw their chance to establish a new nursing profession under this transformation. The content of this new nursing profession was understood as the redirection of German nursing toward the

---

630 Wolf and Vogd, "Professionalisierung der Pflege, Deprofessionalisierung der Ärzte," 151–73.
631 For the Canadian context, see the study of Marie L. Campbell. She revealed that with the introduction of managerial strategies, situations emerged in which "nurses [exerted] power against physicians, in a way and on issues that they have been powerless to do before. At the same time, it is important to notice that the power of nurses to influence physicians in these examples is mediated by an intervening factor: the hospital's central concern about costs" (M. L. Campbell, "Nurses Professionalism in Canada: A Labor Process Analysis," *International Journal of Health Services* 22, no. 4 (1992), 751–65: 760).
632 Ritzer and Walczak, "Rationalization and the Deprofessionalization of Physicians," 7.
633 Bollinger and Hohl, "Auf dem Weg von der Profession zum Beruf," 440–64; Ritzer and Walczak, "Rationalization and the Deprofessionalization of Physicians," 1–22.

WHO's concept of health and the implementation of health education with the empowered healthy patient as the desired outcome. As I showed in chapter 7, the focus on lifestyle is a characteristic of neoliberal rationality, which aims to construct a self-responsible patient-subject who decides and acts based on rational calculations. By doing that, this economized subject is health conscious and understands his or her health as being part of human capital. Hence, with providing such a nursing service, nurses have apparently even become drivers of the neoliberal agenda. This is likely why nurses themselves have already incorporated the neoliberal rationale and perceive themselves (rightly) as agents in these newly constituted healthcare services.

This emerging neoliberal rationale was also accompanied by calls for an effective and efficient nursing service, which nurses appreciated because it was connected to the hope of making the nursing vocation autonomous. The cybernetic logic of the nursing process, that is, thinking about nursing as a process of input, output, and feedback, made nursing phenomena calculable. Nursing work could be structured in calculable terms which could then be connected to costs and profits. However, the transformation of nursing care into an accountable, calculable, and traceable nursing service subordinated the nursing vocation to economic logic. The nursing process, as an accounting tool, promoted the introduction of a managerial and economic logic into nursing practice and defined the frame in which nurses were able to work. Nurses themselves argued that their vocation needed to demonstrate effectiveness in the healthcare setting. The management of nursing service in accordance with economic criteria nurses also perceived as part of their professionalism.

Hence, thinking about a distinct scope of practice in the terms and logic of an accounting tool such as the nursing process situates the nursing vocation and its service within an accounting framework. It makes the nursing vocation calculable and helps to introduce economization strategies into nursing service. Hence, autonomy in nursing care is constrained by external forces in two ways: First, nurses need to make their work transparent and understandable to managers or organizations outside of the nursing vocation. Second, they have to successfully show that their work has a positive impact on the patient. This appears to be a self-fulfilling prophecy, for this is what Detlef Hohlin had declared in 1977, that autonomy in nursing could only be possible within economic structures (see chapter 7.1.1).[634]

As to the results of this study, German nursing scientist Doris Schaeffer is right when she speaks about "tendencies of de-professionalization" brought about by the introduction of economic strategies in nursing, such as the striving for

---

634 Hohlin, "Notwendigkeit der Adaption der Krankenhäuser," 287–90.

profit.⁶³⁵ But although she acknowledges this phenomenon, she still argues that the nursing vocation should show "that nursing performs a valuable although underrated contribution to an effective and efficient healthcare service. [...] Only through connecting professional intentions with the intentions of health policy can the newly begun professionalization be continued."⁶³⁶

---

635 "Deprofessionalisierungtendenzen" (Doris Schaeffer, "Professionalisierung der Pflege [Professionalization of Nursing]," in *Dienstleistungsqualität und Qualität des Arbeitslebens im Krankenhaus*, ed. André Büssing and Jürgen Glaser (Göttingen, Bern, Toronto, Seattle: Hogrefe-Verlag, 2003), 227–43: 234; my translation).
636 "... dass Pflege einen wertvollen, in seiner Bedeutung unterschätzten Beitrag zu einer effektiven und effizienten Gesundheitsversorgung zu leisten vermag", da "nur durch Verknüpfung professions- und gesundheitspolitischer Intentionen [...] die begonnene Professionalisierung erfolgreich vorangetrieben werden [kann]" (Schaeffer, "Professionalisierung der Pflege," 241; my translation).

Chapter 9:
Conclusion

In this study, I aimed to analyze a discourse in German nursing that emerged in the second half of the 20th century and which could be understood as the starting point for professionalization in German nursing. It seems to be quite ironic that the German nursing vocation enthusiastically believed in and argued for the process of its professionalization at a point in time in which professionalism (based on the understanding of the sociology of professions) started to decline. Using the approach of the history of the present, I tried to reveal why German nurses today believe that they have already achieved some progress towards professionalization, while at the same time experiencing huge economic shortcuts in the nursing workplace, constraints in their ability to decide how to organize and provide nursing care, increasing burnout, painful nursing shortages, and a high number of dropouts.

Using the nursing process, I analyzed the connection between the arguments praising the nursing process as an instrument of professionalization and the potential of the nursing process to consequently restructure nursing into a calculable activity. I wanted to understand the connection between the proposed professionalization of German nursing and the increasing pressure on it to legitimize nursing services. The nursing process promised to be an appropriate example: first, the nursing process, a cybernetic process of input, process, output, and feedback, is now understood as a central concept of the German nursing profession. However, based on the perspective of governmentality, the classic understanding of enclosed professions is that they are perceived as obsolete and even as obstacles in today's existing rationale of neoliberalism. Second, the nursing process was implemented with the hope of professionalizing German nursing at exactly the same time as the German Ordoliberal[637] rationale became dominant and the understanding of how to govern a society became based on the mode of economy.

---

637 Ordoliberalism is the German neoliberal variant (see chapter 5.2.1).

The first part of this last chapter brings together the trend towards making nursing accountable and economic as well as its struggle towards professionalization. I will show that together they become a hybrid discourse in the healthcare system that nurses accept even if somewhat blindly. In the second part, I will discuss the frame within which this study can be understood, what it does not answer, and where it might not be adequate. The relevance and implications of this study will be presented in the third part.

9.1 Summary

By the second half of the 20th century, healthcare costs in many nation states were increasingly problematic. Narratives such as "cost-explosion" were used to argue for the introduction of cost-containment strategies and the restructuring of national healthcare systems. The WHO was especially active in pushing for these strategies. With managerial technologies and mechanisms such as cybernetic logic or output-orientation, healthcare services would become calculable and reconstituted as market commodities.

This neoliberal understanding of how a society should function could also be found in the German context. Ordoliberalism as the German variant of neoliberalism called for free competition in all areas of society and a strong state to guarantee it. The argument of cost-explosion in the healthcare system and the need to instil economic behaviour in healthcare workers emerged in the 1960s and 1970s in Germany. The implementation of the nursing process in Germany can be understood as an answer to the problematization of the way healthcare in general, and nursing care in particular, was delivered and measured. The nursing process was one of the strategies to establish this cost-conscious behaviour and to focus on the effectiveness of nursing service.

The Nursing Process as Accounting Tool

To analyze how the nursing process reconstituted nursing service and the perception of nurses themselves, I used the theoretical approach of critical accounting. It helped to explain the impact of an accounting tool such as the nursing process. The logic, techniques, and discursive underpinnings that go along with the nursing process were able to introduce new structures and meanings into healthcare organizations, particularly in nursing services, and make them open to calculation and economization. As an accounting tool, the nursing process is a powerful instrument that is hard to criticize. It produces apparently neutral, rational, and scientific knowledge, which both restructures the organization it derives knowledge from and legitimizes nursing actions that are based on this knowledge. As an apparently neutral accounting tool, the power of the nursing process to transform practices has hardly been acknowledged in healthcare organizations. For example, several nurses perceived the nursing process not as a new understanding of nursing but as something that nurses regularly would do.

From the perspective of critical accounting, accounting tools do not create an exact image of what they are applied to but rather constitute a new reality. This new reality is structured by the logic and language of the respective accounting tool. Hence, the nursing process constituted a new nursing vocation based on the logic of accounting and calculability. Throughout the 1970s and 1980s, the nursing process seems to have been more and more understood as synonymous with professional nursing care. This became obvious in different nursing articles in which professional nursing was defined by the steps of the nursing process.[638]

The nursing process thus opened the nursing vocation to the rationale of neoliberalism. It conceptualizes nursing in such a way that nursing interventions can be transparent, quantified, and thereby measurable. Individual performances can be compared for their efficiency. Hence, the nursing process makes nursing interventions calculable in economic terms, and, therefore, transforms nursing interventions into market commodities.

Based on the logic of the nursing process and its underlying concept of health, nurses and patients were constituted as responsible for attempting to decrease hospital admissions and healthcare costs, and to keep people functioning in society. This is consistent with the German Ordoliberal's claim to change consumer behaviour and thus help prevent certain avoidable expensive illnesses.

Accompanying the perception that professional nursing is nursing care within the structure of the nursing process is that it is automatically rational, accountable, and hence controllable. Therefore, only nursing components that can be verbalized in a rational way can be integrated into the nursing process. Non-verbalizable "goings-on" in nursing care contradict the logic of the nursing process and consequently disappear from nursing's official scope of practice. In other words, when nursing care becomes constituted as the sum of distinct, well-defined single activities in the structure of a cybernetic process, all non-verbalizable activities in nursing (such as emotional work or com-

---

638 E.g. Dorothy C. Hall, "Überlegungen zum Krankenpflegeberuf [Considerations About the Nursing Vocation]," *Krankenpflege* 31, no. 2 (1977), 40–42; Rosemarie Weinrich, "Gedanken zum Berufsbild Krankenpflege [Thoughts About the Vocation Nursing]," *Krankenpflege* 36, no. 1 (1982), 2–3; Renate Reimann, "Pflegeplanung – Was bedeutet geplante Pflege in der Berufspraxis [Nursing Care Plan: The Meaning of Planned Nursing Care in Daily Professional Practice]," *Krankenplege* 33, no. 5 (1979), 154–57; Nicole Delmotte, "Der Krankenpflegeprozeß in Belgien. Erfahrungen mit der WHO-Studie [The Nursing Process in Belgum: Experiences with the WHO Study]," *Krankenpflege* 40, no. 1 (1986), 32–35.

forting patients by being at their side) cannot be considered – neither objectively nor financially – as part of nursing service. If nurses still want to execute these activities, they have to do it on top of their "actual" work.

In 1987, Virginia Henderson, who had promoted the nursing process as an important nursing concept throughout the70s,[639] criticized that the nursing process had become synonymous with nursing work. According to her, the focus on the nursing process devalued the perception of nursing as an art and ignored creativity, intuition, and other ways of thinking, acting, and recognizing that went beyond the nursing process.[640] However, nurses appreciated the introduction of the nursing process and actively participated in the transformation of the German healthcare system into a market place entity in which healthcare services were offered and chosen based on their effectiveness and efficiency. As I showed in the last part of this study, this can be explained with the narrative German nurses developed in their striving for professionalization.

The Hybrid Discourse and the De-professionalization in Nursing

The nursing process was advertised as a concept of professional nursing and also as a component to a new nursing vocation that was able to meet economic demands. The introduction of the nursing process into the nursing vocation changed the discourse in nursing in such a way that a hybrid discourse was established. That is, with the integration of a new logic and language derived from accounting, the discourse in nursing was reconstituted as an accounting-nursing discourse. In this hybrid discourse, it is increasingly difficult to determine where nursing knowledge ends and accounting knowledge begins. Nursing knowledge and accounting knowledge merged in such a way that their two different logics became one. Hence, the newly reconstituted nursing vocation could not be considered outside of accountable nursing.[641] The "mechanization of nursing" or computerization in nursing is one example of this discourse.[642]

---

639 Virginia Henderson, *Principles and Practice of Nursing*, ed. Gladys Nite and Bertha Harmer, 6th ed. (New York: Macmillan, 1978); Virginia Henderson, "The Concept of Nursing," *Journal of Advanced Nursing* 3, no. 2 (1978), 113–30.
640 Virginia Henderson, "Nursing Process: A Critique," *Holistic nursing practice* 1, no. 3 (1987), 7–18.
641 See Thomas Foth, Jette Lange, and Kylie Smith, "Nursing History as Philosophy: Towards a Critical History of Nursing," *Nursing Philosophy* 19, no. 3 (2018), e12210.
642 Manfred Hülsken-Giesler, *Der Zugang zum Anderen. Zur theoretischen Rekonstruktion von Professionalisierungsstrategien pflegerischen Handelns im Spannungsfeld von Mimesis und Maschinenlogik [Access to and Approach of the Other: For a Theoretical Reconstruction of Professionalization Strategies of Nursing Care in the Tension between Mimesis and Machine Logic]*, ed. Hartmut Remmers, vol. 3, Pflegewissenschaft und Pflegebildung (Göttingen: V&R unipress, 2008).

This hybrid discourse constitutes a new image and understanding of nursing. A socially and politically accepted German nursing vocation is based on the principles, which have to be proven, of rationality, effectiveness, and efficiency. However, it seems that this newly developed understanding of nursing lacks some of the aspects that were included in the former understanding of nursing, such as having time available for being with patients or for activities that cannot be captured in a rational, hence measurable (or even scientific) language.

Seeing nursing as a profession in this hybrid discourse, as well as in the new neoliberal rationale, is not necessary and is even perceived as contrary to the neoliberal agenda. I argue these developments in German nursing should be understood more as a form of de-professionalization in the nursing vocation.

Why then, has so much of the literature praised professionalization in German nursing since the 1970s? The professionalization project in German nursing seems to be as diffuse as the understanding and use of the notion of "profession."[643] The hopes nurses had for the professional status of their vocation were in line with different theoretical approaches of the sociology of professions, the main aspect of which was connected to the attempt for autonomy in nursing service. However, the strategies German nurses were using to achieve this status encouraged nursing's reconstruction under a neoliberal agenda and the introduction of accounting mechanisms. In their hopes for professionalization, nurses themselves implemented the nursing process and argued for its necessity in order to make nursing transparent, accountable, and professional. For example, cost-saving measurements that were especially criticized by nurses were actually implemented themselves.[644]

Understanding the nursing process as a strategy to professionalize made nurses eager to implement a language and logic of accounting and the principle

---

[643] Eva-Maria Krampe, "Professionalisierung der Pflege im Kontext der Ökonomisierung [Professionalization of Nursing in the Context of Economization]," in *20 Jahre Wettbewerb im Gesundheitswesen. Theoretische und empirische Analysen zur Ökonomisierung von Medizin und Pflege*, ed. Alexandra Manzei and Rudi Schmiede, Gesundheit und Gesellschaft (Wiesbaden: Springer Fachmedien, 2014), 179–97; Marianne Schmidbaur, *Vom "Lazaruskreuz" zu "Pflege Aktuell": Professionalisierungsdiskurse in der deutschen Krankenpflege 1903-2000 [From "Lazaruskreuz" to "Pflege Aktuell": Discourses on Professionalization in German Nursing Care 1903–2000]* (Königstein: Helmer, 2002).

[644] See the example of the calculation of nursing personnel based on patients' needs (Detlef Hohlin, "Werden Anhaltszahlen durch neue Berechnungsmethoden abgelöst? Teil I [Will Reference Data Soon Be Replaced by New Methods of Calculation? Part I]," *Krankenpflege* 40, no. 3 (1986), 102–04; Detlef Hohlin, "Werden Anhaltszahlen durch neue Berechnungsmethoden abgelöst? Teil II [Will Reference Data Soon Be Replaced by New Methods of Calculation? Part II]," *Krankenpflege* 40, no. 4 (1986), 142–43; Detlef Hohlin, "Werden Anhaltszahlen durch neue Berechnungsmethoden abgelöst? Teil III [Will Reference Data Soon Be Replaced by New Methods of Calculation? Part III]," *Krankenpflege* 40, no. 5 (1986), 189–90, 207).

of economy that came along with the nursing process. In this hybrid nursing discourse, nurses value increasing accountability as the foundation for a more recognized and professional position in German society. In the time of its implementation, the WHO and politically active nurses argued that the nursing process would be a key component in providing high-quality nursing care on the basis of planned care. Moreover, the implementation of the nursing process promised a new direction for nursing, a new and distinct scope of practice, making nurses more independent of the medical profession. The nursing process apparently was a solution to the question of how to separate nursing from the medical profession and build an autonomous scope of practice. Constituting a new nursing vocation within the frame of accounting and the logic of economy opened it to hospital management and administration. Identifying themselves with the aims and logics of their organization constituted a new space in which nurses might act independently. As nursing scientist Eva-Maria Krampe argued in regard to the academization of German nursing, the increasing dominance of managerialism in healthcare opened a space for new responsibilities in nursing such as using nursing research to find possibilities for rationalization in healthcare.[645]

However, this broad hybrid discourse carried the desire and promise of professional nursing only on its surface. The newly established nursing vocation differs profoundly from a traditional understanding of professionalism and from the hopes of autonomy that nurses ascribed to their professionalization project. Hence, the strategy of professionalization as it was perceived and fostered by nurses needs to be understood as a strategy of de-professionalization from within the perspective of neoliberal governmentality.

Still relying on this traditional understanding of professions and holding to that while calling for an accountable nursing profession seems to be a "doublethinking" of nurses – being autonomous and being accountable. Here, however, this doublethinking is more than just the acceptance of two contrary concepts. It is the connection of those contrary concepts in the manner of causality: When we as nurses are accountable then we are able to work autonomously. In consequence, this is can be understood as a de-professionalization in the name of professionalization.[646]

---

645 Eva-Maria Krampe, *Emanzipation durch Professionalisierung: Akademisierung des Frauenberufs Pflege in den 1990er Jahren; Erwartungen und Folgen [Emancipation through Professionalization: The Academization of a Female Vocation in the 1990s; Expectations and Consequences]* (Frankfurt am Main: Mabuse-Verlag, 2009).
646 See Mirko Noordegraaf, "From "Pure" to "Hybrid" Professionalism: Present-Day Professionalism in Ambiguous Public Domains," *Administration & Society* 39, no. 6 (2007), 761–85.

9.2 Limitations

In this study, I aimed to reveal and analyze a large nursing discourse that emerged in the second half of the 20th century in West Germany, focusing especially on the decades of the 1970s and 1980s. To complete this analysis and capture this discourse in-depth, other sources wait for analysis, such as material from Catholic nursing associations, from the union ÖTV, or from managers in healthcare in general. Moreover, focusing only on the 1970s and 80s is a short time frame for such a large hybrid discourse. Attempts to restructure hospital care in Germany can be found earlier in the 1960s and deserve a closer analysis.

Furthermore, this study focuses on the West German context where a unique nursing vocation existed. This nursing vocation was and still is highly influenced by its former Christian foundation even if many nurses do not recognize this and even if this Christian tradition is often criticized. The question is, therefore, whether the findings of this study can be transferred to other Western countries. Moreover, the eurocentrism underlying most scientific research in Western countries also has to be considered. It guided the acknowledgement of the problem in the German nursing vocation, influenced the analysis of discursive structures and shifts, and impacted the conclusions I draw.

The theoretical and methodological framing of this study I consider both a weakness and a strength at the same time. Using the epistemological perspective of the history of the present means neglecting a discoverable unique reality based on hard facts. Rather, with this perspective, I wanted to develop another narrative about the professionalization project of the German nursing vocation, although it is just another option to understand the impact of past developments on how we perceive reality today. Hence, it has to be seen as a piece of a newly created (and criticizable) knowledge about the past, about societal and economic developments, and about the position of the nursing vocation within a society. Additionally, the combination of different perspectives and theories, that is, the historical stance, the perspective on governmentality, and the approaches of critical accounting on professionalization and on de-professionalization, made the framework of this study very complex and sometimes hard to structure, considering that I am neither a historian nor an accounting expert. However, all the knowledge and techniques I derived from those sciences and approaches helped me in the analysis of the developments in German nursing care and in the understanding of this new nursing discourse.

9.3 Relevance and Implication

"Professionalization in nursing" has become a "plastic" notion in German nursing with hardly any concrete meaning. It is used to argue for the implementation of different strategies like Evidence-Based Nursing (EBN) or university nursing study programs. However, what is understood by professionalism is mostly not consciously defined nor is there a concrete connection articulated between the specific concept or technology and the proposed professional status that should be achieved with it. Therefore, establishing a critical philosophy for nursing sciences as well as for the German nursing vocation in general would enable more critical reflection on those concepts and the role the nursing vocation plays in society.

This study aims to deepen questions regarding ongoing processes in German nursing. It demonstrates how theoretical approaches of critical accounting can be applied to the nursing field in order to understand the impact of seemingly pure nursing concepts such as the nursing process. And it offers a new explanation and understanding of the developments in German nursing in the last five decades. Rather than accepting the general narrative of professionalization, I argue that this study helps to explain the paradox of experiencing unsatisfactory working conditions in daily nursing care while simultaneously declaring progress towards the professionalization of the nursing vocation itself.

It is my hope that the results of this research have the potential to develop a new self-understanding of and self-confidence in the German nursing vocation. Nurses need to acknowledge their agency in political and social forces and to understand that they are powerful actors who – every day – use their power in nursing practice. Comprising the largest vocational group in the healthcare system, nurses are the ones who implement new strategies and drive organizational change. By constantly working within the frame of the nursing process, for example, they reinforce the economization of nursing service. And they bring those political rationales and agendas to the sick, as one of the weakest parts of society, who rely heavily on the decisions and perceptions of nurses. Being self-conscious of their powerful position in the healthcare system and over their patients would be a revolutionary and truly professional characteristic of nurses. Nurses need to thus develop a critical and emancipatory perspective on societal developments and their impact on nursing service. Change does not occur when nurses use their power only to keep the system running.

Bibliography

Abbott, Andrew Delano. *The System of Professions: An Essay on the Division of Expert Labor*. Chicago: University of Chicago Press, 1988.

Albert, Martin. "Krankenpflege auf dem Weg zur Professionalisierung [Nursing on Its Way to Professionalization]," 1998. http://phfr.bsz-bw.de/files/12/93_1.pdf.

American Nurses Association. *Nursing: Scope and Standards of Practice*, edited by Inc Ovid Technologies. 2 ed. Silver Spring, Md.: American Nurses Association, 2010.

Ammende, Rainer, Frank Arens, Ingrid Darmann-Finck, Roswitha Ertl-Schmuck, Brigitte von Germeten-Ortmann, Gertrud Hundenborn, Barbara Knigge-Demal, Uwe Machleit, Christine Maier, Sabine Muths, and Anja Walter. "Rahmenpläne der Fachkommission nach § 53 PflBG [Frameworks for Nursing Education]," 2019, https://www.bibb.de/dokumente/pdf/geschst_pflgb_rahmenplaene-der-fachkommission.pdf.

Andresen, Knut, Ursula Bitzegeio, and Jürgen Mittag. "Arbeitsbeziehungen und Arbeitswelt(en) im Wandel: Problemfelder und Fragestellungen [Work Relations and Working Environment(s) in Transition: Problems and Questions]." In *"Nach dem Strukturbruch"? Kontinuität und Wandel von Arbeitsbeziehungen und Arbeitswelt(en) seit den 1970er Jahren*, edited by Knut Andresen, Ursula Bitzegeio and Jürgen Mittag, 7–23. Bonn: Verlag J. H. W. Dietz Nachf. GmbH, 2011.

Andrzejak, Marita. "Krankenpflege als Dienstleistung [Nursing as Service]." *Krankenpflege* 36, no. 3 (1982): 82–84.

Andrzejak, Marita, Christine Morenz-Geis, Gesche Popp-Sennewald, and Maria Schwertl-Staubach. "Konzeptionen zur Betriebsgestaltung auf der Grundlage des Berufsbildes Krankenpflege des DBfK [Conception for Business Organization Based on the Professional Image of Nursing Released by the Dbfk]." *Krankenpflege* 40, no. 3 (1986): 125.

Annandale, Ellen. "Proletarianization or Restratification of the Medical Profession? The Case of Obstetrics." *International Journal of Health Services* 19, no. 4 (1989): 611–34.

Ansmann, Lena, and Holger Pfaff. "Providers and Patients Caught between Standardization and Individualization: Individualized Standardization as a Solution. Comment on '(Re) Making the Procrustean Bed? Standardization and Customization as Competing Logics in Healthcare'." *International Journal of Health Policy and Management* 7, no. 4 (2017): 349–52.

Ashworth, Pat, Agnes Bjørn, Geneviève Déchanoz, Nicole Delmotte, Elisabeth Farmer, Anna Bulanda Kordas, Elsa Kristiansen, Helen Kyriakidou, Majda Slajmer-Japelj, Maija

Sorvettula, and Marta Stankova., *People's Needs for Nursing Care: A European Study.* edited by World Health Organization Copenhagen: World Health Organization, 1987.

August, Vincent. *Technologisches Regieren. Der Aufstieg des Netzwerk-Denkens in der Krise der Moderne. Foucault, Luhmann und die Kybernetik [Technological Governing. The Rise of Network-Thinking During the Crisis of Modernity. Foucault, Luhmann, and Cybernetics].* Bielefeld: transcript Verlag, 2021.

Barnum, Barbara Stevens. "The Nursing Process Worldwide: What Is Its Future?" In *The Nursing Process: A Global Concept*, edited by Monika Habermann, Leana R. Uys and Barbara Parfitt, 155–67. Edinburgh; New York: Elsevier/Churchill Livingstone, 2006.

Barry, Andrew, Thomas Osborne, and Nikolas Rose. "Introduction." In *Foucault and Political Reason: Liberalism, Neo-Liberalism and Rationalities of Government*, edited by Andrew Barry, Thomas Osborne and Nikolas Rose, 1–17. Chicago: The University of Chicago Press, 1996.

Bartholomeyczik, Sabine. "Arbeitsplatz Krankenbett [Bedside Workplace]." *Krankenpflege* 41, no. 5 (1987): 158–61.

–. "Gesundheit als Voraussetzung patientenorientierter Krankenpflege [Health as Precondition for Patient-Oriented Nursing Care]." *Krankenpflege* 40, no. 5 (1986): 178–80.

Bayern. "Mitgliederversammlung am 9.11.1974 [General Meeting on November 9th, 1974]." *Krankenpflege* 28, no. 12 (1974): 521.

Beedholm, Kirsten, Kirsten Lomborg, and Kirsten Frederiksen. "Ruptured Thought: Rupture as a Critical Attitude to Nursing Research." *Nursing Philosophy* 15, no. 2 (2014): 102–11.

Beer, Stafford. "Cybernetics: A Systems Approach to Management." *Personnel Review* 1, no. 2 (1972): 28–39.

Begerow, Anke, and Uta Gaidys, "COVID-19 Pflege Studie. Erfahrung von Pflegenden während der Pamdemie – erste Teilergebnisse [COVID-19 Nursing Study. Experiences of Nurses during the Pandemic – First Results]." *Pflegewissenschaft Sonderausgabe, April* (2020): 33–36

Behr, Thomas, Gerd Dielmann, Rolf Höfert, Michael Huneke, Bjørn Kähler, Stefan Neumann, Petra Selg, and Claudia Stiller-Wüsten. "Positionspapier: Pflege raus aus dem Abseits – Empfehlungen zu einer Refokussierung auf den Kernprozess der Pflege [Position Paper: Nursing Away from the Offset: Recommendations for Re-Focussing on the Core Process of Nursing]." In *Aufbruch Pflege*, edited by Thomas Behr, 61–81. Wiesbaden: Springer Fachmedien, 2015.

Benner, Patricia, and Christine Tanner. "Clinical Judgement: How Expert Nurses Use Intuition." *American Journal of Nursing* 87, no. 1 (1987): 23–31.

Berg, Marc. "Practices of Reading and Writing: The Constitutive Role of the Patient Record in Medical Work." *Sociology of Health & Illness* 18, no. 4 (1996): 499–524.

Bernet, Brigitta. "Vom "Berufsautomaten" zum "Flexiblen Mitarbeiter". Die Krise der Organisation und der Umbau der Personallehren um 1970 [From the "Occupational Machine" to the "Flexible Employee"]." In *Wertewandel in der Wirtschaft Und Arbeitsweltarbeit, Leistung Und Führung in den 1970er und 1980er Jahren in der Bundesrepublik Deutschland*, edited by Bernhard v. Dietz and Jörg Neuheiser. Wertewandel im 20. Jahrhundert, 31–54. Berlin: De Gruyter Oldenbourg, 2016.

Berridge, Virginia. "Medizin, Public Health und die Medien in Großbritannien von 1950 bis 1980 [Medicine, Public Health and the Media in Britain from the 1950s to the 1970s]." In

Das präventive Selbst. Eine Kulturgeschichte moderner Gesundheitspolitik, edited by Martin Lengwiler and Jeannette Madarász, 205-28. Bielefeld: transcript Verlag, 2010.
Bischoff-Wanner, Claudia. "Pflege im historischen Vergleich [Nursing in Historical Comparison]." In *Handbuch Pflegewissenschaft*, edited by Doris Schaeffer and Klaus Wingenfeld, 19-36. Weinheim und Basel: Beltz Juventa, 2014.
Bischoff, Claudia. *Frauen in der Krankenpflege: Zur Entwicklung von Frauenrolle und Frauenberufstätigkeit im 19. und 20. Jahrhundert [Women in Nursing: About the Development of the Female Role and Female Employment in the 19th and 20th Century]*. Vol. 3rd, Frankfurt am Main; New York: Campus-Verlag, 1997.
–. "Krankenpflege als Frauenberuf [Nursing as a Female Vocation]." *Das Argument/ Sonderband* 86 (1982): 13-27.
Bischoff, Claudia, and Bernd Wanner. "Krankenpflege an der Hochschule? [Nursing at University?]." *Krankenpflege* 38, no. 2 (1984): 64-66.
Blumenstock, Jan. "Das Märchen von der Kostenexplosion im Gesundheitswesen [The Fairytale About the Cost Explosion in the Health Care System]." *Krankenpflege* 34, no. 7/8 (1980): 248-49.
BMG. "Konzertierte Aktion Pflege [Concerted Action Nursing]," Bundesministerium für Gesundheit, 2019, https://www.bundesgesundheitsministerium.de/en/service/begriffe-von-a-z/k/konzertierte-aktion-pflege.html.
Böhm, Franz. "Die Idee des Ordo im Denken Walter Euckens [The Idea of Ordo in the Mindset of Walter Eucken]." *ORDO Jahrbuch für die Ordnung von Wirtschaft und Gesellschaft* 3 (1950): XV-LXIV.
Bollinger, Heinrich, and Joachim Hohl. "Auf dem Weg von der Profession zum Beruf: Zur Deprofessionalisierung des Ärzte-Standes [On the Way from a Profession to a Vocation: About the Deprofessionalization of the Physicians]." *Soziale Welt* 32, no. 4 (1981): 440-64.
Braun, Bernard. "Auswirkung der DRGs auf die Versorgungsqualität und Arbeitsbedingungen im Krankenhaus [Impact of DRGs on the Quality of Care and Working Conditions in the Hospital]." In *20 Jahre Wettbewerb im Gesundheitswesen. Theoretische und empirische Analysen zur Ökonomisierung von Medizin und Pflege*, edited by Alexandra Manzei and Rudi Schmiede, 91-113. Wiesbaden: Springer Fachmedien, 2014.
Brown, Wendy. *Undoing the Demos: Neoliberalism's Stealth Revolution*. New York: Zone Books, 2015.
Brunner, Leni, and Sabine Goedeckemeyer. "Modellversuch einer Pflegeplanung auf zwei Stationen – Protokoll (1. Folge) [Pilot Project of a Nursing Care Plan on Two Wards: Protocol (1st Part)]." *Krankenpflege* 34, no. 2 (1980): 46-48.
–. "Modellversuch einer Pflegeplanung auf zwei Stationen – Protokoll (2. Folge) [Pilot Project of a Nursing Care Plan on Two Wards: Protocol (2nd Part)]." *Krankenpflege* 34, no. 3 (1980): 87-90.
–. "Modellversuch einer Pflegeplanung auf zwei Stationen – Protokoll (3. Folge Und Schluß) [Pilot Project of a Nursing Care Plan on Two Wards: Protocol (3rd Part and End)]." *Krankenpflege* 34, no. 4 (1980): 122-24.
–. "Teil der Pflegeplanung – Das Erstgespräch (1. Teil) [Part of the Nursing Care Plan: The Initial Meeting (1st Part)]." *Krankenpflege* 35, no. 4 (1981): 152-54.

Büchner, Edith, and Wilhelm Thiele. "Untersuchungen über Patientenversorgung und Pflegequalität [Research on Patient Care and Nursing Quality]." *Das Krankenhaus* 76, no. 9 (1984): 401–03.
Bulechek, Gloria M., Howard Karl Butcher, and Joanne McCloskey Dochterman. *Nursing Interventions Classification (NIC)*. 5th ed. St. Louis: Mosby/Elsevier, 2008.
Büssing, André, and Jürgen Glaser. "Arbeitsbelastungen, Burnout und Interaktionsstress im Zuge der Reorganisation des Pflegesystems [Workload, Burnout, and Interaction Stress in the Course of the Reorganization of Nursing Systems]." In *Dienstleistungsqualität und Qualität des Arbeitslebens im Krankenhaus*, edited by André Büssing and Jürgen Glaser, 101–29. Göttingen, Bern, Toronto, Seattle: Hogrefe-Verlag, 2003.
Buus, Niels, and Michael Traynor. "The Nursing Process: Nursing Discourse and Managerial Technologies." In *The Nursing Process: A Global Concept*, edited by Monika Habermann, Leana R. Uys and Barbara Parfitt, 31–46. Edinburgh; New York: Elsevier/Churchill Livingstone, 2006.
Campbell, M. L. "Nurses Professionalism in Canada: A Labor Process Analysis." *International Journal of Health Services* 22, no. 4 (1992): 751–65.
Carr-Saunders, Alexander M., and Paul A. Wilson. *The Profession*. London: Frank Cass & Co. Ltd., 1964.
Castel, Robert. ""Problematization" as a Mode of Reading History." In *Foucault and the Writing of History*, edited by Jan Goldstein, 237–52, 303–04. Cambridge, Massachusetts: Basil Blackwell Ltd, 1994.
Chaaban, Taghrid, Rola Hallal, Karen Carroll, and Monique Rothan-Tondeur. "Cybernetic Communications: Focusing Interactions on Goal-Centered Care." *Nursing Science Quarterly* 34, no. 1 (2021): 30–32.
Chapman, Christopher S., David J. Cooper, and Peter B. Miller. "Linking Accounting, Organizations, and Institutions." In *Accounting, Organizations, and Institutions: Essays in Honour of Anthony Hopwood*, edited by Christopher S. Chapman, David J. Cooper and Peter B. Miller, 1–29. New York: Oxford University Press, 2009.
Chua, Wai Fong. "Experts, Networks and Inscriptions in the Fabrication of Accounting Images: A Story of the Representation of Three Public Hospitals." *Accounting, Organizations and Society* 20, no. 2 (1995): 111–45.
Clark, Elizabeth A. *History, Theory, Text. Historians and the Linguistic Turn*. Cambridge, Mass.: Harvard University Press, 2004.
Cocks, Geoffrey, and Konrad Hugo Jarausch. *German Professions, 1800–1950*. New York: Oxford University Press, 1990.
Council Directive 77/452/EEC. "Council Directive of 27 June 1977 concerning the Mutual Recognition of Diplomas, Certificates and Other Evidence of the Formal Qualifications of Nurses Responsible for General Care, Including Measures to Facilitate the Effective Exercise of the Right of Establishment and Freedom to Provide Services (77/452/Eec)." edited by Council of the European Communities, 1977.
Cueto, Marcos, Theodore M. Brown, and Elizabeth Fee. *The World Health Organization. A History*. Cambridge: Cambridge University Press, 2019.
Darmann-Finck, Ingrid, and Heiner Friesacher. "Editorial zu Professionalisierung in der Pflege [Editorial on the Professionalization of Nursing]." *ipp info* 5, no. 07 (2009): 1–2.
DBfK. "Bayern Fortbildung – Systematische Planung der Pflege [Further Education in Bavaria: Systematic Planning of Nursing Care]." *Krankenpflege* 34, no. 3 (1980): 92.

–. "Berufsbild Krankenpflege [Job Description: Nursing]." *Krankenpflege* 34, no. 2 (1981): 64–66.
–. "Bremen, Hamburg und Schleswig-Holstein [Bremen, Hamburg and Schleswig-Holstein]." *Krankenpflege* 33, no. 4 (1979): 132.
–. "Fortbildungstage [Training Days]." *Krankenpflege* 35, no. 3 (1981): 119.
–. "Großveranstaltung zum Tag der Krankenpflege [Major Event at the Day of Nursing]." *Krankenpflege* 32, no. 3 (1978): 99.
DBfK Gesamtverband/Redaktion KRANKENPFLEGE. "Die Krankenpflege von heute und morgen – Arbeitspapier des Weltbundes der Krankenschwestern und Krankenpfleger – ICN [Nursing of Today and Tomorrow: Working Paper of the International Council of Nurses – ICN]." *Krankenpflege* 40, no. 9 (1986): 353–56.
Delmotte, Nicole. "Der Krankenpflegeprozeß in Belgien. Erfahrungen mit der WHO-Studie [The Nursing Process in Belgum: Experiences with the WHO Study]." *Krankenpflege* 40, no. 1 (1986): 32–35.
Dittrich, Friederike. "Der Terminal auf der Station [The Computer on the Ward]." *Krankenpflege* 38, no. 9 (1984): 278–79.
–. "Pflege ist Leistung – Dokumentation ist Beweis [Nursing Is a Service: Documentation Is the Proof]." *Krankenpflege* 38, no. 4 (1984): 142–44.
DKG. "DKG-Vorstand verabschiedet Muster einer Pflegedokumentation und Anpassung des Zeitaufwandes für Apothekenpersonal [Board of the German Hospital Society Passes the Draft of a Nursing Documentation and Adaption of the Expenditure of Time for Pharmacy Staff]." *Das Krankenhaus* 77, no. 6 (1985): 236–37.
–. "Struktur und Organisation des pflegerischen Dienstes im Krankenhaus [Structure and Organization of the Nursing Service in the Hospital]." *Krankenpflege* 38, no. 9 (1984): 306–07.
–. "Wir stellen vor: Die Deutsche Krankenhausgesellschaft [We Present: The German Hospital Society]." *Krankenpflege* 37, no. 3 (1983): 106–07.
Doering-Manteuffel, Anselm. "Langfristige Ursprünge und dauerhafte Auswirkungen [Long-Term Origins and Lasting Effects]." In *Das Ende der Zuversicht? Die siebziger Jahre als Geschichte*, edited by Konrad H. Jarausch, 313–29: Göttingen: Vandenhoeck & Ruprecht, 2008.
Doering-Manteuffel, Anselm, and Lutz Raphael. "Nach dem Boom [After the Boom]." In *Vorgeschichte der Gegenwart. Dimensionen des Strukturbruchs nach dem Boom*, edited by Anselm Doering-Manteuffel, Lutz Raphael and Thomas Schlemmer, 9–34. Göttingen: Vandenhoeck & Ruprecht, 2016.
–. *Nach dem Boom. Perspektiven auf die Zeitgeschichte seit 1970 [After the Boom: Perspectives on Contemporary History since 1970]*. 3rd ed. Göttingen: Vandenhoeck & Ruprecht, 2012.
Donley, Rosemary. "The Need for Rationality, Conceptualization, and Problem Solving." In *Human Needs 3 and the Nursing Process*, edited by Helen Yura and Mary B. Walsh, 85–116. Norwalk, Conn.: Appleton-Century-Crofts, 1983.
Drees, Annette. *Die Ärzte auf dem Weg zu Prestige und Wohlstand. Sozialgeschichte der württembergischen Ärzte im 19. Jahrhundert [Physicians on Their Way to Prestige and Prosperity: A Social History About the Physicians of Württemberg in the 19th Century]*. Studien zur Geschichte des Alltags. edited by Hans J. Teuteberg and Peter Borscheid. Vol. 9, Münster: F. Coppenrath Verlag, 1988.

Dreißiger, Regina. "Information im Pflegedienst [Information in Nursing Services]." *Krankenpflege* 32, no. 6 (1978): 200–04.
Dreyfus, Hubert L., and Paul Rabniow. *Beyond Structuralism and Hermeneutics. With an Afterword by and an Interview with Michel Foucault*. 2nd ed. Chicago: The University of Chicago Press, 1983.
Drogendijk, Arie C. "Gesundheit, Krankheit und Kybernetik [Health, Illness, and Cybernetic]." *Elektromedizin* 7, no. 3 (1962): 160–71.
EC. "Council Directive of 27 June 1977 Concerning the Coordination of Provision Laid Down by Law, Regulation or Administrative Action in Respect of the Activities of Nurses Responsible for General Care (77/453/Eec)." Official Journal of the European Communities, 1977.
Editors of the History of the Present. "Introducing History of the Present." *History of the Present: A Journal of Critical History* 1, no. 1 (2011): 1–4.
Eichhorn, Friedrich. "Grundgedanken zur Rationalisierung des Pflegedienstes [Basic Ideas on the Rationalization of Nursing Service]." *Die Agnes-Karll-Schwester* 11, no. 3 (1957): 78–82.
Eichhorn, Siegfried. "Die betriebswirtschaftlichen Aspekte der Leistungssteigerung durch Zusammenarbeit [Economic Aspects to Increase Performance through Collaboration]." *Das Krankenhaus* 58, no. 8 (1966): 315–23.
–. *Krankenhausbetriebslehre: Theorie und Praxis des Krankenhausbetriebes Band 1 [Business Operation of Hospitals: Theory and Practice of the Hospital Administration. First Volume]*. Schriften des Deutschen Krankenhausinstituts E. V. Düsseldorf Band 11. 3rd ed. Köln: Verlag W. Kohlhammer, 1975.
–. "Zielkonflikte zwischen Leistungsfähigkeit, Wirtschaftlichkeit und Finanzierung der Krankenversorgung [Conflicts of Objectives between Performance, Efficiency and Financing of Health Care]." *Das Krankenhaus* 66, no. 5 (1974): 186–96.
Ellrich, Manfred. "Kommunikationsbeziehungen im Pflegebereich und ihre Auswirkungen auf technische Rufsysteme [Communication Relations in Nursing Service and Their Impact on Technical Call Systems]." *Das Krankenhaus* 75, no. 1 (1983): 8–10.
Ermarth, Elizabeth Deeds. "The Closed Space of Choice: A Manifesto on the Future of History." In *Manifestos for History*, edited by Keith Jenkings, Sue Morgan and Alun Munslow, 50–66. London, New York: Routledge Taylor & Francis Group, 2007.
Etzioni, Amitai. *The Semi-Professions and Their Organization: Teachers, Nurses, Social Workers*. New York: Free Press, 1969.
Eucken, Walter. "Das ordnungspolitische Problem [The Regulative Problem]." *ORDO Jahrbuch für die Ordnung von Wirtschaft und Gesellschaft* 1 (1948): 56–90.
Europäische Krankenpflegevereinigung. "Memorandum zur Grundausbildung in der Krankenpflege [Memorandum on the Basic Vocational Training in Nursing]." *Krankenpflege* 41, no. 7/8 (1987): 278–80.
Eversberg, Dennis. "Destabilisierte Zukunft [De-Stabilized Future]." In *Vorgeschichte der Gegenwart*, edited by Anselm Doering-Manteuffel and Lutz Raphael, 451–74. Göttingen: Vandenhoeck & Ruprecht, 2016.
Evetts, Julia. "A New Professionalism? Challenges and Opportunities." *Current Sociology* 59, no. 4 (2011): 406–22.
Fejes, Andreas. "Governing Nursing through Reflection: A Discourse Analysis of Reflective Practices." *Journal of advanced nursing* 64, no. 3 (2008): 243–50.

Fiechter, Verena, and Martha Meier. *Pflegeplanung. Eine Anleitung für die Praxis [Nursing Care Plan: An Instruction for Practice].* Basel: RECOM, 1987.
Fischer, Renate. *Berufliche Identität als Dimension beruflicher Kompetenz: Entwicklungsverlauf und Einflussfaktoren in der Gesundheits- und Krankenpflege [Vocational Identity as Dimension of Vocational Competence: Development and Influencing Factors in Nursing].* Bielefeld: Bertelsmann, 2013.
Foth, Thomas. *Caring and Killing: Nursing and Psychiatric Practice in Germany, 1931-1943.* Göttingen: V&R unipress, 2013.
Foth, Thomas, and Dave Holmes. "Governing through Lifestyle: Lalonde and the Biopolitical Managemnt of Public Health in Canada." *Nursing Philosophy* 19, no. 4 (2018): 1-11.
Foth, Thomas, Jette Lange, and Kylie Smith. "Nursing History as Philosophy: Towards a Critical History of Nursing." *Nursing Philosophy* 19, no. 3 (2018/07/01 2018): e12210.
Foucault, Michel. "Afterword. The Subject and Power." In *Michel Foucault: Beyond Structuralism and Hermeneutics. With an Afterword by and an Interview with Michel Foucault*, edited by Hubert L. Dreyfus and Paul Rabinow. Chicago: The University of Chicago Press, 1983.
-. *The Archaeology of Knowledge and the Discourse of Language*, edited by Michel Foucault. New York: Vintage Books, 2010.
-. *The Birth of Biopolitics: Lectures at the Collège De France, 1978-79.* Basingstoke, New York: Palgrave Macmillan, 2008.
-. "Body/Power." In *Power/Knowledge: Selected Interviews and Other Writings 1972-1977*, edited by Colin Gordon, 55-62. New York: Harvester Press, 1980.
-. *Discipline and Punish: The Birth of the Prison.* Vol. 2. New York: Vintage Books, 1995.
-. "Governmentality." In *The Foucault Effect: Studies in Governmentality: With Two Lectures by and an Interview with Michel Foucault*, edited by Graham Burchell, Colin Gordon and Peter Miller, 87-104. Chicago: University of Chicago Press, 1991.
-. "Nietzsche, Genealogy, History." In *The Foucault Reader*, edited by Paul Rabinow, 76-100. New York: Pantheon Books, 1984.
-. "Orders of Discourse." *Social Science Information* 10, no. 2 (1971): 7-30.
-. "Polemics, Politics and Problematizations. An Interview with Michel Foucault." In *The Foucault Reader*, edited by Paul Rabinow, 381-90. New York: Pantheon Books, 1984.
-. "The Politics of Health in the Eighteenth Century." In *Power/Knowledge: Selected Interviews and Other Writings 1972-1977*, edited by Colin Gordon, 166-82. New York: Harvester Press, 1980.
-. "The Politics of Health in the Eighteenth Century." *Foucault Studies* 18 (2014): 113-27.
-. "Questions of Method." In *The Foucault Effect: Studies in Governmentality: With Two Lectures by and an Interview with Michel Foucault*, edited by Graham Burchill, Colin Gordon and Peter Miller, 73-86. Chicago: University of Chicago Press, 1991.
-. *"Society Must Be Defended" Lectures at the College De France 1975-76.* New York: Picador, 2003.
-. *""*Society Must Be Defended," Lectures at the Collège De France, March 17, 1976." Chap. 2 In *Biopolitics: A Reader*, edited by Timothy C. Campbell and Adam Sitze, 61-81. Durham: Duke University Press, 2013.
-. "Two Lectures." In *Power/Knowledge: Selected Interviews and Other Writings 1972-1977*, edited by Colin Gordon, 78-108. New York: Harvester Press, 1980.

Fraser, Nancy. "From Discipline to Flexibilization? Rereading Foucault in the Shadow of Globalization." *Constellations* 10, no. 2 (2003): 160–71.

Freidson, Eliot. *Professionalism: The Third Logic*. Chicago: University of Chicago Press, 2001.

Friesacher, Heiner. "Segen oder Fluch für die Pflege? Pflegediagnosen und Pflegeklassifikationssysteme [Boon and Bane for Nursing? Nursing Diagnoses and Nursing Classification Systems]." *Padua* 2, no. 4 (2007): 43–47.

–. *Theorie und Praxis pflegerischen Handelns [Theory and Practice of Nursing Action]*. Göttingen: V&R unipress, 2008.

–. "Wider die Abwertung der eigentlichen Pflege [Against the Devaluation of Actual Care]." *intensiv* 23, no. 4 (2015): 200–14.

Fritsche, Wolfgang, and Wolfgang F. Meyer. "Gesundheitserziehung und Gemeindepflege [Health Education and Parish Nursing]." *Die Agnes-Karll-Schwester* 22, no. 1 (1968): 3–6.

Fritsche, Wolfgang, and Christa Topfmeier. "Gedanken zu Inhalt und Methodik der Gesundheitserziehung [Thoughts Upon Content and Method of Health Education]." *Die Agnes-Karll-Schwester* 21, no. 4 (1967): 133–35.

Garland, David. "What Is a "History of the Present"? On Foucault's Genealogies and Their Critical Preconditions." *Punishment & Society* 16, no. 4 (2014): 365–84.

Geschwilm, Renate. "Pflegeplanung [Nursing Care Plan]." *Krankenpflege* 31, no. 9 (1977): 293–94.

Gilbert, Tony. "Reflective Practice and Clinical Supervision: Meticulous Rituals of the Confessional." *Journal of Advanced Nursing* 36, no. 2 (2001): 199–205.

Gilbert, Tony P. "Trust and Managerialism: Exploring Discourses of Care." *Journal of Advanced Nursing* 52, no. 4 (2005): 454–63.

Goode, William J. "Encroachment, Charlatanism, and the Emerging Profession: Psychology, Sociology, and Medicine." *American Sociological Review* 25, no. 6 (1960): 902–65.

–. "The Theoretical Limits of Professionalization." In *The Semi-Professions and Their Organization: Teachers, Nurses, Social Workers*, edited by Amitai Etzioni, 266–313. New York: Free Press, 1969.

Gordon, Colin. "Afterword." In *Power/Knowledge: Selected Interviews and Other Writings 1972–1977*, edited by Colin Gordon, 229–59. London, New York: Harvester Press, 1980.

Grauhan, Antje. "Berufsethische Normen in der Krankenpflege [Ethical Norms in Nursing]." *Krankenpflege* 39, no. 7–8 (1985): 231–33.

Grauhan, Antje, and fellows. "Mittelfristiges WHO-Programm für Krankenpflege- und Hebammenwesen in Europa [Middle-Term Program of the WHO Concerning Nursing and Midwifery in Europe]." *Krankenpflege* 32, no. 2 (1978): 67–68.

Gronemeyer, Reimer, and Charlotte Jurk. "Entprofessionalisieren wir uns! Über die Sprache der Versorgungsindustrie: Wie Plastikwörter die Sorge um andere infizieren und warum wir uns davon befreien müssen [We Should De-Professionalize! About the Language of the Supply Industry: How Plastic Words Contaminate the Care for the Other and Why We Need to Free Ourselves from It]." In *Entprofessionalisieren wir uns! Ein kritisches Wörterbuch über die Sprache in Pflege und Sozialer Arbeit*, edited by Reimer Gronemeyer and Charlotte Jurk, 9–12. Bielefeld: transcript Verlag, 2017.

Grote, Norbert and Bernd Tews, "Der Pflegenotstand ist längst da. Die Sicherstellung der pflegerischen Versorgung muss wieder gewährleistet werden [The Nursing Shortage

already exists. Ensuring Nursing Care Needs to be Guaranteed]." *bpa Magazin* 12, no. 4 (2022): 12–14.
Habermann, Monika. "The Nursing Process: Developments and Issues in Germany." In *The Nursing Process: A Global Concept*, edited by Monika Habermann, Leana R. Uys and Barbara Parfitt, 95–105. Edinburgh; New York: Elsevier/Churchill Livingstone, 2006.
Habermann, Monika, and Leana R. Uys. *The Nursing Process: A Global Concept*. Edinburgh, New York: Elsevier/Churchill Livingstone, 2006.
Hacking, Ian. "Biopower and the Avalanche of Printed Numbers." *Humanities in Society*, no. 5 (1982): 279–95.
Hagner, Michael. "Vom Aufstieg und Fall der Kybernetik als Universalwissenschaft [On the Rise and Fall of Cybernetics as a Universal Science]," In *Die Transformation des Humanen. Beiträge zur Kulturgeschichte der Kybernetik*, edited by Michael Hagner and Erich Hörl, 2nd ed., 38–71, Frankfurt am Main: Suhrkamp, 2018.
Hall, Dorothy C. "A Position Paper on Nursing." *Journal of Advanced Nursing* 2, no. 3 (1977): 327–28.
–. "Probleme der Krankenpflegeausbildung in Europa [Problems of Nursing Education in Europe]." *Krankenpflege* 29, no. 10 (1976): 292, 301–03.
–. "Überlegungen zum Krankenpflegeberuf [Considerations About the Nursing Vocation]." *Krankenpflege* 31, no. 2 (1977): 40–42.
Hämel, Kerstin, and Doris Schaeffer. "Who Cares? Fachkräftemangel in der Pflege [Who Cares? Shortage of Professional Nurses]." *Zeitschrift für Sozialreform* 59, no. 4 (18.12. 2013 2013): 413–31.
Hamm, Walter. "Programmierte Unfreiheit und Verschwendung: Zur überfälligen Reform der gesetzlichen Krankenversicherung [Programmed Bondage and Dissipation: On the Overdue Reform of the Statutory Health Insurance]." *ORDO Jahrbuch für die Ordnung von Wirtschaft und Gesellschaft* 35 (1984): 21–42.
–. "Verschwendung in Krankenhäusern durch falsche Anreize [Wastefulness in Hospitals Because of False Incentives]." *ORDO Jahrbuch für die Ordnung von Wirtschaft und Gesellschaft* 33 (1982): 363–368.
Hampton-Robb, Isabel. "The Nurse and the Public." *The Canadian Nurse* 1, no. 1 (1905): 9–11.
Harpine, Frances H. "Assessing the Needs of the Patient." In *The Nursing Process; Assessing, Planning, Implementing, and Evaluating; The Proceedings of the Continuing Education Series Conducted at the Catholic University of America, March 2 through April 27, 1967*, edited by Helen Yura and Mary B. Walsh, 21–43. Washington: Catholic University of America Press, 1968.
Harris, L. Barbara. "Becoming Deprofessionalized: One Aspect of the Staff Nurse's Perspective on Computer-Mediated Nursing Care Plans." *Advances in Nursing Science* 13, no. 2 (1990): 63–74.
Haug, Marie R. "The Deprofessionalization of Everyone?" *Sociological Focus* 8, no. 3 (1975): 197–213.
Heartfield, Marie. "Nursing Documentation and Nursing Practice: A Discourse Analysis." *Journal of Advanced Nursing* 24, no. August (1996): 98–103.
Henderson, Virginia. "The Concept of Nursing." *Journal of Advanced Nursing* 3, no. 2 (1978): 113–30.
–. "Nursing Process: A Critique." *Holistic Nursing Practice* 1, no. 3 (1987): 7.

–. *Principles and Practice of Nursing*. edited by Gladys Nite and Bertha Harmer. 6th ed. New York: Macmillan, 1978.

Heuwer, Karin, and Helga Laurinat. "Qualitätssicherung medizinischer und pflegerischer Leistungen im Gesundheitsdienst [Quality Assurance of Medical and Nursing Performance in the Health Care Service]." *Krankenpflege* 39, no. 7-8 (1985): 238-?

Hofmann, Irmgard. "Die Rolle der Pflege im Gesundheitswesen. Historische Hintergründe und heutige Konfliktkonstellationen [The Role of the Nursing Vocation in the Health Care System: Historical Background and Recent Conflicts]." *Bundesgesundheitsblatt - Gesundheitsforschung - Gesundheitsschutz* 55, no. 9 (2012): 1161-67.

Hohlin, Detlef. "Neue Horizonte für die Krankenpflege [New Horizons for Nursing Care]." *Krankenpflege* 30, no. 1 (1976): 13-14.

–. "Notwendigkeit der Adaption der Krankenhäuser an Strukturänderungen aus pflegerischer Sicht [A Nursing Perspective on the Necessity of Hospitals Adapting to Structural Changes]." *Krankenpflege* 31, no. 9 (1977): 287-90.

–. "Werden Anhaltszahlen durch neue Berechnungsmethoden abgelöst? Teil I [Will Reference Data Soon Be Replaced by New Methods of Calculation? Part I]." *Krankenpflege* 40, no. 3 (1986): 102-04.

–. "Werden Anhaltszahlen durch neue Berechnungsmethoden abgelöst? Teil II [Will Reference Data Soon Be Replaced by New Methods of Calculation? Part II]." *Krankenpflege* 40, no. 4 (1986): 142-43.

–. "Werden Anhaltszahlen durch neue Berechnungsmethoden abgelöst? Teil III [Will Reference Data Soon Be Replaced by New Methods of Calculation? Part III]." *Krankenpflege* 40, no. 5 (1986): 189-90, 207.

Holmes, Dave, Amélie Perron, and Patrick O'Byrne. "Evidence, Virulence, and the Disappearance of Nursing Knowledge: A Critique of Evidence-Based Dogma." *Worldviews on Evidence-Based Nursing* 3, no. 3 (2006): 95-102.

Hölzel-Seipp, Liselotte. "Der praktische Krankenpflegeprozeß [The Practical Nursing Process]." *Die Agnes-Karll-Schwester, der Krankenpfleger* 23, no. 5 (1969): 201-03.

Huerkamp, Claudia. *Der Aufstieg der Ärzte im 19. Jahrhundert vom gelehrten Stand zum professionellen Experten: Das Beispiel Preußens [The Rise of Physicians in the 19th Century from the Rank of Intellectuals to the Professional Expert: The Example of Prussia]*. Kritische Studien zur Geschichtswissenschaft. edited by Helmut Berding, Jürgen Kocka and Hans-Ulrich Wehler. Vol. 68, Göttingen: Vandenhoeck & Ruprecht, 1985.

Hülsken-Giesler, Manfred. *Der Zugang zum Anderen. Zur theoretischen Rekonstruktion von Professionalisierungsstrategien pflegerischen Handelns im Spannungsfeld von Mimesis und Maschinenlogik [Access to and Approach of the Other: For a Theoretical Reconstruction of Professionalization Strategies of Nursing Care in the Tension between Mimesis and Machine Logic]*. Pflegewissenschaft und Pflegebildung, edited by Hartmut Remmers. Vol. 3, Göttingen: V&R unipress, 2008.

Hunt, Jennifer. "Pflegeforschung – Bringt sie etwas? [Nursing Research: Is It Helpful?]." *Krankenpflege* 38, no. 7-8 (1984): 227-31.

Illig, Falk. *Gesundheitspolitik in Deutschland. Eine Chronologie der Gesundheitsreformen der Bundesrepublik [Health Politics in Germany: A Chronology of Health Reforms of the Federal Republic]*. Wiesbaden: Springer VS, 2017.

Isfort, Michael. "Prozessuale Pflege – Oder die nächste Fahrt geht rückwärts! [Processural Nursing Care: Or the Next Turn Is Backwards]." *Die Schwester Der Pfleger* 44, no. 6 (Sonderdruck 7/05) (2005): 1–10.
Isfort, Michael, Frank Weidner, Andrea Neuhaus, Sebastian Kraus, Veit-Henning Köster, and Danny Gehlen. "Pflege-Thermometer 2009. Eine bundesweite Befragung von Pflegekräften zur Situation der Pflege und Patientenversorgung im Krankenhaus [NursingThermometer: A Federal Survey of Nurses About the Situation of Nursing and Patient Care in the Hospital]," 2009. Deutsches Institut für angewandte Pflegeforschung e.V. (dip), https://www.researchgate.net/profile/Michael_Isfort/publication/288897767_Zur_Situation_des_Pflegepersonals_in_deutschen_Krankenhausern_-_Ergebnisse_des_Pflege-Thermometers_2009/links/56b47c6608aecddf26b573a9.pdf.
Jansen, Wilma. "Überblick über die wesentlichen Referate [Overview of Essential Presentations]." *Krankenpflege* 32, no. 6 (1978): 197–200.
Jarausch, Konrad H. "Verkannter Strukturwandel [Misunderstood Structural Change]." In *Die siebziger Jahre als Geschichte*, edited by Konrad H. Jarausch, 9–26: Göttingen: Vandenhoeck & Ruprecht, 2008.
Jarrard, Jenny K. "Engineered Standards in Hospital Nursing: Management Engineers Can Give Reinforcement and Correction to Problem Solving." *Nursing Management* 14, no. 4 (1983): 29–32.
Jessen, Ralph. "Bewältigte Vergangenheit – blockierte Zukunft? [Mastered Past: Blocked Future?]." In *Das Ende der Zuversicht? Die siebziger Jahre als Geschichte*, edited by Konrad H. Jarausch, 177–95: Göttingen: Vandenhoeck & Ruprecht, 2008.
Johnson, Terry. "Governmentality and the Institutionalization of Expertise." In *Health Professions and the State in Europe*, edited by Terry Johnson, Gerald Larkin and Mike Saks, 7–24. London, New York: Routledge, 1995.
Jung, Karl. "Führt Kostendämpfung im Gesundheitswesen zu einem Dilemma in der Krankenpflege? [Does Cost Containment in the Health Care System Lead to a Dilemma in Nursing?]." *Krankenpflege* 32, no. 2 (1978): 49–51.
Kellner, Anne. *Von der Selbstlosigkeit zur Selbstsorge. Eine Genealogie der Pflege [From Selflessness to Self-Care: A Genealogy of Nursing]*. Pflege und Gesundheit. edited by Regina Lorenz-Krause. Vol. 4, Berlin: LIT Verlag Dr. W. Hopf, 2011.
Kelly, Daniel. "Opening New Discourses in Nursing: The History of the Nursing Process in the UK." In *The Nursing Process: A Global Concept*, edited by Monika Habermann, Leana R. Uys and Barbara Parfitt, 15–29. Edinburgh, New York: Elsevier/Churchill Livingstone, 2006.
Kennihan, Mary, Tatheer Zohra, Radha Devi, Chitra Srinivasan, Josefina Diaz, Bradley S. Howard, and Susan S. Braithwaite. "Individualization through Standardization: Electronic Orders for Subcutaneous Insulin in the Hospital." *Endocrine Practice: Official Journal of the American College of Endocrinology and the American Association of Clinical Endocrinologists* 18, no. 6 (2012): 976–87.
Kesselring, Annemarie. "Psychosoziale Pflegediagnostik: Eine interpretativ-phänomenologische Perspective [Psycho-Social Nursing Diagnosis: An Interpretative-Phenomenological Perspective]." *Pflege* 12, no. 4 (1999): 223–28.
Klein, Walter. "'Sie sehen mir alle mit freundlichen Gesichtern entgegen' Die Beziehung zwischen Patienten und Krankenschwestern im Saarbrücker Bürgerhospital in der Mitte des 19. Jahrhunderts ['They All Look at Me with Friendly Faces': The Relationship

between Patientes and Nurses in the Public Hospital of Saarbrücken in the Middle of the 19th Century]." *Medizin, Gesellschaft, und Geschichte: Jahrbuch des Instituts für Geschichte der Medizin der Robert Bosch Stiftung* 21 (2002): 63-90.

Kraft, Stephanie, and Matthias Drossel. "Untersuchung des sozialen, beruflichen und gesundheitlichen Erlebens von Pflegekräften in stationären Krankenpflegeeinrichtungen – Eine qualitative Analyse [Study About the Social, Vocational, and Health-Related Experiences of Nurses in Stationary Nursing Care Organizations]." *HeilberufeScience* 10, no. 3 (2019/11/01 2019): 39-45.

Kramer, Nicole. "Neue soziale Bewegungen, Sozialwissenschaften und die Erweiterung des Sozialstaats. Familien- und Altenpolitik in den 1970er und 1980er Jahren [New Social Movements, Social Sciences and the Expansion of the Social State: Politics for Families and Elderly in the 1970s and 1980s]." *Archiv für Sozialgeschichte* 52 (2012): 211-30.

Krampe, Eva-Maria. *Emanzipation durch Professionalisierung: Akademisierung des Frauenberufs Pflege in den 1990er Jahren; Erwartungen und Folgen [Emancipation through Professionalization: The Academization of a Female Vocation in the 1990s; Expectations and Consequences]*. Frankfurt am Main: Mabuse-Verlag, 2009.

–. "Professionalisierung der Pflege im Kontext der Ökonomisierung [Professionalization of Nursing in the Context of Economization]." In *20 Jahre Wettbewerb im Gesundheitswesen. Theoretische und empirische Analysen zur Ökonomisierung von Medizin und Pflege*, edited by Alexandra Manzei and Rudi Schmiede. Gesundheit und Gesellschaft, 179-97. Wiesbaden: Springer Fachmedien, 2014.

Kreutzer, Susanne. *Arbeits- und Lebensalltag evangelischer Krankenpflege. Organisation, soziale Praxis und biographische Erfahrungen, 1945-1980 [Daily Work and Life in Protestant Nursing: Organization, Social Practice, and Biographical Experiences, 1945-1980]*. Göttingen: V&R unipress, 2014.

–. "'Before, We Were Always There – Now, Everything Is Separate': On Nursing Reforms in Western Germany." *Nursing History Review* 16 (2008): 180-200.

–. "Conflicting Christian and Scientific Nursing Concepts in West Germany, 1945-1970." In *Routledge Handbook on the Global History of Nursing*, edited by Patricia D'Antonio, Julie A. Fairman and Jean C. Whelan, 151-64. London, New York: Routledge, 2016.

–. "'Hollywood Nurses' in West Germany: Biographies, Self-Images, and Experiences of Academically Trained Nurses after 1945." *Nursing History Review* 21 (2013): 33-54.

–. "Krankenbeobachtung. Zur Entwertung einer pflegerischen Schlüsselkompetenz in der Bundesrepublik und Schweden nach 1945 [Patient Observation: On the Devaluation of a Key Competence in Nursing in the Federal Republic of Germany and Sweden after 1945]." In *Gesundheit/Krankheit. Kulturelle Differenzierungsprozesse um Körper, Geschlecht und Macht in Skandinavien*, edited by Lill-Ann Körber and Stefanie von Schnurbein. Berliner Beiträge zur Skandinavistik, Bd. 16. Berlin: Nordeuropa-Institut, 2010.

–. "Rationalization of Nursing in West Germany and the United States, 1945-1970." In *Critical Approaches in Nursing Theory and Nursing Research*, edited by Thomas Foth, Dave Holmes, Manfred Hülsken-Giesler, Susanne Kreutzer and Hartmut Remmers, 209-27. Göttingen: Universitätsverlag Osnabrück im V&R unipress GmbH, 2017.

–. "Sorge für Leib und Seele – Arbeits- und Lebensalltag evangelischer Krankenpflege, 1950er bis 1970er Jahre [Caring for Body and Soul: Daily Work and Life in Protestant Nursing, 1950s to 1970s]." In *Entwicklungen in der Krankenpflege und in anderen*

Gesundheitsberufen nach 1945. Ein Lehr- und Studienbuch, edited by Sylvelyn Hähner-Rombach and Pierre Pfütsch, 91–119. Frankfurt am Main: Mabuse-Verlag, 2018.
- —. *Vom "Liebesdienst" zum modernen Frauenberuf: Die Reform der Krankenpflege Nach 1945 [From "Labor of Love" to a Modern Female Profession: Nursing Reform after 1945]*. Reihe Geschichte und Geschlechter. Vol. 45, Frankfurt am Main u. a.: Campus-Verlag, 2005.
- Kroeker, Lore. "Aktuelles aus der Hauptgeschäftsstelle [News from the Headquaters of the Dbfk]." *Krankenpflege* 33, no. 1 (1979): 13–14.
- —. "Klinische Pflegepraxis. Ermittlung, Entwicklung und Auswertung [Clinical Nursing Practice: Ascertaining, Development, and Evaluation]." *Krankenpflege* 37, no. 2 (1983): 53–54.
- —. "Referentenentwurf eines Gesetzes zur Neuordnung der Krankenfinanzierung vom 16. 7. 1984. Anhörung beim Bundesministerium für Arbeit und Sozialordnung am 31. 7. 1984 – Kurzbericht [Draft of a Law for the Rearrangement of Health Care Financing, July 16th, 1984. Official Hearing in the Federal Ministry for Work and Social Order, July 31st, 1984]." *Krankenpflege* 38, no. 9 (1984): 289.
- Krohwinkel, Monika. *Der Pflegeprozess am Beispiel von Apoplexiekranken: Eine Studie zur Erfassung und Entwicklung ganzheitlich-rehabilitierender Prozeßpflege [The Nursing Process Using the Example of Patients with Strokes: A Study to Capture and Develop Holistic-Rehabilitative Nursing Care in a Process]*. Schriftenreihe des Bundesministeriums für Gesundheit. edited by Bundesministerium für Gesundheit. Vol. 16, Baden-Baden: Nomos Verlagsgesellschaft mbH & Co. KG, 1993.
- —. "Krankenpflegeforschung in Europa [Nursing Research in Europe]." *Krankenpflege* 33, no. 3 (1979): 83–85.
- —. "Krankenpflegeforschung in Europa. 2. Arbeitstagung europäischer Krankenpflegeforscher in Kopenhagen [Nursing Research in Europe: Second Work Day of European Nursing Researchers in Copenhagen]." *Krankenpflege* 34, no. 1 (1980): 15.
- —. "Krankenschwestern arbeiten gemeinsam an der Verbesserung der Krankenpflege in Europa. Eine Orientierungshilfe zur Forschungskomponente des mittelfristigen Programms der Weltgesundheitsorganisation für das Krankenpflege- und Hebammenwesen in Europa [Nurses Collaborate to Improve Nursing in Europe]." *Krankenpflege* 34, no. 6 (1980): 195–97.
- —. "Pflegeforschung und ihre Auswirkung in der Praxis im Zusammenhang mit Pflege [Nursing Research and Its Impact on Practice Regarding Nursing]." *Krankenpflege* 38, no. 7–8 (1984): 224–27.
- —. "Pflegepersonal setzt sich für bessere Gesundheit ein [Nurses Campaign for Better Health]." *Krankenpflege* 38, no. 5 (1984): 138–40.
- —. "Wie kann Krankenpflegeforschung uns helfen, besser zu pflegen? [How Can Nursing Research Help Us to Provide Better Nursing Care?]." *Krankenpflege* 34, no. 1 (1980): 14–15.
- KrPflAPrV. "Ausbildungs- und Prüfungsverordnung für die Berufe in der Krankenpflege vom 16. Oktober 1985 [Regulation for Education and Examination in the Occupations of Nursing from October 16th, 1985]." In *Z 5702 A*, edited by Bundesgesetzblatt, 1985.
- KrPflG. "Krankenpflegegesetz vom 16. Juli 2003 (Bgbl. I S. 1442), das zuletzt durch Artikel 1a des Gesetzes vom 17. Juli 2017 (Bgbl. I S. 2581) geändert worden ist [Nursing Act 2003]." 2003.

Krüger, Helga. "Professionalisierung von Frauenberufen – Oder Männer für Frauenberufe interessieren? Das Doppelgesicht des arbeitsmarktlichen Geschlechtersystems [Professionalization of Female Vocations: Or Making Men Interested in Female Vocations?]." In *Feministische Forschung – Nachhaltige Einsprüche*, edited by Kathrin Heinz and Barbara Thiessen. Studien Interdisziplinäre Geschlechterforschung, 123–43. Wiesbaden: VS Verlag für Sozialwissenschaften, 2003.

Kühn, Hagen. "Ethische Probleme der Ökonomisierung von Krankenhausarbeit [Ethical Problems of the Economization of Hospital Work]." In *Dienstleistungsqualität und Qualität des Arbeitslebens im Krankenhaus*, edited by André Büssing and Jürgen Glaser, 77–98. Göttingen, Bern, Toronto, Seattle: Hogrefe-Verlag, 2003.

Kurunmaki, Liisa. "A Hybrid Profession:The Acquisition of Management Accounting Expertise by Medical Professionals.(Author Abstract)." *Accounting, Organizations and Society* 29, no. 3 4 (2004): 327.

Lalonde, Marc. "A New Perspective on the Health of Canadians. A Working Document." Minister of Supply and Services Canada, 1974. http://www.phac-aspc.gc.ca/ph-sp/pdf/perspect-eng.pdf.

Landwehr, Achim. "Die Kunst, sich nicht allzu sicher zu sein: Möglichkeiten kritischer Geschichtsschreibung [The Art of Being Uncertain: Options in Writing Critical History]." *Werkstatt Geschichte* Sonderdruck Esseypreis 2012 (2012): 3–12.

–. *Historische Diskursanalyse [Historical Discourse Analysis]*. 2nd ed. Frankfurt am Main: Campus-Verlag, 2009.

Lange, Jette, Susanne Kreutzer, and Thomas Foth. "Pflege berechenbar machen – Der Pflegeprozess als Accounting Technology in historischer Perspektive [Making Nursing Accountable: The Nursing Process as Accounting Technology in a Historical Perspective]." In *Neue Technologien in der Pflege – Grundlegende Reflexionen und Pragmatische Befunde*, edited by Manfred Hülsken-Giesler, Susanne Kreutzer and Nadin Dütthorn, 2022. Göttingen: V&R unipress, 231–253.

Lanig, Jörg, and Günther Hanke. "PIK – Ein Bund-Länder EDV-Verfahren für den Pflegedienst im Krankenhaus [PIK – A Federal-Länder Computing Procedure for Nursing Service in the Hospital]." *Das Krankenhaus* 82, no. 3 (1990): 131–34.

Larson, Magali Sarfatti. *The Rise of Professionalism: A Sociological Analysis*. Berkeley: University of California Press, 1977.

Laurinat, Helga. "Bericht über die 7. Delegiertenversammlung [Report of the 7th Delegates Meeting]." *Krankenpflege* 34, no. 6 (1980): 207.

Lemke, Thomas. *Eine Kritik der politischen Vernunft: Foucaults Analyse der modernen Gouvernementalität [A Critique of Political Reason: Foucault's Analysis of Modern Governmentality]*. Vol. 6., Berlin: Argument Verlag, 2014.

–. *Gouvernementalität und Biopolitik [Governmentality and Biopolitics]*. Vol. 2., Wiesbaden: VS Verlag für Sozialwissenschaften, 2008.

Lengwiler, Martin, and Jeannette Madarász. "Präventionsgeschichte als Kulturgeschichte der Gesundheitspolitik [Prevention History as Cultural History]." In *Das präventive Selbst. Eine Kulturgeschichte moderner Gesundheitspolitik*, edited by Martin Lengwiler and Jeannette Madarász, 11–28. Bielefeld: transcript Verlag, 2010.

Levá, Sirkka. "Eine gute Krankenpflege. Was ist damit gemeint, und wie ist sie zu erreichen? [Good Nursing Care: What Are We Talking About, and How Can It Be Achieved]. *Die Agnes-Karll-Schwester* 11, no. 2 (1957): 54 & 56.

Lingenberg, Erika. "Gruppenpflege – Ergebnis eines Arbeitsgesprächs [Nursing Care in Groups: Results of a Working Meeting]." *Krankenpflege* 34, no. 4 (1980): 118–22.
Ludwig, Annemarie. "3. Delegiertenversammlung des DBfK am 24./25. Sept. 1976 im Bildungszentrum Essen [Third Meeting of Dbfk Delegates, September 24th/25th, 1976 in the Training Center Essen]." *Krankenpflege* 30, no. 11 (1976): 327–29.
Lukes, Steven. *Power. A Radical View*. 2nd ed. Hampshire, New York: Palgrave Macmillan, 2005.
Lundgreen, Peter. "Wissen und Bürgertum. Skizze eines historischen Vergleichs zwischen Preußen/Deutschland, Frankreich, England und den USA, 18.–20. Jahrhundert [Knowledge and Bourgeoisie. Outline of a Historical Comparision between Prussia/Germany, France, England, and the USA, 18th-20th Century]." In *Bürgerliche Berufe. Zur Sozialgeschichte der Freien und Akademischen Berufe im internationalen Vergleich*, edited by Hannes Siegrist, 106–24. Göttingen: Vandenhoeck & Ruprecht, 1988.
Manzei, Alexandra, and Rudi Schmiede. "Über die neue Unmittelbarkeit des Marktes im Gesundheitswesen – Wie durch die Digitalisierung der Patientenakte ökonomische Entscheidungskriterien an das Patientenbett gelangen [On the New Immediacy of the Market in the Health Care System: How Economic Criteria for Decision Making Came to the Bedside Via Digitalization of Patient Records]." In *20 Jahre Wettbewerb im Gesundheitswesen. Theoretische und empirische Analysen zur Ökonomisierung von Medizin und Pflege*, edited by Alexandra Manzei, 219–39. Wiesbaden: Springer Fachmedien, 2014.
Manzeschke, Arne. "Privatisierung von Krankenhäusern. Ethische Erwägungen zum moralischen Status eines öffentlichen Gutes [Privatization of Hospitals: Ethical Considerations on the Moral Status of a Public Good]." *Pflege und Gesellschaft* 14, no. 1 (2009): 24–38.
Mattes, Monika. "Krisenverliererinnen? Frauen, Arbeit und das Ende des Booms [Losers of the Crisis? Women, Work and the End of the Boom]." In *"Nach dem Strukturbruch"? Kontinuität und Wandel von Arbeitsbeziehungen und Arbeitswelt(en) seit den 1970er Jahren*, edited by Knut Andresen, Ursula Bitzegeio and Jürgen Mittag, 127–40. Bonn: Verlag J. H. W. Dietz Nachf. GmbH, 2011.
Mattheis, Dr. "Die Rolle der Krankenpflege im Gesundheitswesen [The Role of Nursing in Health Care]." *Krankenpflege* 34, no. 3 (1980): 80.
McKinlay, John B., and Joan Arches. "Towards the Proletarianization of Physicians." *International Journal of Health Services* 15, no. 2 (1985): 161–95.
Merkel, Christa. "Können Arbeitserleichterungen im Pflegebereich durch verbesserte Informationsweitergabe (EDV) erwartet werden? [Can an Ease of Work Be Expected in Nursing Thanks to a Better Information Flow (Computing)?]." *Krankenpflege* 38, no. 9 (1984): 282–84.
Methoden zur Humanisierung des Krankenhauses. "Methoden zur Humanisierung des Krankenhauses: Individuelle Pflege I [Methods to Humanize the Hospital: Individual Nursing Care, Part I]." *Krankenpflege* 27, no. 6 (1974): 252.
Metzler, Gabriele. "Staatsversagen und Unregierbarkeit in den siebziger Jahren? [Government Failure and Ungovernability in the 1970s?]." In *Das Ende Der Zuversicht? Die siebziger Jahre als Geschichte*, edited by Konrad H. Jarausch, 243–60: Göttingen: Vandenhoeck & Ruprecht, 2008.

Meyer, John W., and Ronald L. Jepperson. "The "Actors" of Modern Society: The Cultural Construction of Social Agency." *Sociological Theory* 18, no. 1 (2000): 100-20.
Mieg, Harald A. "Professionalisierung [Professionalization]." In *Handbuch Berufsbildungsforschung*, edited by Felix Rauner, 342-49. Bielefeld: Bertelsmann, 2005.
Miller, Peter. "Calculating Economic Life." *Journal of Cultural Economy* 1, no. 1 (2008): 51-64.
—. "The Margins of Accounting." *The Sociological Review* 46, no. 1_suppl (1998): 174-93.
Miller, Peter, and Michael Power. "Accounting, Organizing, and Economizing: Connecting Accounting Research and Organization Theory." *Academy of Management Annals* 7, no. 1 (2013/06/01 2013): 557-605.
Miller, Peter, and Nikolas Rose. "Governing Economic Life." [In en]. *Economy and Society* 19, no. 1 (28 Jul 2006 1990): 1-31.
—. "Political Power Beyond the State: Problematics of Government." In *Governing the Present: Administering Economic, Social and Personal Life*, edited by Peter Miller and Nikolas Rose, 53-83. Cambridge, Malden: Polity Press, 2008.
Mills, Sara. *Michel Foucault*. London; New York: Routledge, 2003.
Mirowski, Philip, and Dieter Plehwe. *The Road from Mont Pe`Lerin: The Making of the Neoliberal Thought Collective*. Cambridge, Mass.: Harvard University Press, 2009.
Mischo-Kelling, Maria. "Gesundheit – Ein pflegerisches Paradigma und Maßstab für Pflegequalität [Health: A Nursing Paradigm and Benchmark for Nursing Quality]." *Krankenpflege* 41, no. 2 (1987): 52-54, 63-64.
—. "Gesundheit und Lebensqualität – Ein Anliegen der Pflege für die Zukunft [Health and Quality of Life: A Concern of Nursing for the Future]." *Krankenpflege* 40, no. 5 (1986): 180-84.
Moers, Martin, and Doris Schaeffer. "Pflegetheorien [Nursing Theories]." In *Handbuch Pflegewissenschaft*, edited by Doris Schaeffer and Klaus Wingenfeld, 37-66. Weinheim und Basel: Beltz Juventa, 2014.
Moorhead, Sue. *Nursing Outcomes Classification (NOC)*. 4th ed. St. Louis: Mosby Elsevier, 2008.
Morsey, Rudolf. *Die Bundesrepublik Deutschland, Entstehung und Entwicklung bis 1969 [The Federal Republic of Germany, Its Formation and Development until the Year 1969]*. München: De Gruyter Oldenbourg, 2007.
Mrda, Rada, and Josef Göbbels. "Kontrolle – Zur Diskussion gestellt [Control: An Issue for Discussion]." *Krankenpflege* 31, no. 4 (1977): 136-37.
Müller-Groeling, Hubertus. "Zur ökonomischen Problematik der gesetzlichen Krankenversicherung [About the Economic Problems of the Statutory Health Insurance]." *ORDO Jahrbuch für die Ordnung von Wirtschaft und Gesellschaft* 19 (1968): 485-98.
Nelson, Sioban, and Suzanne Gordon. "The Rhetoric of Rupture: Nursing as a Practice with a History?" *Nursing Outlook* 52, no. 5 (2004): 255-61.
Neumann, Marita. "Berufsspezifische Entwicklung der Pflege – Vom Helfer zur Profession [Vocational Development of Nursing: From Assistant to Profession]." In *Case Management: Praktisch und effizient*, edited by Christine von Reibnitz, 3-18. Berlin, Heidelberg: Springer, 2009.
Neumeister, Heddy. "Autoritäre Sozialpolitik [Authoritarian Social Policy]." *ORDO Jahrbuch für die Ordnung von Wirtschaft und Gesellschaft* 12 (1961): 187-252.

Nightingale, Florence. *Notes on Nursing: What It Is and What It Is Not.* New York: Dover Publications, Inc., 1969/1860.

Nolte, Karen. "Pflege von Sterbenden im 19. Jahrhundert. Eine ethikgeschichtliche Annäherung [Caring for the Dying in the 19th Century: An Ethic-Historical Approach]." In *Transformationen pflegerischen Handelns. Institutionelle Kontexte und soziale Praxis vom 19. bis 21. Jahrhundert,* edited by Susanne Kreutzer, 87–107. Göttingen: V&R unipress, 2010.

Noordegraaf, Mirko. "From "Pure" to "Hybrid" Professionalism: Present-Day Professionalism in Ambiguous Public Domains." *Administration & Society* 39, no. 6 (2007): 761–85.

Nuffield Provincial Hospitals Trust. *The Work of Nurses in Hospital Wards: Report of a Job-Analysis [Job-Analysis Team Director, H.A. Goddard].* London: Nuffield Provincial Hospitals Trust, 1953.

Oelke, Uta. "Projektbericht - Akademisierung von Pflege [Project Report: The Academization of Nursing]", 1994 http://serwiss.bib.hs-hannover.de/files/51/oelke_1994a.pdf.

Oevermann, Ulrich. "Theoretische Skizze einer revidierten Theorie professionalisierten Handelns [Theoretical Outline of a Revised Theory of Professional Action]." In *Pädagogische Professionalität: Untersuchungen zum Typus pädagogischen Handelns,* edited by Arno Combe and Werner Helsper, 70–182. Frankfurt am Main: Suhrkamp Verlag, 1996.

Orlando, Ida Jean. *The Dynamic Nurse-Patient Relationship: Function, Process, and Principles.* New York: Putnam, 1961.

Ossen, Peter, and Anja Wunsch. "Am Puls der Zeit. Interview: Perspektiven des DKI 60 Jahre nach seiner Gründung [In Pace with the Times. Interview: Perspectives of the German Hospital Institute (DKI) 60 Years after Its Foundation]." *Das Krankenhaus,* no. 2 (2014): 110–14.

Parkin, Paul A. C. "Nursing the Future: A Re-Examination of the Professionalization Thesis in the Light of Some Recent Developments." *Journal of Advanced Nursing* 21, no. 3 (1995): 561–67.

Parsons, Talcott. "Professions." In *International Encyclopedia of the Social Sciences,* edited by David L. Sills, 536–47. London: Crowell Collier and McMillan, Inc., 1968.

–. "The Professions and Social Structure." *Social Forces* 17, no. 4 (1939): 457–67.

Participants of a continuing education course. "EDV in der Krankenpflege – Chance oder Bedrohung [Computing in Nursing: Chance or Threat?]." *Krankenpflege* 38, no. 9 (1984): 304–06.

PflBRefG. "Gesetz zur Reform der Pflegeberufe (Pflegeberufereformgesetz) vom 17. Juli 2017 [Law for the Reformation of the Occupations in Nursing from July 17th, 2017]." In *Teil I Nr. 49,,* edited by Bundesgesetzblatt, 2581–614. ausgegeben zu Bonn am 24. Juli 2017, 2017.

Pieper, Marianne, and Encarnación Gutiérrez Rodríguez. "Einleitung [Introduction]." In *Gouvernementalität: Ein sozialwissenschaftliches Konzept in Anschluss an Foucault,* edited by Marianne Pieper and Encarnación Gutiérrez Rodríguez, 7–21. Frankfurt am Main [u. a.]: Campus-Verlag, 2003.

Preston, Alistar M. "The Birth of Clinical Accounting: A Study of the Emergence and Transformations of Discourses on Costs and Practices of Accounting in U.S. Hospitals." *Accounting Organizations and Society* 17, no. 1 (1992): 63–100.

Ptak, Ralf. *Vom Ordoliberalismus zur Sozialen Marktwirtschaft [From Ordoliberalism to Social Market Economy]* [in German]. Wiesbaden: VS Verlag für Sozialwissenschaften, 2004.

Radek, Monika Elisabeth. *Weltkultur am Werk? Das globale Modell der Gesundheitspolitik und seine Rezeption im nationalen Reformdiskurs am Beispiel Polens [World Culture at Work? The Global Model of Health Policy and Its Reception in the National Reform Discourse: The Example of Poland]* [in German]. Bamberg: University of Bamberg Press, 2011.

Ramge, Carola. "Effizienzverbesserung im Pflegedienst durch Umstrukturierung der pflegerischen Versorgung [Improvment of Efficiency in Nursing Service through Restructuring Nursing Care]." *Das Krankenhaus* 66, no. 5 (1974): 200–04.

Reimann, Renate. "Information im Dienst des Kranken [Information at Patients' Service]." *Krankenpflege* 33, no. 7/8 (1979): 249–53.

–. "Krankenpflege zwischen Tradition und Forderung [Nursing between Tradition and Demand]." *Krankenpflege* 36, no. 1 (1982): 5–7.

–. "Pflegeplanung – Was bedeutet geplante Pflege in der Berufspraxis [Nursing Care Plan: The Meaning of Planned Nursing Care in Daily Professional Practice]." *Krankenplege* 33, no. 5 (1979): 154–57.

–. "Probleme der Bestimmung und Messung von Pflegequalität [The Problems of Determination and Measurement of Quality in Nursing]." *Krankenpflege* 32, no. 5 (1978): 166, 79–80.

–. "Stagnation oder Fortschritt in der Entwicklung der Pflegeberufe? [Stagnation or Progress in the Development of Nursing Occupations?]." *Krankenpflege* 35, no. 1 (1981): 20 & 37.

–. "Teil II: Das Bildungsangebot für zukunftsorientierte Krankenpflege [Part II: The Educational Program for a Future-Oriented Nursing Care]." *Krankenpflege* 31, no. 5 (1977): 160–61.

Remmers, Hartmut. *Pflegerisches Handeln. Wissenschafts- und Ethikdiskurse zur Konturierung der Pflegewissenschaft [Nursing Action: Scientific and Ethical Discourses to Outline Nursing Science]*. Reihe Pflegewissenschaft. Bern: Verlag Hans Huber, 2000.

Ridic, Goran, Suzanne Gleason, and Ognjen Ridic. "Comparisons of Health Care Systems in the United States, Germany and Canada." *Materia socio-medica* 24, no. 2 (2012): 112–20.

Ringelhann, Rupert. "Eindrücke von der Interhospital '85 in Düsseldorf [Impressions from the Interhospital '85 in Dusseldorf]." *Krankenpflege* 39, no. 7–9 (1985): 236–38.

Ritzer, George, and David Walczak. "Rationalization and the Deprofessionalization of Physicians." *Social Forces* 67, no. 1 (1988): 1–22.

Rödder, Andreas. *Die Bundesrepublik Deutschland 1969-1990 [The Federal Republic of Germany 1969-1990]*. Oldenbourg Grundriss der Geschichte, edited by Lothar Gall, Karl-Joachim Hölkeskamp and Hermann Jakobs. Vol. 19 A, München: R. Oldenbourg Verlag, 2004.

Romano, Carol, Kathleen A. McCormick, and Linda McNeely. "Nursing Documentation: A Model for a Computerized Data Base." *Advances in Nursing Science*, no. 1 (1982): 43–56.

Rose, Nikolas. "Expertise and the Government of Conduct." *Studies in Law, Politics, and Society* 14 (1994): 359–97.

—. "Government, Authority and Expertise in Advanced Liberalism." *Economy and Society* 22, no. 3 (1993): 283–99.
—. "Medicine, History and the Present." In *Reassessing Foucault: Power, Medicine and the Body. Studies in the Social History of Medicine*, edited by Colin Jones and Roy Porter, 48–72. London, New York: Routledge, 1994.
Rosenbrock, Rolf, and Thomas Gerlinger. *Gesundheitspolitik. Eine systematische Einführung [Health Policy. A Systematic Introduction]*. 3rd ed. Bern: Verlag Hans Huber, 2014.
Salvage, Jane. "Professionalization Or Struggle for Survival? A Consideration of Current Proposals for the Reform of Nursing in the United Kingdom." *Journal of Advanced Nursing* 13, no. 4 (1988): 515–19.
Sarasin, Philipp. *Geschichtswissenschaft und Diskursanalyse [History and Discourse Analysis]* [in German]. 4th ed. Frankfurt am Main: Suhrkamp Verlag, 2014.
Sauer, Dieter. "Permanente Reorganisation [Permanent Re-Organization]." In *Vorgeschichte der Gegenwart. Dimensionen des Strukturbruchs nach dem Boom*, edited by Anselm Doering-Manteuffel, Lutz Raphael and Thomas Schlemmer, 37–56. Göttingen: Vandenhoeck & Ruprecht, 2016.
Schaeffer, Doris. "Professionalisierung der Pflege [Professionalization of Nursing]." In *Dienstleistungsqualität und Qualität des Arbeitslebens im Krankenhaus*, edited by André Büssing and Jürgen Glaser, 227–43. Göttingen, Bern, Toronto, Seattle: Hogrefe-Verlag, 2003.
Schattat, Barbara. "Bericht über meine ersten Monate in USA im Rahmen des Schwestern-Austauschprogramms [Report on My First Months During a Nurse Exchange in the USA]." *Die Agnes-Karll-Schwester* 15, no. 8 (1961): 263–64.
Schellenberg, Margit. "Die Bedeutung einer patientenorientierten Pflegeplanung [The Importance of a Patient-Oriented Nursing Care Plan]." *Krankenpflege* 31, no. 9 (1977): 291–93.
Schildt, Axel. "Das letzte Jahrzehnt der Bonner Republik. Überlegungen zur Erforschung der 1980er Jahre [The Last Decade of the Bonner Republic: Considerations for the Investigation of the 1980s]." *Archiv für Sozialgeschichte* 52 (2012): 21–46.
—. *Die Sozialgeschichte der Bundesrepublik Deutschland bis 1989/90 [The Social History of the Federal Republic of Germany until 1989/90]*. Enzyklopädie Deutscher Geschichte. edited by Lothar Gall. Vol. 80, München: R. Oldenbourg Verlag, 2007.
Schmidbaur, Marianne. *Vom "Lazaruskreuz" zu "Pflege Aktuell": Professionalisierungsdiskurse in der deutschen Krankenpflege 1903–2000 [From "Lazaruskreuz" to "Pflege Aktuell": Discourses on Professionalization in the German Nursing Care 1903–2000]*. Königstein: Helmer, 2002.
Schomburg, Ingo. "Pflegeplanung und ganzheitliche Pflege im Stationsalltag – Pflegemodellstation und Arbeiten mit dem Krankenpflegeprozeß [Nursing Care Plan and Holistic Care in the Daily Routine of the Ward: Training Ward and Working with the Nursing Process]." *Krankenpflege* 38, no. 7–8 (1984): 231, 236–38.
Schulte, Josefia. "Betriebliche Steuerung Aufgabe des Krankenpflegepersonals? Modelle zur Stellenbeschreibung – 1. Teil [Operational Administration Task Nursing Personnel? Models for a Job Description – 1st. Part]." *Das Krankenhaus* 75, no. 1 (1983): 23–26.
Seibring, Anne. "Die Humanisierung des Arbeitslebens in den 1970er-Jahren: Forschungsstand und Forschungsperpektiven [Humanization of Work Life in the 1970s: State of and Perspectives on Research]." In *"Nach dem Strukturbruch"? Kontinuität und*

Wandel von Arbeitsbeziehungen und Arbeitswelt(en) seit den 1970er Jahren, edited by Knut Andresen, Ursula Bitzegeio and Jürgen Mittag, 107–26. Bonn: Verlag J. H. W. Dietz Nachf. GmbH, 2011.

Send, Cornelia. "Mittel für die Durchführung der individuellen Pflege (I) [Instruments for Providing Individual Nursing Care I]." *Krankenpflege* 29, no. 7 (1975): 274.

–. " Mittel für die Durchführung der individuellen Pflege (II) [Instruments for Providing Individual Nursing Care II]." *Krankenpflege* 29, no. 8 (1975): 324.

–. " Mittel für die Durchführung der individuellen Pflege (III) [Instruments for Providing Individual Nursing Care III]." *Krankenpflege* 29, no. 9 (1975): 368.

–. " Mittel für die Durchführung der individuellen Pflege (IV) [Instruments for Providing Individual Nursing Care IV]." *Krankenpflege* 29, no. 10 (1975): 409.

SGB V. "Sozialgesetzbuch. Fünftes Buch. Gesetzliche Krankenversicherung [Social Legislation Book. Book Five. Statutory Health Insurance]." 2019.

Siebers, Hedi. "Krankenpflegeausbildung der achtziger Jahre. Auszüge eines Vortrags [Nursing Education in the 1980s: Extracts of a Presentation]." *Krankenpflege* 34, no. 2 (1980): 65–66.

Siepmann, Maren, and David A. Groneberg. "Der Arztberuf als Profession – Deprofessionalisierung [The Medical Vocation as Profession: Deprofessionalization]." *Zentralblatt für Arbeitsmedizin, Arbeitsschutz und Ergonomie* 62 (2012): 288–92.

Simon, Irmgard. "Ein bayrischer Gruß an alle Fortbildungs-Muffel [A Bavarian Salute to All Continuing Education Grumps]." *Krankenpflege* 33, no. 1 (1979): 15–16.

Simon, Michael. *Das Gesundheitssystem in Deutschland. Eine Einführung in Struktur und Funktionsweise [the Health Care System in Germany. An Introduction in Structure and Functionality]*. 4th ed. Bern: Verlag Hans Huber, 2013.

–. "Die ökonomischen und strukturellen Veränderungen des Krankenhausbereichs seit den 1970er Jahren [The Economic and Structural Changes of the Hospital Setting since the 1970s]." In *Mutationen des Krankenhauses: Soziologische Diagnosen in organisations- und gesellschaftstheoretischer Perspektive*, edited by Ingo Bode and Werner Vogd, 29–45. Wiesbaden: Springer Fachmedien, 2016.

–. *Krankenhauspolitik in der Bundesrepublik Deutschland. Historische Entwicklung und Probleme der politischen Steuerung stationärer Krankenversorgung [Hospital Policy in the Federal Republic of Germany: Historical Developments and Problems of Political Control Stationary Health Care]*. Studien zur Sozialwissenschaft Band 209. Wiesbaden: Springer Fachmedien, 2000.

Southgate, Beverley. "Postmodernism." In *A Companion to the Philosophy of History and Historiography*, edited by Aviezer Tucker, 540–49. Chichester: Blackwell Publishing Ltd., 2009.

Steinbrück, Margarete. *Schwesternarbeit auf der Station: Bericht über eine englische Arbeitsstudie [Nurses' Work on the Ward: Report on an English Working Study]* [in German]. edited by Bd. 1. Schriften des Deutschen Krankenhausinstituts e.V. Karlsruhe/Baden: Braun, 1954.

Steppe, Hilde. "Das Selbstverständnis der Krankenpflege in ihrer historischen Entwicklung [Self-Conception of Nursing in Its Historical Development]." *Pflege – Die wissenschaftliche Zeitschrift für Pflegeberufe* 13 (2000): 77–83.

Stichweh, Rudolf. "Professionen in einer funktional differenzierten Gesellschaft [Professions in a Functionally Differentiated Society]." In *Pädagogische Professionalität:*

Untersuchungen zum Typus pädagogischen Handelns, edited by Arno Combe and Werner Helsper, 49-69. Frankfurt am Main: Suhrkamp Verlag, 1996.

Stolberg, Michael. "Heilkundige: Professionalisierung und Medikalisierung [Healers: Professionalization and Medicalization]." In *Medizingeschichte: Aufgaben, Probleme, Perspektiven*, edited by Norbert Paul and Thomas Schlich, 69-86. Frankfurt am Main, New York: Campus-Verlag, 1998.

Storch, Janet L., and Shirley M. Stinson. "Concepts of Deprofessionalization with Application to Nursing." In *Political Issues in Nursing: Past, Present, and Future*, edited by Rosemary White, 33-44. Chichester: John Wiley & Sons Ltd, 1988.

Stratmeyer, Peter. "Ein historischer Irrtum der Pflege. Plädoyer für einen kritisch-distanzierten Umgang mit dem Pflegeprozess [A Historical Error in Nursing: A Plea for a Critical and Distanced Attitude Towards the Nursing Process]." *Dr. med. Mabuse* 106 (1997): 34-38.

Süß, Dietmar. "Der Sieg der grauen Herren? [The Victory of the Men in Grey]." In *Vorgeschichte der Gegenwart*. 109-28: Vandenhoeck & Ruprecht, 2016.

Süß, Dietmar, and Meik Woyke. "Schimanskis Jahrzehnt? Die 1980er Jahre in historischer Perspektive [Schimanski's Decade? The 1980s in a Historical Perspective]." *Archiv für Sozialgeschichte* 52 (2012): 3-20.

Süß, Winfried. "Der bedrängte Wohlfahrtsstaat. Deutsche und europäische Perspektiven auf die Sozialpolitik der 1970er-Jahre." *Archiv für Sozialgeschichte* 47 (2007): 95-126.

—. "Umbau am "Modell Deutschland". Sozialer Wandel, ökonomische Krise und wohlfahrtsstaatliche Reformpolitik in der Bundesrepublik "Nach dem Boom" [Rebuildings on "Model Germany": Social Change, Economic Crisis and Reform Policy of the Welfare State of the Federal Republic "after the Boom"]." *Journal of Modern European History* 9, no. 9 (2011): 215-40.

Taubert, Johanna. *Pflege auf dem Weg zu einem neuen Selbstverständnis: Berufliche Entwicklung zwischen Diakonie und Patientenorientierung [Nursing on Its Way to a New Self-Concept: Occupational Development between Diaconry and Patient Orientation]*. 2nd ed. Frankfurt am Main: Mabuse-Verlag, 1994.

The Nuffield Provincial Hospital Trust. *The Work of Nurses on Hopsital Ward: Report of a Job Analysis*. London: Nuffield Lodge, 1953.

Thiel, Sabine. "Pflegeplanung und Pflegedokumentation [Nursing Care Plan and Nursing Documentation]." *Krankenpflege* 40, no. 1 (1986): 9-12.

Thießen, Malte. "Praktiken der Vorsorge als Ordnung des Sozialen: Zum Verhältnis von Impfungen und Gesellschaftskonzepten im "langen 20. Jahrhundert" [Practices of Prevention as Social Order: On the Relationship of Vaccinations and Societal Concepts in the "Long 20th Century"]." In *Geschichte der Prävention. Akteure, Praktiken, Instrumente*, edited by Sylvelyn Hähner-Rombach, 203-27. Stuttgart: Franz Steiner Verlag, 2015.

Thompson, J. N. "Der Krankenpflegeprozeß – Mit Vorsicht zu behandeln! [The Nursing Process: Treat Carefully!]." *Krankenpflege* 34, no. 7/8 (1980): 243-44.

Tietze, Ingrid. "10. Fortbildungskongreß für Krankenschwestern/-pfleger in Berlin [10th Congress for Further Education for Nurses in Berlin]." *Krankenpflege* 33, no. 7/8 (1979): 282.

Timmermann, Carsten. "Risikofaktoren: Der scheinbar unaufhaltsame Erfolg eines Ansatzes aus der amerikanischen Epidemiologie in der deutschen Nachkriegsmedizin

[Risk Factors: The Apparently Unstoppable Success of an Approach from American Epidemiology in the German Postwar Period]." In *Das präventive Selbst. Eine Kulturgeschichte moderner Gesundheitspolitik*, edited by Martin Lengwiler and Jeannette Madarász, 251–77. Bielefeld: transcript Verlag, 2010.

Trill, Roland. "Anforderungen an ein EDV-gestütztes Kommunikationssystem für den Pflegebereich [Requirements for a Computing-Based Communication System in Nursing]." *Krankenpflege* 40, no. 9 (1986): 342–44.

—. "Grundlagen Der EDV – Eine Einführung für Krankenpflegekräfte [Basics of Computing: An Introduction for Nurses]." *Krankenpflege* 38, no. 9 (1984): 279–81.

—. "Qualitätssicherung in der Krankenpflege [Quality Assurance in Nursing]." *Das Krankenhaus* 78, no. 9 (1986): 380–84.

Trockel, Birgit, and Irmgard Knäuper Notthoff, Margret. *Who Is Who in der Pflege. Deutschland – Schweiz – Österreich [Who Is Who in Nursing? Germany – Switzerland – Austria]*. Bern, Göttingen, Toronto, Seattle: Verlag Hans Huber, 1999.

Vaubel, Roland. "Die deutschen Staatsausgaben: Wende oder Anstieg ohne Ende? [The German Government Expenditures: Turning Point or Recession without Ending?]." *ORDO Jahrbuch für die Ordnung von Wirtschaft und Gesellschaft* 35 (1984): 3–19.

Veldhorst-Groenewegen, J. G., and G. van der Reep. "EVA – Ein patientenorientiertes Instrumten für Pflegeadministration [EVA: A Patient-Oriented Tool for Nursing Administration]." *Krankenpflege* 38, no. 9 (1984): 301–04.

Wallenstein, Sven-Olov. "Introduction: Foucault, Biopolitics, and Governmentality." In *Foucault, Biopolitics, and Governmentality*, edited by Jakob Nilsson and Sven-Olov Wallenstein, 7–34. Stockholm: Södertörn Philosophical Studies, 2013.

Walsh, Mary B., and Helen Yura. *Human Needs and the Nursing Process*. New York: Appleton-Century-Crofts, 1978.

WCPT. "Position Statement of the World Confederation for Physical Therapy." 2007. https://www.wcpt.org/sites/wcpt.org/files/files/WCPT_Description_of_Physical_Therapy-Sep07-Rev_2.pdf.

Weber, Marianne. "Der Krankenpflegeprozeß in der Schweiz: Ergebnisse eines Forschungsprojektes und seine Folgen [The Nursing Process in Switzerland: Results of a Research Project and Its Consequences]." *Krankenpflege* 40, no. 1 (1986): 30–32.

Weber, Max. *Grundriss der Sozialökonomie. III. Abteilung Wirtschaft und Gesellschaft [Layout of Social Economy: Third Division Economy and Society]*. Tübingen: Verlag von J. C. B. Mohr (Paul Siebeck), 1922.

Wehrenpfennig, Werner. "Krankenhäuser an zwei Fronten engagiert. Gedanken zum Hauptthema des vierten deutschen Krankenhaustages "Leistungssteigerung im Krankenhaus durch Zusammenarbeit" [Hospitals Engaged on Two Frontiers: Thoughts on the Topic of the Fourth German Hospital Day "Increasing Performance in the Hospital through Collaboration"]." *Das Krankenhaus* 58, no. 5 (1966): 168–70.

Weinrich, Rosemarie. "Arbeitsbericht der Hauptgeschäftsführerin für das Jahr Oktober 1977 – September 1978, vorgelegt auf der 5. Delegiertenversammlung des DBfK – gekürzt [Working Report of the General Manager for the Year October 1977 – September 1978. Presented at the Fifth Meeting of the DBfK Delegates – Shortened]." *Krankenpflege* 32, no. 11 (1978): 378–80.

—. "Ausblick auf die Arbeit des DBfK in den 80er Jahren [Outlook on the Work of the DBfK in the 80s]." *Krankenpflege* 35, no. 1 (1981): 16–18.

–. "Bedeutung und Stellenwert der Krankenpflege in unserer Gesellschaft [Role and Importance of Nursing Care in Our Society]." *Krankenpflege* 38, no. 1 (1984): 2–3.
–. "Der Wandel im bisher üblichen Verständnis von Krankenpflege [The Change in the Common Perception of Nursing]." *Krankenpflege* 35, no. 4 (1981): 156–58.
–. "Gedanken zum Berufsbild Krankenpflege [Thoughts About the Vocation of Nursing]." *Krankenpflege* 36, no. 1 (1982): 2–3.
–. "Kurz berichtet aus der Hauptgeschäftsstelle [Brief Report of the Essentials of the Head Office]." *Krankenpflege* 30, no. 2 (1976): 49–50.
–. "Rechtsnormen und ethische Normen in der Krankenpflege [Legal Norms and Ethical Norms in Nursing]." *Krankenpflege* 39, no. 7–8 (1985): 234–36.
–. "Sitzung des Rates der Ländervertreter – 18. internationaler Krankenpflegekongreß in Tel Aviv [Meeting of the Council of the Representatives of the Countries – 18th International Nursing Congress in Tel Aviv]." *Krankenpflege* 39, no. 9 (1985): 298–301.
–. "Stellungnahme zum Entwurf einer Ausbildungs- und Prüfungsverordnung für die Berufe der Krankenpflege – (KrPflAPrO) [Commentary on the Draft of the Training and Examination Regulations of the Nursing Occupations]." *Krankenpflege* 36, no. 10 (1982): 321–22.
–. "Wichtiges in Kürze aus der Hauptgeschäftsstelle [Brief Overview of the Essentials of the Head Office]." *Krankenpflege* 30, no. 6 (1976): 183–84.
–. "Zusammengefasster Arbeitsbericht der Hauptgeschäftsstelle vom 26.4.1980–25.4.1981 [Summarized Working Report of the Head Office from April 26th, 1980 to April 25th, 1981]." *Krankenpflege* 35, no. 6 (1981): 251–54.
Weir, George Moir. *Survey of Nursing Education in Canada*. Toronto: University of Toronto Press, 1932.
Wetterer, Angelika. *Arbeitsteilung und Geschlechterkonstruktion. "Gender at Work" in theoretischer und historischer Perspektive [Division of Labor and Gender Construction. "Gender at Work" in a Theoretical and Historical Perspective]*. Theorie und Methode. Vol. 19, Köln: Herbert von Halem Verlag, 2002/2017.
WHO. "Declaration of Alma-Ata. International Conference on Primary Health Care, Alma-Ata, Ussr, 6–12 September 1978." 1978. https://www.who.int/publications/almaata_declaration_en.pdf.
–. "The First Ten Years of the World Health Organization." Geneva: World Health Organization, 1958.
–. "The Fourth Ten Years of the World Health Organization 1978–1987." Geneva: World Health Organization, 2011.
–. "Global Strategy for Health for All by the Year 2000." 1981, https://iris.wpro.who.int/bitstream/handle/10665.1/6967/WPR_RC032_GlobalStrategy_1981_en.pdf.
–. "Organizational Study on "Methods of Promoting Development of Basic Health Services". Report of the Working Group, 16 January 1973." World Health Organization, 1973.
–. "Proposed Programme Budget for 1976 and 1977." In *No. 220*, 1974.
–. "Regional Committee for Europe. Report on the Twenty-Fourth Session." In *EB55/26*, 1974.
–. "Report of the Nineteenth Session of the Regional Committee for Europe 9–13 September." Budapest: World Health Organization, 1969.

–. "The Second Ten Years of the World Health Organization 1958–1967." Geneva: World Health Organization, 1968.
–. "The Third Ten Years of the World Health Organization 1968–1977." Geneva: World Health Organization, 2008.
Wiemeyer, Joachim. "Die Konzertierte Aktion im Gesundheitswesen nach dem Krankenversicherungs-Kostendämpfungsgesetz [Concerted Action in the Health Care System after the Cost-Containment Act for Health Insurance]." *Jahrbuch für Christliche Sozialwissenschaften* 20 (1979): 251–88.
Wiener, Norbert. *Cybernetics or Control and Communication in the Animal and the Machine*. Vol. 2nd edition, Fourth Printing, Cambridge, Massachusetts: The M.I.T. Press, 1985.
Wilensky, Harold L. "The Professionalization of Everyone?" *American Journal of Sociology* 70, no. 2 (1964): 137–58.
Wilkesmann, Maximiliane, Birgit Apitzsch, and Caroline Ruiner. "Von der Deprofessionalisierung zur Reprofessionalisierung im Krankenhaus? Honorarärzte zwischen Markt, Organisation und Profession [From De-Professionalization to Re-Professionalization in the Hospital? Fee-Based Physicians between the Market, Organization, and Profession]." *Soziale Welt* 66, no. 3 (2015): 327–46.
Wismar, Matthias. *Gesundheitswesen im Übergang zum Postfordismus [The Health Care System in Transistion to Post-Fordism]*. Frankfurt am Main: VAS – Verlag für akademische Schriften, 1996.
Wittmann, Luise. "Die Pflegeplanung in der Intensivpflege [The Nursing Care Plan in Intensive Care]." *Krankenpflege* 31, no. 5 (1977): 178–80.
Witz, Anne. *Professions and Patriarchy*. London, New York: Routledge, 1992.
Wolf, Julian, and Werner Vogd. "Professionalisierung der Pflege, Deprofessionalisierung der Ärzte oder vice versa? [Professionalization of Nursing, Deprofessionalization of Physicians, or Vice Versa?]." In *Professionskulturen – Charakteristika unterschiedlicher professioneller Praxen*, edited by Silke Müller-Hermann, Roland Becker-Lenz, Stefan Busse and Gudrun Ehlert, 151–73. Wiesbaden: Springer Fachmedien, 2018.
Wolff, Horst-Peter, and Jutta Wolff. *Geschichte der Krankenpflege: Mit 5 Tabellen [History of Nursing: With 5 Charts]*. Basel [u. a.]: RECOM-Verlag, 1994.
–. *Krankenpflege: Einführung in das Studium ihrer Geschichte [Nursing Care: Introduction in the Study of Its History]*. Vol. 2nd, Frankfurt am Main: Mabuse-Verlag, 2011.
Wong, Woon Hau. "Caring Holistically within New Managerialism." *Nursing Inquiry* 11, no. 1 (2004): 2–13.
Yura, Helen, and Mary B. Walsh. *The Nursing Process: Assessing, Planning, Implementing, and Evaluating. The Proceedings of the Continuing Education Series Conducted at the Catholic University of America, March 2 through April 27, 1967*. Washington: Catholic University of America Press, 1968.
Yura, Helen, Mary B. Walsh, and Dorothy Ozimek. *Nursing Leadership: Theory and Process*. 2nd ed. New York: Appleton-Century-Crofts, 1981.
Zacharias, Siegfried. "Dekor-Design auf Porzellangeschirr ist nicht Selbstzweck [Decor Design on Procelain Dishes Is Not an End in Itself]." *Das Krankenhaus* 72, no. 7 (1980): 215–16.